A HISTORY OF DANCE
IN AMERICAN HIGHER EDUCATION

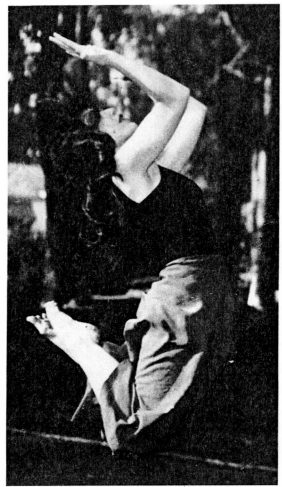

Frontispiece: Detail of "Modern Dance"
Photograph, courtesy of F.W. Olin Library
Mills College.

A HISTORY OF DANCE
IN AMERICAN HIGHER EDUCATION
Dance and the American University

Thomas K. Hagood

Studies in Dance
Volume 1

The Edwin Mellen Press
Lewiston•Queenston•Lampeter

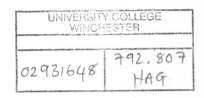
Library of Congress Cataloging-in-Publication Data

Hagood, Thomas K.
   A history of dance in American higher education : dance and the American university /
Thomas K. Hagood.
      p. cm. -- (Studies in dance ; v. 1)
   Includes bibliographical references and index.
   ISBN 0-7734-7799-3
   1. Dance--Study and teaching (Higher)--United States--History. I. Title. II. Series.

GV1589 .H33   2000
792.8'071'173--dc21

00-020262

This is volume 1 in the continuing series
Studies in Dance
Volume 1 ISBN 0-7734-7799-3
SD Series ISBN 0-7734-7742-X

A CIP catalog record for this book is available from the British Library.

Author's Cover Photograph: Photo by James E. Graham, Mills College, Oakland, CA.

The Edwin Mellen Press
Box 450
Lewiston, New York
USA 14092-0450

The Edwin Mellen Press
Box 67
Queenston, Ontario
CANADA L0S 1L0

The Edwin Mellen Press, Ltd.
Lampeter, Ceredigion, Wales
UNITED KINGDOM SA48 8LT

Printed in the United States of America

Dedication

To my teachers

Contents

Origins of the University in Western Culture
The Early School as an Environment for Learning
The Medieval Period: Teaching Societies, Avaricious Chancellors,
    and Introduction of the "Universitas"
Seeking the License of "Jus Ubique Docendi"
Regional Difference in University Organization
Developments in American Higher Education: 1636-1910
The College Curriculum: "Telling Ourselves Who We Are"
Changes in American Culture 1820-1870: Effects on the University
Immigration and the German Influence on the University
Physical Culture, Hygiene, and the Normal School: Early Physical Education
    Programs in Higher Education
The Academic Revolution: 1870-1910
The University as a Social Laboratory

Dance in 19th Century America: Social Grace, Sinful Pleasure
Popular Interest in Antiquity: Resurgent Classic Ideals in a Modern Age;
    Impact on Physical Education and Dance
Progressive Education: Origins and Principles
John Dewey's Influence on Programs in Physical Education: Traditional
    v Progressive Education
Progressive Education in Retrospect: A Critical Perspective
Anderson, Sargent and Gulick: Three Pioneers for Physical Education
    and Dance
American Pageantry: Dance for a Democratic Community
World War 1 and the "New" Gymnastics

Dance in America – 1895-1925; Becoming Art and Business; First
    Programs in Higher Education
Isadora Duncan
Ruth St. Denis and Ted Shawn
Dance: First Programs in Higher Education
Gertrude Colby and Margaret H'Doubler - University Programs in Dance:
    1913-1926

Dance and Higher Education in the 1950s: Modern Dance in Higher Education
The 1950s - Dance as Art, Dance as Exercise: A Continuing Struggle
    for Identity
Impulse: A West Coast Annual
Cultural Factors Influencing Dance in America in the 1950s
Regional Activity in the Arts and Dance

America in the 1960s: A Culture in Transition - New Developments in the Arts
Implementing the Arts in Higher Education
Dance in Higher Education: 1960-1970
The Dance as a Discipline Conference - 1965
College Dance: Aesthetic v Professional
The Developmental Conference on Dance 1966-1967
The American Dance Symposium: 1968

The 1970s: The "Dance Boom" in Higher Education
American College Dance Festival
The Council of Dance Administrators

From "Boom" to "Bust": The Struggle for Survival in a Corporate University
Dance in the Corporate University: 1980-1990

Dance Scholarship in Transition: A Post Modern Aesthetic
Dance Scope: Exploring Dance as an Aesthetic Discipline
The Committee on Research in Dance: Organized Action for Dance Research
Academic Research in Dance
Dance Scholarship and Pedagogy in Transition: A "Post-Modern Aesthetic"
The Discipline Revisited: Multiculturalism and Changing Demographics

Experiments with Change in the Dance Program
Organized Activity: New Specialization in the Field
Educating Tomorrow's Dancer: Some Thoughts from the Field
Projections for the Future

Illustrations

Cover Illustration. "Party in the Sky-A Revival Hymn," Choreography by Marian Van Tuyl, 1939. Photograph, courtesy of R.W. Olin Library, Mills College.

Frontispiece. Detail of "Modern Dance": student demonstrating Modern Dance at Mills College, circa 1940.

Figures

TABLES
Number and Title

Preface

I was extremely pleased to be asked to review this book and then to write the preface. I had selfishly wanted to get my hands on this manuscript from the moment I knew it was being produced because of my interest in and passion (like Tom's) for dance in American higher education.

Dr. Hagood has provided the dance and higher education world with a volume that has never before been published. He has managed to consolidate, contextualize, and encapsulate the very broad topic of a history of dance in American higher education into comprehensive and meaningful chapters. He is an expert in his topic having studied, explored, and researched dance in higher education for many years; now he shares his valuable knowledge. Readers will be rewarded with carefully documented research from numerous and well respected sources in the fields of dance education, physical education, history, psychology, and sociology.

While America is a young country relative to its Asian and European neighbors, a rich history of dance in American education has been carefully woven for the readers of this comprehensive book. The chapters travel on a chronological pathway taking us from the earliest beginnings of the development of higher education efficiently through several centuries ultimately arriving at prospects for the 21st Century. Each period of history discussed eloquently ties dance and higher education together with aesthetics, arts, business, culture, economics, education, and politics. A broad-based discussion occurs throughout the book, but Dr. Hagood never loses his focus on dance in higher education.

According to Dr. Hagood, his book is "an account of a struggle for cultural, academic, and artistic clarification and meaning for dance as this has been waged behind ivied walls." In this account he shares a fascinating array of details about dance and its development in higher education including information about many dance education pioneers, their contributions, and their struggles. Some of these pioneers include Isadora Duncan, Ruth St. Denis, Ted Shawn, Gertrude Colby, Margaret H'Doubler, Martha Graham, Louis Horst, Doris Humphrey, Charles Weidman, Hanya Holm, and John Martin, along with many others who danced, taught, critiqued, and wrote on behalf of dance in higher education.

Landmark conferences such as the Dance as a Discipline conference in 1965, the Developmental Conference on Dance 1966-1967, and the American Dance Symposium in 1968 are discussed and analyzed concerning their importance and contributions toward assimilation of dance into higher education. A variety of dance organizations are presented in light of support and direction that they have provided for dance in higher education.

The historical development of dance in higher education is carefully traced. Academic research in dance, dance scholarship, and dance pedagogy surface in the book to help illustrate the fact that dance is an academic discipline and, without a doubt, has a legitimate place in higher education in both theory and practice.

The future can only be a projection, a speculation of things to come as the last chapter indicates. Often we predict the future in terms of what we hope reality will be; this is especially true of dance in higher education. We (dance educators in higher education), hope it will be properly nourished, respected, valued, and hold a secure place in the higher education curriculum. We continually hope that dance will be used to positively change and enrich the lives of all who come in contact with it, including the higher education community. Each day is a new challenge for us in dance in higher education; we must continue to work diligently to make these hopes become reality.

After reading this book, I realized that it subtly provides hope and encouragement for today's dance educators based on historical viewpoints that dance truly belongs in the academic curriculum in higher education. Dance education pioneers left a foundation for all of us to build upon for each new generation. We in dance education have a tremendous responsibility to continue "waging the battle behind the ivied walls for higher education" for dance, dance, and more dance. I place my bricks on the foundation provided for me by generations of dance educators.

Thanks, Tom, for giving me the privilege of reading your book, and inspiring me.

Marcia L. Lloyd, Ed. D.
Professor of Dance
Idaho State University
Pocatello, Idaho 83209

INTRODUCTION

Dance and the American University, began as dissertation research at the University of Wisconsin-Madison in 1986. Upon entering the doctoral program in dance at Wisconsin, my advisor encouraged me to use my first semester to explore, and refine, ideas for my research topic. Knowing that I had always had a particular interest in the 'how' and 'why' of dance in higher education, I enrolled in a graduate seminar in the Department of Educational Administration titled: *Organization and Governance in Higher Education.* My experiences in that seminar led me toward the subject of my dissertation, and eventually to the subject and writing of this book. I am grateful to have begun this research while a student at Wisconsin, where dance found its first recognition as an academic discipline in 1926.

That dance has evolved into an academic discipline of substance is still quite surprising to many, both in and outside of the university. In the short time that dance has enjoyed academic recognition in higher education the task of the university dance educator has been to work around, over, and through ambiguous and fragmented meanings in order to clarify the nature of dance as an art and academic discipline. Over the years, most college dance educators have worked to infuse the dance curriculum with a sense of academic and artistic rigor. Yet, while these efforts have helped dance become a major program in over 200 of our nation's colleges and universities, the fact remains that for many of our students and colleagues, the meanings and contexts for appreciating dance often remain poorly, and even oddly, defined and understood.

My hope is that this book will appeal to those who wish to refine their understanding of dance in the American university. To that end, and to help situate the interested reader who may know little about dance, let us first consider how dance is generally understood and defined in American culture. Understanding the academic history of dance is, in part, contingent on understanding dance as a contemporary cultural phenomenon. Popular conceptions of dance shape the landscape for dance in the academy. For many readers, issues and notions surrounding "art-dance," "social dance," "educational dance," "dance and gender," and even "dance and sin," frame their understanding of the topic of this book. To contextualize the subsequent matter of the history of dance in the university, I begin with common definitions for dance, like those found in a typical English dictionary.

The American Heritage Dictionary defines dance as a verb, with the following primary definitions: "1. to move rhythmically to music, using prescribed or improvised steps and gestures, 2. to leap or skip about excitedly; caper, 3. to bob up and down." [1] The first definition seems clear enough; dance is movement, and most often dance movement is rhythmic, involving a set of prescribed or improvised steps and/or gestures. However, definitions two and three seem much more ambiguous: To bob up and down? To caper? At least moving rhythmically to music, "using prescribed or improvised steps and gestures," suggests aspects of the experience of dance. But the notions of excited skipping and the caper seem dated, and sort of silly. As far as the topic of this book is concerned, a major limitation of the definitions provided is that they do little to indicate that dance is something one might study, and study at no less of a place than the university.

Dance is also held in check by broader cultural constraints, old and deeply rooted in a societal consciousness that shapes our cultural norms. European biases tie dance to the erotic, to a "low" intellect, to drunkenness, sin, and debauched behavior. Roman intellectual disdain for dance was well illustrated by Cicero's remark: "Nemo fere saltat sobrius - no sober person dances." [2] In Roman culture dance evolved over time toward the pantomimic, and strong sexual content

2

in dance was very evident by the Empire's decline. Early Christian/Catholic dogma reviled the dance as a fast track toward corporal sin. Protestant theology took this several steps further, and even today, as Ann Wagner notes in her text *Adversaries of Dance: From the Puritans to the Present*, conservative religious groups, most of these of Protestant affiliation, distribute anti-dance tracts and evangelical colleges require their students to sign contracts of behavior that include prohibitions on dance. [3]

For much of European and American history dance has suffered the effects of being caught within a curious web of social/sexual contexts. Strung between the realms of sex and beauty and form and fornication, dance is simultaneously a symbol and physical manifestation of both the accepted and the deviant, the envied and the reproachable. Dance is a metaphor for all that is located on the continuum of the social-sexual; in terms of orientation, presentation, and practice.

Dance has much to contend with as it is referenced, managed, and negotiated culturally. Society's rules for dance; the "who, what, when, where, and how" of dance, are a complex and slippery set of regulations that are deeply woven into the matrix of our lives. The explicit and implicit social contexts for bobbing and excited skipping are legion, and are specific to a wide range and variety of contexts. There are many rules for dance - for the range of kinds of dance included in different events, for the individuals who dance, for the groups who dance; in divers situations, and in ordinary and extraordinary circumstances - that making sense of their meaning and impact is difficult, and often quite humorous. To illustrate an example of this consider the subject of children and dance.

Simply put, kids will dance at the drop of a hat. They move rhythmically, caper, bob, and skip, frequently, and find a certain delight in expressing themselves through creative movement invention. Children dance to demonstrate feeling, to augment their developing vocabulary, and to show their interest in communicating with others. As children we respond with dance-like movements at the slightest notion of joy, of anticipation, anxiety, or at moments of discovery, and this is socially acceptable until around the age of five. From about the age of six on our dancing becomes fraught with an increasingly complex set of social ramifications; rules that are buried in the opaque contexts of what is appropriate behavior for little boys and girls, "young ladies," and "young gentlemen." As childhood wanes dance looses its comfortable place in our set of devices for expression and communication and becomes trapped as a behavior whose experiential and expressional context must be appropriate.

Yet even though the "who, what, when, where, and how" of dance becomes more Byzantine with age and cultural acquiescence, a vestige of the innocent spontaneity in the dance we know and are allowed as children stays with most of us throughout life. This vestigial dance surfaces from time to time, particularly when we experience sudden floods of feeling. Bursts of dance spew forth at opportune and inopportune moments, sometimes charming to others, other times embarrassing the dancer. Rhythmic vertical bobbings, capers that escape our vigilant desire to act accordingly, and the desire to express life through non-utilitarian movement, seem to be innate, some might suggest important, manifestations and characteristics of our humanity. As an expression of our humanness, dance is in us, it is around us, it passes through us; it is us.

The enigmatic, controversial, and seemingly vestigial presence of dance in our lives makes it slippery subject matter for scholarly inquiry. Dance is difficult to pin down, or handle empirically, because it is so omnipresent, subjectively interpreted, and so ambiguously defined: Adjudicate a bob? Measure a caper? How does one separate the purely utilitarian from the non-utilitarian in human movement? How does one measure movement designed to please aesthetic tastes, or fulfill a social contract? Dance remains hard for some academics to take seriously because of its subjective, aesthetic, and broadly defined social nature. But, for those seeking to understand the phenomenon of dance, the hope persists that someday we may come to terms with its pervasive, ambiguous, and yet fecund nature. This book is written toward that end.

Dance and the American University acquaints the reader with an aspect of dance history that, prior to this volume, has not been documented in a comprehensive manner. This is an account of the struggle for cultural, academic, and artistic clarification and meaning for dance as this has been waged behind ivied walls. In this century the university has played an enormously important role in peeling back the ill-defined and, to some, distasteful cultural trappings of dance. Higher education came to this function slowly and with some trepidation, yet the fact remains that when the university became a place to dance, dance began an intellectual and academic journey out of the shadows and away from ambiguity toward greater recognition and understanding. The history of dance in higher education is a fascinating story full of odd twists, fitful starts and stops, remarkable coincidences, and steel-willed personalities. Arguably the first of the arts, dance was the last to find acceptance and a place in our educational systems. Educationally, dance grew from the top down, finding an academic home in the university before its art-related presence was considered in our schools. The struggle for meaning and understanding in dance continues today, within the academy and outside in the world of art-dance, sport-dance, social-dance, ritual-dance, metaphoric- dance, and even virtual-dance. *Dance and the American University* is written because it is through higher education that many in 20th century American society have come to know dance as an art, as a discipline, and as a human experience that is worthy of our considered attention.

The text of *Dance and the American University* begins with an overview of the events that led to the creation of the university in Western culture. The creation of a morally and socially relevant learning community in medieval Europe set the stage for the scope and depth of higher education in the present; of which dance is a part. Here, in the evolution of the centrality and importance of liberal learning in Western culture, and in a valuing of society's obligation to educate its citizens, the seeds for thinking of the university as a cultural repository bloomed. The beginnings of the university also represent the origin of the idea that advanced

5

education is education in preparation for the individual's career and adult contribution to society.

Beginning in the 11th century, the history of the creation of the university first involved Papal and then royal actions meant to secure and manage the allegiance of medieval scholar guilds. At first a purely abstract legal notion of corporate singularity, the "universitas" led to the notion of the "college" as a place to acquire an education in the seven liberal arts, and the "university" as the place to acquire advanced education in theology, law, and medicine. The evolution of European nationalism and the subsequent Protestant Reformation led to royal charters for colleges and universities and the infusion of a corresponding secularism in higher education. After this history is reviewed, a discussion of the organizational characteristics of Europe's universities is followed by a discussion of the transplantation of higher education to the New World in the 17th century.

The story of American higher education begins with the founding of Harvard University in 1636. Post-colonial higher education is then explored for its characteristics, one of which was a slow but important trend toward university studies as professional-vocational preparation. Issues of immigration, mechanization, the effects of Jacksonian egalitarianism, and some important policy positions in the first decades of the 19th century are reviewed for their impact on ante-bellum higher education. The Academic Revolution of 1870 - 1910 is next considered. The influences of a rapidly developing industrial-consumer culture, a turn toward the German model in university research and professionalism, and infusion of the German concepts of "lehrfreiheit" and "lernfreiheit" are considered and contextualized to provide a sense of the nature of the impact of the Academic Revolution on higher education in America. This section of the history is augmented by a review of the cultural evolution of dance in America leading up to the beginning of the 20th century. Admittedly, the history of the university is a full and complex one. The inclusion of the history of American culture and higher education 1636 - 1910 is provided to offer context for

6

a better understanding of the circumstances that led to the eventual inclusion of dance in academia in the first decades of the 20th century.

Here, at the beginning of the last century of the millennium, the text of *Dance and the American University* turns fully toward its topic. Beginning with an assessment of the first university dance programs, I then include a separate chapter on the dance educator who initiated the first major curriculum for dance in higher education; Margaret H'Doubler. The story of Margaret H'Doubler's great contribution to a philosophy for dance in higher education is followed by a telling of the story of Martha Hill and Mary Josephine Shelly, architects of the "Bennington Experience," a seminally important event for dance in higher education. From Bennington a subsequent turn toward professional standards in dance curricula emerged. An overview of discourse on the matter of dance in the university setting, including its affiliation with physical education, is followed by a chapter on the beginnings of the first national organization for dance educators, the National Section on Dancing of the American Physical Education Association. The struggle between the liberal and professional nature of dance in higher education framed the discussion for dance in the university for three decades; 1934 - 1966.

Following the cultural upheaval of World War II, dance emerges in the 1950's as a program in search of an independent academic identity. The idea of dance as a discipline came to the fore in the 1960's, and the cultural and academic events that comprise this decade of development are reviewed for their contribution to the evolution and substance of dance in higher education. Organized activity in dance advocacy, and the Dance Boom in program enrollments are dealt with in the 1970's, with the activities and story of the Council of Dance Administrators and the creation of a National Association of Schools of Dance central to this part of the history.

As the story of *Dance in the American University* moves towards the present I consider the events and contingencies of the Reagan Revolution and the notion of the "corporate university" on dance programs in the 1980's.   A

7

discussion of the evolution of dance scholarship and the issues of diversity and multiculturalism on dance program development brings this history to the present decade. Finally, I attempt to frame discussion on dance in higher education in the 1990's, and conclude this text with a final section on Projections for the Future.

Understanding the myriad of events, circumstances, and contingencies that combine to provide history with substance, presents the historian with the task of making choices. In *Dance and the American University* I have chosen not to write about individual programs but rather to focus on points of view, policy making, position statements, and the work of organized groups. This is a first attempt at contextualizing the history of dance *with* the history of higher education, and at contextualizing the history of dance *in* higher education.

The fact that much of the history of this latter context is of the recent past presents this writer with a unique set of considerations. What I did here an hour ago is "history," but even in my own mind these actions have not become that "which was." Like looking out over a deep and wide landscape, description of the distance, "that which was," suffers from my limited ability to "see" all the discreet elements that make up that landscape. Much of the story of dance in higher education grows dusty on shelves in college studios, or resides in the memories of people who have either passed away, or who are advanced in age and difficult to reach. Conversely, the closer I come to describing that which exists in my immediate presence, "that which has recently been," there is the risk of becoming enamored with individual aspects of the present environment to the possible exclusion of considering the whole; things are just too close. With that said, I have attempted to delve into the past and address the present through reference to the historical scholarship of others, through the use of documents contemporaneous to the event discussed whenever possible, and to oral and written histories, either previously recorded or solicited for the purposes of this study. I hope the reader understands that in presenting this history there is a chance in missing something that may be important. It is here that the history of the story of dance in the American university is ripe for additional exploration.

8

CHAPTER 1

The story of organized education in Western culture is a rich and complex one. Out of the "Studium Generale" (general school) of the early medieval period emerged the university and a philosophy for education that was unique to European culture. The purpose of education was meant to accomplish three central objectives; 1. to develop the individual's ability to contribute to society, 2. to push back the boundaries of knowledge, and 3. to forward the cultural legacy. From its origins in medieval European culture, to the development of the large, research universities of 20th century America the story of higher education in the West provides contexts for better understanding the historical development of all contemporary academic disciplines. This fact is no less true for dance.

Elementary learning in the West was organized around the first of the three objectives listed above; to facilitate the individual's constructive participation in society through education. The perspective that the educated had an obligation to apply their knowledge for the betterment of society was a unique characteristic of the medieval school. Education in the classical world of antiquity did not consider an ethical obligation to use knowledge in this way. Secondary education, from which the university evolved, took into consideration the second and third objectives through advanced studies. All three of these objectives framed the development of the university in its philosophy and in its resulting organization and governance. These notions represent the seeds from which grew educational contexts for attending to matters of science and the humanities, and later, to art and the body in higher education. And, while the connecting philosophical thread

9

of why we educate our citizens has taken many courses in its evolution, the foundations of learning are the well-spring from which the thinking and rationales of early dance educators evolved.

The following chapter does not attempt to include dance or dancing in the context of discussing the historic development of the university between the 13th and 19th centuries. Popular notions of medieval scholars pondering the number of angels that could dance on the head of a pin notwithstanding, dance does not begin to play a substantial role in higher education until the 19th century. This introductory chapter is meant to help situate the reader in understanding how the university evolved first in Europe and then in America. The development of higher education in a democratic and industrial society set the stage for the university's attention to the arts.

Origins of the University in Western Culture

Intellectual culture in the early years of western Europe came from Rome and the Catholic church carried the Roman intellectual tradition forward into the thousand years that comprise the Middle Ages (the period in European history between the years AD. 476 to AD. 1453). One of the first tasks of the nascent Church was the education of a largely pagan Europe. The practice of educating converts to Catholicism was conflicted by the fact that while the Church was the chief remnant of Roman civilization, it also greatly feared the substance of Roman intellectual discourse. Catholic educators struggled with the necessity of preserving the language and literature of Roman civilization while simultaneously exposing those aspects of Roman culture included in the content of an unedited secular literature. This was no easy task. Catholicism was a religion of ideas and concepts. To be a good Catholic one had to understand and accept the logic that informed the Catholic Articles of Faith. Education ultimately meant exposure to secular writings and speculative thought. [1]

Beyond a basic Catholic education Roman intellectualism became a concern when secular language and readings were necessary for advanced studies. Learning in these contexts meant an increased possibility of student exposure to a provocative and potentially corrupting literature. As one's education progressed, complexity and depth of learning mandated access to realms of knowledge where speculation and critical analysis were common. Speculation often leads one to doubt, and in the Catholic world of religious absolutes, this was a dangerous exercise of mind. In *The Evolution of Educational Thought* , Durkheim (1969) quotes early Church educator Minucius Felix:

> Si quando cogimur litterarum secularium recordari et aliquid ex his discere, nan nostrae sit voluntatis sed, ut its dicam, garvissimae necessitatis.

> [If ever we are compelled to bring to mind secular literature and to learn something from it, let it not be at our desire, but, I would say, under the gravest necessity.] [2]

To manage access to knowledge acceptable areas of inquiry were defined. These represent the early curriculum designed to provide the requisite skills to manage church and social existence. Learning in the early medieval period was organized under the rubrics of the Trivium and the Quadrivium.

The Trivium involved the study of grammar, rhetoric and logic, considered the first and most important areas of knowledge for the young mind to master. From introductory studies in grammar came the term "grammar school," a phrase that is still used to refer to elementary education. Instruction in the Trivium involved temperance of mind, the intellect as revealed through rules of language, and the logic of causal order. Developing language skills, particularly the ability to defend one's intellectual position through logic based argument, dominated higher learning in the West well into the 19th century. The Quadrivium focused on the more refined, applied, and potentially dangerous areas of arithmetic, geometry, astronomy, and music. The Trivium was the bedrock of education, the Quadrivium was reserved for scholars. Together, the Trivium and Quadrivium were equated with the divine by the Catholic scholar Cassiodorus (c. 490 - 585), who imparted a scriptural significance to their study by identifying the three subjects of the Trivium, and the four subjects of the Quadrivium, as the "Seven

Liberal Arts"; the number seven having a special significance in early Christian mysticism: 3

> The whole of human knowledge was divided into seven branches, or seven fundamental disciplines; these are the *septum artes liberales* [grammar, rhetoric, logic, arithmetic, geometry, astronomy, and music], which name was used as a title for the great works of Cassiodorus. This division into seven reaches back to the latter days of classical antiquity; we find it for the first time in *Martianus Capella*, at the beginning of the 6th century....[For] centuries it was to remain as the basis of education. In this way it took on in the eyes of the people of the time a kind of mystical character. The seven arts were compared with the seven pillars of wisdom, the seven planets, the seven virtues. The number seven itself was deemed to have a mystical meaning.
> The seven arts did not all enjoy equal status; they were divided into two groups whose educational significance was very different, and which the Middle Ages always distinguished from one another with the greatest care. 4

The Early School as an Environment for Learning

Catholic religious doctrine involved an active renunciation and rejection of worldly (e.g. material, physical) pleasures. In a spirit of focused and transcendent learning, facilities for education were either located in remote areas or in proximity to cathedrals and churches where the distractions and temptations of daily life could best be monitored and controlled. Here, faculty and students delved into the substance of a religious education in an undisturbed, communal, and pious atmosphere. Students seeking an education were not expected to enter church service upon completion of their formal studies, however all were expected to use their knowledge to improve the lives of their fellow Christians. The communal nature of the educational environment, and the idea that scholars would serve the needs of the larger population were important developments in education. In the Greco-Latin world of antiquity learning had not involved participation in an organized or morally focused intellectual community. Teachers taught their students independently and most often in their own homes. There was no tradition of the educated having an obligation to serve society. Education in medieval Europe bred a sense of relatedness between members of the community and emphasized the individual's intellectual and spiritual obligation to the cultural good that existed outside the walls of the school:

The school as we find it at the beginning of the Middle Ages does indeed constitute a great and important innovation. It is distinguished by characteristics wholly alien to everything the ancients called by the same name. Of course, as we have said, it borrowed from paganism the subject matter of what was taught there; but this subject matter was expounded in a brand new way and from this exposition something quite new resulted....[M]oreover it can be argued that it is only during this period that school, in the real sense of the term, emerged. For a school is not simply a place where a teacher teaches; it has a moral life of its own, a moral environment, which envelops the teacher no less than the pupils. Antiquity knew nothing like this. It had teachers, but it did not have genuine schools. [5]

The Medieval Period: Teaching Societies, Avaricious Chancellors, and Introduction of the "Universitas"

As the medieval period evolved, European culture became complex in its organization. Systems for facilitating cooperative action among similarly skilled peoples became increasingly necessary. Those with a common occupation banded together to create "guilds," an early manifestation of present day corporations. Scholars, like tradesmen and other specialists of the day, organized to protect their rights, and to insure that those who joined their ranks had the requisite skill to practice their profession. Scholarly guilds and teaching societies were located in residence at a church or abbey or traveled about the countryside teaching and lecturing as requests for their services warranted.

In the latter medieval period the social and political organization of European culture became increasingly complex and sophisticated. Political life was unsettled as authority over the myriad petty kingdoms, duchies, municipalities, and bishoprics passed to and fro as the vicissitudes of war, marriage, death, or birth required. Meanwhile the demand for the practical and stabilizing services of learned societies increased. Greater demand for the services of scholars inevitably led to their crossing royal, municipal, religious, and intellectual borders. Factious politicians and religious leaders were quick to use the service of scholars to support political or cultural agendas. They also had few qualms about charging exorbitant fees of license for the privilege of teaching. Guild members struggled to protect themselves from greedy or ruthless local authorities. Scholars wanted the right to certify their colleagues and have this privilege universally recognized. The need for a standardized curriculum, protection from the vagaries of local politics, and the rights of teaching societies to award and use degrees, became increasingly necessary and emerged over time.

Throughout the eleventh and twelfth centuries, European Catholicism was at war with Middle Eastern Islam in the Crusades. As the Crusades progressed the Roman Catholic Pope and the Germanic Holy Roman Emperor dominated Europe's developing political culture. Each recognized the changing political and intellectual mood of Europe. Between the traditional political notions of a Catholic-universal and a feudal-local Europe emerged a new political-cultural model, largely based on common use of language. Following the Crusades, European culture began to evolve toward the secular-state, although the trend toward identifying oneself as 'English' or 'French' took many generations of intrigue, marriage, and civil war to firmly establish. As the twelfth century came to a close national identity was beginning to replace feudal or Catholic political identification in Europe. The university was born and tempered at the edge of the growing chasm between state and church.

Europe's early royal families settled in capital cities such as London, Paris, Madrid, and Vienna to facilitate their accumulation of political and military power. Schools associated with political centers accumulated an enhanced social and intellectual cache. These were called Studium Generale, a general school were all students were received. According to Rashdall (1895), the Studium Generale was the direct precursor to the creation of the university and the term came into broad usage at the beginning of the 13th century. The Studium Generale had three characteristics, 1. the school attracted students from all regions, 2. it was a place where at least one of the professions of theology, law, or medicine was taught, and 3. subjects were taught by a "considerable number" of Masters. [6] The Holy Roman Emperor Frederick Barbarossa was the first monarch to encourage students to congregate to his domains in an Imperial Bull (proclamation) delivered in 1158. Schachner (1938), writes that the Emperor Barbarossa's Bull *Habita*, was "the first general charter of privileges for students anywhere." [7] In Paris, the

Ecole de Paris shared in the prestige that the city itself was acquiring. Durkheim states that: "...it [the Ecole de Paris] had an attraction which was incomparably greater than that of other schools in the kingdom and even in neighboring countries." [8]

Seeking the license of "Jus Ubique Docendi"

During the first centuries of the medieval period, the custom of credentialing and recognizing the rights of educators to teach was assigned to regional Bishops through their award of a *licentia docendi* (teaching license). As teachers became more numerous and attention to their needs became more time consuming, the Bishops relegated the authority of degree conferral to their Cathedral Chancellor. Cathedral Chancellors were not always selected from the ranks of the educated, and in many cases were not above avarice. By the beginning of the 12th century the scholarly guilds were struggling with the ·Chancellors for control over the conferral of degrees, licensing of teachers, and to bring an end to the rampant graft that had become increasingly common. Scholars sought a license of *jus ubique docendi* (universal license to teach) - the right, once credentialed, to teach anywhere without having to pass new examinations and pay new fees. They turned to the Pope for help, and in their defense a series of Papal Bulls were issued in the first decades of the 13th century. In 1212, a Papal Bull mandated that Cathedral Chancellors award degrees to candidates judged worthy by a certain number of teachers and in 1220, the Pope forbade Chancellors the right to excommunicate members of a scholarly society without Papal authorization. [9]

Pope Innocent IV afforded comprehensive Catholic protection to the growing number of Studium Generale in a Bull he issued in 1243. Innocent recognized the benefits of this action for both its social and political advantages. Schachner (1938), writes that: "By heaping benefits and favors on the struggling universities, by protecting them against even kings and avaricious churchmen, they [the Church] bound all grateful scholars to them with bonds of steel." [10]

15

Innocent's stewardship of the Church coincided with changes in the political evolution of royal prerogative in European culture. Bishops had little recourse in challenging or countering the potential threat of a burgeoning royal will, should their actions and allegiance be viewed as rebellious. Catholicism profited from the benefits of a centralized, and strengthened Papal dominance in education. Innocent's Papal Bull of 1243 went beyond the petty concerns of whether the Cathedral Chancellor or the local scholars would be granted final say in the conferral of academic degrees. Socially, Papal recognition of the pre-eminence of the scholar's guilds in certifying and licensing teachers meant the guilds would have a continued stake in accepting and supporting Rome's interests in education. Politically, Catholic authority and influence in education helped consolidate and buttress the Pope's position dealing with the growing influence and strength of Europe's royal families.

To justify this strengthening of Church control over higher education, Innocent's legal scholars borrowed a concept from Roman civil law - the idea of the "universitat," or "free corporation." In Roman law, the universitat was an abstract legal notion of singularity where separate and independent legal identity was granted to an aggregate of persons based on recognition of their function in society: a universitas of scholars or a universitas of teaching masters. The universitas was a corporate entity and was not associated with a location or series of buildings. The term 'college' was originally used to identify the buildings that housed members of the universitas. Over time the terms 'college' and 'university' became associated with lower and upper divisions of higher education. The college housed instruction in the liberal arts, the university focused on the professions of theology, law, and medicine. According to Rashdall:

> It is mere accident that the term 'university' came to be restricted to a particular kind of guild or corporation: just as the terms convent, corps, congregation, and college, have similarly been restricted to certain kinds of associations....[T]he term university was generally in the Middle Ages used distinctly of the scholastic body whether of teachers or scholars, not of the place in which such a body was established, or even of its collective schools. [11]

Innocent's Bull had far reaching implications. Not only did his proclamation frame the legal construction of the university, the idea of legal recognition for a group's activity also represents the beginnings of the modern corporation. Groups of scholars or religious orders (Dominican or Franciscan) could be recognized as 'universitas'; and thereby legally separate in the eyes of canon and civil law. Universitas were authorized to perform their functions for society and the church in perpetuity. Separate legal status meant an end to the guild system for education and much greater academic freedom and independence from the whims of local control. It also meant greater Papal influence over what the curriculum would include, the religious affiliation of the faculty, and the manner in which subjects would be taught.

The leading Studium Generale of Europe were recognized as universitas under the authority of Rome. Important university centers were established in Paris, France; Bologna, Italy; and in Cambridge and Oxford, England. Appropriating this idea, Europe's royal and political families began to establish universities of their own. New centers for higher learning were created where the resources of a state, city, or family afforded the establishment of a university. By the latter years of the 13th century the Holy Roman Emperor Frederick II was competing with Pope Gregory IX in granting license of authorization to universities. The original reason for Papal protection of the Scholars had become moot by the middle of the 14th century as royal and city charters for universities became more common. [12] Non-Catholic control of the university increased in northern Europe following the advent of the Protestant Reformation in the 16th century. [13]

The university curricula evolved in tandem with developments in the organization and governance of higher learning. Acceptance into professional study was contingent upon successful completion of college education in the liberal arts; the student had to pass college exams before being allowed entrance

17

into the university. The remnant of this curricular model is evidenced in today's general education requirement within the context of the undergraduate experience.

Regional Differences in University Organization

Universities in southern and northern Europe developed differently in terms of their governance and organizational characteristics. In northern Europe the University of Paris assumed a pre-eminent position among institutions of higher learning. The University became entangled in the French religious-civil wars of the 16th and 17th centuries with the coming of the Protestant Reformation. Protestant (Huguenot) scholars were permitted into the ranks of the university when politically secure and tolerant monarchs occupied the French throne. Diversity in the religious affiliation of professors stimulated the intellectual environment of the French university. Yet Protestant scholars were also persecuted when political circumstances were less stable. The whole-sale slaughter of French Protestants in the Massacre of St. Bartholomew's Day during the regency of Catherine de Medici, and the Draggonade during the reign of Louis XIV, were two such events. [14]

England accepted the Protestant Reformation when King Henry VIII broke off relations with the Catholic Church in the 16th century. Protestant scholars fleeing Catholic persecution on the continent contributed greatly to the intellectual vitality of the English university. Following the break with Rome, English universities were recognized by a royal charter of incorporation. Royal charters established perpetual succession in management and allowed the Masters of the college great latitude in developing their own rules of governance. Provisions for the privilege of royal review were necessary to obtain a charter. The boards that conducted review for the King however, were managed by a staff appointed by the professoriate. [15]

In Italy, higher education evolved much less formally in academic organization. The Catholic Church continued to dominate the substance of the Italian curriculum, but the organizational structure of the Italian university was quite unique. In the early years of the Italian university the students managed the masters, directing their education as they independently contracted with scholars for instruction. The degree to which scholars worked together in an academic community was quite limited. Over time, the Italian city-states of the late renaissance began to compete for the best scholars and developed a sort of bidding war that kept scholars on the move. With cities competing for the best faculty, families and institutions funding universities demanded greater control over how their monies were spent. This eliminated the hiring power of students. Municipal committees, forerunners of the civic governing boards common in American higher education today, were formed to guard the financial and political interests of university funders.

The creation of the university was an extraordinarily important step in the evolution of culture and thought in the western world. Its organization may be traced to the religious and intellectual tidal pool that settled and shaped itself following the cultural storms surrounding the fall of Rome. Out of this cauldron emerged the substance of first a Catholic, and later a nationalistic-European culture, with the university playing a central role in cultural development and retention. The story of higher education shifts gears when transplanted to the New World in the 17th century. Here the American university takes on new and unique characteristics and traits as the academy reflects the circumstances and contingencies of an emergent democratic and industrial society.

Developments in American Higher Education: 1636 - 1910

Throughout the colonial period of 1620 - 1776, higher education in North America was modeled after the English-Scottish tradition where the liberal arts and the professions were taught within a Protestant theological framework. This is referred to as the classic curriculum. Harvard, founded in Cambridge, Massachusetts in 1636 was the first chartered university in America. Almost six decades later the College of William and Mary was established in Williamsburg, Virginia in 1693. Both Harvard and William and Mary modeled their organization after the royal charters for England's Oxford and Cambridge Colleges. Yale College was begun in New Haven, Connecticut in 1701. The founders of Yale asked the colonial legislature to authorize a single, non-academic board of governance. The externally organized Yale Corporation, reminiscent of the municipal managers of the Italian university, became the subsequent model of choice for governance by private and state supported colleges and universities in America.

The number and kinds of colleges in America slowly grew in the years leading up to the Revolutionary War. The majority of these were independent colleges founded by religious groups, but as external control of colleges became more common some were created that were more secular in their origins. The curricula that developed in America's colleges gradually began to reflect discreet differences, although most remained alike. Colleges framed higher learning around the classic curriculum. Women were not included. Only after successful completion of examinations in the classics were students permitted to proceed to the university to prepare for the profession of choice. Professional field training after college was done as apprentice to a practitioner. There were no state licenses for medicine or law. Those fortunate enough to attend college were from the upper classes and a large part of their educational experience was devoted to establishing networks to reinforce their place in the social order. The curriculum in colonial America was reflective of the times. As the years passed and the political atmosphere in the colonies became more contentious and fluid, so too did the atmosphere in the universities. The evolution of American higher education toward academic and intellectual diversity was a response to the interests and needs of a developing democratic society. This evolution ultimately led to the inclusion of dance in higher education.

The first attempt at expanding the components of the classic curriculum was initiated by Benjamin Franklin and the Reverend William Smith when they established the College of Philadelphia (later renamed the University of Pennsylvania), in 1740. Franklin and Smith designed a curriculum that included studies in history, politics, trade, and economics. The sciences were also included with courses offered in physics and zoology. [16] Mabel Lee (1983), writing in her text *A History of Physical Education and Sports in the U.S.A.*, states that Franklin was "...the first recorded promoter of physical education." Franklin offered "detailed instructions and advice on setting up a physical-activity school program. He even gave instructions on the techniques of teaching some of the activities, most notably swimming." [17]

Following the upheaval of the Revolutionary War the pace for change in American higher education quickened. The idea of a university education began to take on a new and more practical character. State sponsored universities were formed in Georgia (1785), North Carolina (1789), Vermont (1789), South Carolina (1801), Ohio (1804) and Virginia (1819). In the public university regular innovation in the curriculum first took hold on a broad scale. [18] Academic historian Frederick Rudolph (1977), writes that by the early 19th century the university's role as the breeding ground for a small social elite started to change as the nation's economic potential became more apparent. Colleges began accepting members of the growing middle class and emphasized course work designed to prepare students for a career. Although one would not have found radical differences between colleges during the ante-bellum years leading up to the Civil War, the trend in American higher education was toward greater academic choice and vocational preparation. Vocationalism in post-colonial education has its roots in immigration and the developing industrial base of the American economy, and in the politically free and secular environment in which colleges and universities could be established. [19]

The College Curriculum: "Telling Ourselves Who We Are"

> For the curriculum has been an arena in which the dimensions of American culture have been measured, an environment for certifying an elite at one time and for facilitating the mobility of an emerging middle class at another. It has been one of those places where we have told ourselves who we are. It is important territory. [20]

In the first decades of the 19th century, political and economic change and innovation in American culture led toward curricular experimentation and an interest in educational vocationalism. This was a time of legal and philosophical clarification for the role of the university in a democratic society. Soon after the ending of the war of separation from England, the newly formed United States Supreme Court agreed to hear a case that helped define the independent nature of the university and its legal relations with the state.

With the trend toward legislative appointment of university trustees and board's of directors, questions began to arise regarding the degree of influence politicians might hold over private colleges within their jurisdiction. A struggle between legislatures and private colleges partially supported by public monies arose over the matter of control and oversight. Cloaked in the notions of personal freedom and independence that dominated political thinking in the years leading up to the Revolutionary War, some college masters began to question the legal authority of legislatures when they felt institutional rights were being intruded upon by colonial government, e.g. in matters determining curriculum or in the hiring of faculty. College masters argued that the university, as a corporation, enjoyed the legal rights and status of an individual citizen. Following the Revolution, the matter was directed to the newly formed United States Supreme Court under Chief Justice Marshall. The Court decided in the matter of Dartmouth College v Woodward (1817), that the private nature of Dartmouth's corporate status afforded it the same rights in coming to contract with the State as were afforded the State's citizens: therefore a violation of the terms of contract would represent a violation of an individual's freedom as defined by the United States Constitution: "The opinion of the Court, after mature deliberation, is that this is a contract, the obligation of which cannot be impaired without violating the Constitution of the United States." [21]

The Dartmouth decision led to a reexamination of the legal relationship between state and university. As a result of the Court's findings, state funds for private institutions were diverted to public universities under the control of corporations created by the state legislature. This is important to consider in the history of dance in higher education because the turn toward separate funding for public and private institutions led to ends that ultimately helped expand the range and kinds of curricular opportunities offered by the university. Public institutions provided vocational preparation and services to the citizens of the state, and private institutions were free to experiment with original approaches to education subsidized by their patrons. A freer and more fluid educational environment for higher learning emerged from the Dartmouth decision.

Another important conceptual leap for American higher education came about as a result of the Yale Report of 1828. In the years just prior to the beginning of Andrew Jackson's tenure as President of the United States, students at Yale were questioning the faculty's insistence that they master the dead languages of Greek and Latin. Meddling by students in the design of the university curriculum prompted the President of Yale, Jeremiah Day, and Yale's trustees (the "Yale Corporation"), to commission a special report on the university's curriculum. The Yale Report is considered the first American statement on educational philosophy.

For President Day and members of the Yale Corporation, the Report was an important clarification of the appropriateness of the curriculum, and the meaning of university study. Authored by Day and Professor Richard Kinsley (Professor of classics, mathematics, and the history of New England; a good example of the range of expertise expected of faculty in the classic curriculum), the Report was first published in January, 1829 in the *American Journal of Science and Arts*. The Yale Report reaffirmed the value of advanced learning in religion, languages, classic literature, and mathematics, arguing that these areas of knowledge developed the student's lifelong intellectual and moral discipline. [22] Historically, Day's Report has been labeled a reactionary statement of educational policy concerned with nipping the influence of a bourgeois intellectual laxity at the academic bud. Ironically though, in part because of its conservative and authoritarian tone, the Report also acted as a catalyst for continued academic

23

debate regarding curricular experimentation. In the years immediately following the Yale Report, the growing influence of "Jacksonian Democracy," which fostered a political and social egalitarianism in American culture, clashed with the traditional values of exclusiveness and restriction that were the hallmark in admissions and curricular planning in higher education. The result was a decline in enrollments which jeopardized the success of colleges and universities not endowed to the extent as that of Yale. With their very survival at stake, less traditionally bound colleges were further encouraged to develop curricula more in tune with the needs of their communities and an emerging, professionally oriented middle class. [23]

Changes in American Culture 1820-1870: Effects on the University

In the years following the Yale Report, 1830-1860, the United States was expanding in size, embarking on the process of inventing and establishing an enormous industrial capacity and attracting ever increasing numbers of immigrants. The changes associated with geographical expansion, industrialization, and population growth impacted all levels of culture, including organized education. Increasingly, agriculture and engineering, physics, chemistry, and other technical areas of study were included in the college curriculum. Immigrant educators, particularly those with credentials in the sciences from German universities, found teaching positions in American colleges and helped to change the tenor and nature of advanced learning.

Another stimulus for the development of higher education in America came with congressional passage of the Morrill-Land Grant Act in 1862. Essentially a federal give away of acreage to the states, the Morrill-Land Grant Act was designed to help establish state operated universities:

> Long agitation by agricultural societies, farm journals, and other advocates of vocation training for farmers and mechanics-Jonathan Baldwin Turner being the most important-influenced Justin S. Morrill of Vermont to introduce into Congress a bill to aid in the establishment of agricultural and mechanical arts colleges in every state of the Union. The measure passed congress in 1858 but constitutional objections induced President Buchanan to veto it. A similar measure, since called the Morrill Act, was signed by

President Lincoln in 1862. States were offered 30,000 acres of land for each representative and senator they were entitled to in the national legislature, as an endowment for the proposed schools. In some states the lands were given to existing institutions, as in Wisconsin where the state university was the beneficiary; elsewhere they were conveyed to newly established agricultural and technical colleges such as Purdue University or the Illinois Industrial University, now the University of Illinois. [24]

The expanded network of public universities stimulated the trend in higher learning toward curricular experimentation and flexibility. Land Grant colleges and universities successful in attracting students, faculty, and external funding, including newly appropriated government funds for research and development, were imitated for their structure, organization, and curriculum. The competition for a limited applicant pool led to development of the elective and utilitarian/vocational course offering as a very attractive academic lure for students. Out of the Land Grant college's interest in an expanded curriculum emerged their willingness to first incorporate courses in physical education, and later, courses in dance.

Following the conflict of the Civil War, peace meant continued geographic expansion, a rapid return to industrialization, resurgent immigration, and an explosive growth in the American middle class. The profound range of development in industry and commerce in the years 1870 - 1900, led to radical changes at all levels of American culture. Acknowledging the full range of this evolution would lead us far afield from the focus of this text. The creation of a product driven industrial economy, and the public's ready access to commodity, media, and transportation raised people's expectations regarding their standard of living, and raised their expectations about the benefits of education. Increased access to print media in particular stimulated the public's desire to benefit from developments in business, science, and education. [25] The cultural norms of the 19th century were shed and replaced with new paradigms for living. A direct consequence of efficient media distribution stimulated changes in the nature of American education, particularly in higher education. Reform in primary and secondary education was stimulated by national press coverage of the public's demand for change in the school curriculum. Educational reform was

25

conceptualized in teacher training programs and in the new graduate schools of education.

Developments in American politics, industrialization, and the public's interest in commodity also helped redefine the university's place in society. After the Civil War a university education was becoming much less concerned with the certification of gentlemen, and more concerned with adult, middle class issues of career and economic success. The acquisition of skills and full participation in, and benefit from, the fruits of culture became the goal of America's burgeoning middle class. The university was a place to educate the literate and technologically aware graduates, both male and female, that were needed to provide professional expertise, manage business, develop industry, and create other specialized systems for a rapidly evolving consumer culture. Within this larger context were buried myriad other new ways of thinking about higher education, both externally, as the university was perceived by the public, and internally as academics retooled higher education to meet the public's expectations.
26

Immigration and the German Influence on the University

In the 19th century, the tide of immigrants coming to America began to assume flood proportions. Increases in population meant greater demand for the products of culture, and social adaptation to these demands invariably led to educational change: more schools, different kinds of programs, different kinds of outcomes. Some immigrants had been professionals and educators in their home countries and brought unique ideas and perspectives on education. Perhaps the most important of influences were those of German academics with the German philosophy for the university. These had a major impact on American higher education.

American students had been traveling to German universities since the beginning of the 19th century for advanced study. In the 1820's the first wave of German academics migrated to the United States to escape the intellectual repression that followed the defeat of Napoleon and the rise of reactionism in European politics. A second wave of German nationals came to the United States in the 1840's; again largely as a result of political repression:

> In 1848 revolutionary movements swept over Europe, and in Germany the government used a policy of reaction and suppression to meet the demands for a liberal government. The result was the migration of thousands of the best German citizens to the United States. [27]

> During the 19th century more than 9,000 Americans studied at German universities, all but 200 of them after 1850. The Johns Hopkins University, opened in Baltimore in 1876 with an inaugural address by Thomas Huxley, the Darwinian, was an expression of both the English and German influence. The new emphasis implied an increase in the scholar's stature, freedom, and prestige. Inspired more or less by the example of Johns Hopkins, 15 major graduate schools or departments had been established by the end of the century. [28]

German academics brought to America an emphasis on the importance of discipline-based specialization, the use of scientific methods in research, and the importance of research and development to a university's mission. German professionals introduced the academic concepts of "lernfreiheit" and "lehrfreiheit". Lernfreiheit translates as "the freedom of the learner." As a concept lernfreiheit led to independence of thought and to the elective course and freedom of academic choice for students. Lehrfreiheit means "the freedom of the teacher." Lehrfrieheit led to the concept of academic freedom and the professional status of professors. [29]

Student participation in educational decision making, and the specialized, professional academic focusing on discipline based study, were important new perspectives for American higher education. The empowerment of the student in educational choice further opened the door for a greater range of curricular offerings. Viewing the professoriate as the recognized authority in matters related to their area of specialization stimulated the recognition of new disciplines within the curriculum. The concepts of lernfreiheit and lehrfreiheit helped pave the way for the acceptance of new academic disciplines including dance.

Physical Culture, Hygiene, and the Normal School: Early Physical Education Programs in Higher Education

Another important German contribution to American educational life was the German idea of "physical culture", and the subsequent development of the Gymnasium Movement. Throughout the 19th century teachers and administrators in American education had been aware of the need for a systematic approach to student health and physical well being. According to Rice (1926), the first stage of the physical culture movement in America's schools began in the 1830's and was introduced by German trained educators. One or more of the following four basic activities were taught:

1. Exercises derived from military activities (like marching and parades), or manual labor.

2. "Jahn," (or, "German") gymnastics developed by Freidrich Ludwig Jahn.

3. "Ling," (or, "Swedish") gymnastics developed by Per Henrick Ling, or;

4. A type of calisthenics developed specifically for women by Catherine Beecher. [30]

German methods for guiding and structuring physical activity sessions during the school day found ready acceptance in American educational circles. In turn, regularly scheduled physical culture in public schools created a need for specialized teacher training programs.

Williams and Brownell discuss the history of academic and curricular development for physical education in, *The Administration of Health and Physical Education* (1934). In the last decade of the 19th century physical culture was re-labeled "physical training," and when physical training and matters of health and hygiene were blended together the term "physical education" gained prominence. [31] Williams and Brownell, and Rice (1926), write that the first teacher training program for physical educators was founded by Dr. Diocletian Lewis at the Boston Normal Institute for Physical Education in 1861, and for the next several decades Lewis' methods dominated the curriculum. [32] By the end of the 19th century, course work in aesthetic culture, physical training, and hygiene were included in curriculum designs at colleges specifically devoted to teacher preparation termed "Normal Schools."

Due to the lobbying efforts of the Women's Christian Temperance Union (WCTU) in the 1880's curricular attention to hygiene was blended into programs for physical training. Members of the WCTU pressured state legislatures to require the teaching of the effects of alcohol and tobacco use on America's youth. Disease prevention in the schools came to the fore in 1894 with a national Medical Inspection Movement. The first state to mandate curricular attention to the body in the primary grades was Ohio in 1892. In 1899 North Dakota became the first state to require regular periods of physical training and hygiene for grades 1 - 12. [33] According to Williams and Brownell (1934), the Morrill-Land Grant Act also stimulated the development of physical education teacher training as state college programs were designed to serve the needs of the community.

The German contribution to American education's attention to health and well being had an effect both in and outside of the schools. Wherever there was an established German immigrant population physical culture, health, home economics, and practical medicine were taught at local "Turnvereine". In their heyday the local Turnvereine helped citizens lead better, more productive lives. The "Turner Movement" was a very important contributor to developing American interest in regular physical activity and health. [34] Today, some communities in the American mid-west have active Turner Halls. According to Rice:

> The German gymnastic societies, *Turnvereine*, [German name of the society] soon made their appearance where sufficient number [of German immigrants] settled. The Cincinnati *Turngemeinde* was the first one organized in the new country, but was closely followed by the New York *Turngemeinde* ; both were founded in the latter part of 1848. By 1852 twenty-two societies had been organized throughout the North. [35]

The Academic Revolution: 1870 - 1910

While the needs of the body were being attended to in America's grammar schools, and teacher training programs for physical educators were being developed in state colleges and Normal Schools, a more profound revolution of sorts was changing the way in which higher education was structured and managed. Among historians of American higher education, the period from the end of the Civil War and leading up to the first years of the 20th century, has been termed the era of the "Academic Revolution." Between 1870 and 1910, the model for the organization and governance of higher education as we know it today fully emerged. The contemporary organization of the American university emerged from the ante-bellum college. The German attention to scientific method and research, and the concepts of lehrfreiheit and lernfreiheit stimulated new ways of engaging the student in the process of their own education and empowered the professoriate to see themselves as masters of specific areas of knowledge. These ideas also helped frame the subsequent evolution of the university. But the fundamental and pervasive nature of the range of change and reformatting in American higher education between 1870 and 1910 is beyond the introduction of science and new ideas in the student-faculty experience.

The Academic Revolution introduced the use of numbered courses, the unit system of assigning credit, departmental organization, the bureaucratic system of administration and governance, the offices and functions of college president, academic dean, and department chair, elective course offerings, the professional academic, the discipline specific professoriate, even the notion of discipline singularity. All these changes appeared quickly and with little variation among American institutions of higher learning. Vesey (1973), comments that the reasons for the large scale adaptation of a new model for organization and management in the university remain a mystery. [36] There is little in the historic record to suggest why these changes happened so suddenly and so similarly. In an attempt to clarify the suddenness and homogeneity of the Academic

Revolution, scholars have cited the cultural and economic factors previously referenced. The sudden acceptance and manner of the new model for the organization and management of higher education is certainly reflective of a similar trend in American industry and business during the same period. As the Industrial Age came to full bloom, standardization of production, mechanization, and product delivery were influencing the organization of the industrial shop floor. Reform and Progressive political movements were forcing business and government to come to terms with the twin pulls of markets and profit, and consumer and labor protection. Labor and business leaders were both increasingly adamant about what each perceived as fair regarding the distribution of wealth, wages, and reasonable working hours.

As industry and government became more systems oriented, specialized, and bureaucratized, so too did the university. Schools and departments of agriculture, engineering, business, education, and the physical and natural sciences took their place along side traditional academic programs in the arts and humanities. The turn toward bureaucratization and curricular vocationalism in higher education was very much to the advantage of industry and a capitalist economy. From applied studies in science, business, and education, the university solidified its place as the training ground for the experts necessary to address the country's social-educational problems, industrial needs, and economic goals. [37]

Relations between labor and management become more contentious and complicated as America's industrial base expanded in the decades following the Civil War. Business leaders took on public personas as robber barons and fat cats. Voter opinion began to turn toward matters of reform and regulation. The federal anti-trust initiatives of the Roosevelt presidency (such as the *Sherman Anti-Trust Act* of 1890), set an example for state and local political leaders seeking to reform laws and policies that for years had favored the interests of business over those of the individual. [38] Progressive politicians favored self-discipline, duty to family and community, self-reliance, individualism, and a return of political power to the people. Fanning the discourse in public affairs was the growing tabloid press, perhaps best exemplified by Joseph Pulitzer's *New York World*. In an effort to eliminate competition and boost sales, the tabloids were the vehicle for much of the urban population's daily news, sensationalizing by exposing business, government, and even education for inhumane and short sighted practices. [39] Popular, progressive opinion was translated into voter action and this shaped the nature and focus of reform in government and in education.

Reform was driven by the real issues of quality of life for the lower and middle classes. Population centers developing around industrial and transportation hubs had grown quickly and were in need of better and more sophisticated management and planning. Matters of public health and standards of living, directly impacted by low wages for workers, poor city planning, limited access to affordable and clean housing, short food supplies, and antiquated sanitation systems, were taking on a new and heightened importance. The practical matters of daily living reinforced the need for an organized educational approach to matters concerned with the physical health of the individual, the community, and the nation.

The University as Social Laboratory

American higher education was being redefined in many ways by the last decades of the 19th century. Curricular experimentation was indulged in and the idea of the university serving the needs of the citizens of the state gained acceptance. Higher education was increasingly considered the preferred environment for vocational training. The university assumed new responsibilities in research and development, addressed the societal needs of a growing and increasingly urban population, and emerged as the environment for professional, vocational preparation. The university was being recast as the technological, social, and educational laboratory for America. By 1900 the scene was set for innovation and change in higher education on all fronts. In that spirit the American university began to attend to matters of the body and include physical education, and later dance, as independent academic disciplines.

The history of higher education of this period was not, however, simply a matter of development and improved opportunity. Blum et. al. (1989), discuss the sudden bureaucratization and expansion of the university curriculum circa 1900:

> A mistaken conception of democracy led to the assumption of equality among all academic pursuits and justified the teaching of courses in almost any subject, however trivial. Institutions became overexpanded, overcrowded, and absurdly bureaucratized. A misguided deference to the opinions of alumni, sports enthusiasts, and the unlettered public led to an anarchical confusion of values and distortions of academic purpose. For the first time in recorded history institutions of higher learning assumed the function of providing mass entertainment in spectacular sports, particularly football, and the comparative distinction of a university came to depend on its success in pursuing these enterprises. [40]

The university's willingness to teach courses, "in almost any subject, however trivial," was difficult for many conservative members of the faculty and community to reconcile. Justification for new courses and new ways of looking at the university, in part a result of the progressive idea of the service university, ·challenged traditional notions of academic propriety and substance. At the vanguard of state universities serving the public was the University of Wisconsin, where the "Wisconsin Idea of Education", the original plan for the service university, was initiated. It was also at Wisconsin that the idea of dance as an academic major was first realized. This development is fully addressed in Chapter 4.

CHAPTER 2

Dance in 19th Century America: Social Grace, Sinful Pleasure

Until the last decades of the 19th century, dance in America was generally not thought of as an appropriate activity outside strictly controlled social settings. Dance was certainly not considered an art form of any consequence, nor was it recognized for its potential as an educational medium. While dance was not totally vilified in Western culture, its advocates were few, and not much came of their efforts to explain or rationalize dance as an educational medium.

In, *The Rise of the Arts on the American Campus*, author Jack Morrison writes that there were some who saw good in a dance education and wrote of its potential, among them: Sir Thomas Elyot, John Milton, John Locke, and the Reverend John Cotton of the Massachusetts Bay Colony. [1] A few educational programs incorporated dance within the curriculum, and forward thinking individuals such as Thomas Jefferson appreciated dance as "one of the arts that 'embellished life.' "[2] But the fact remained that for most Americans dance education was of little concern and of peripheral interest at best.

In 19th century religious circles there was still considerable opposition to the social ramifications of dance. The idea that dancing between the sexes led to inappropriate social contexts and opportunities was firmly entrenched in the thinking of many conservative clergy and their followers. This was particularly true of Protestant religions of a Puritan tradition, which were pre-eminent in shaping American moral norms. [3] As an example of Puritan thinking on the matter of dance in the early Colonial period, consider the following excerpt from a sermon given by the Reverend Increase Mather to his fellow citizens of the Massachusetts Bay Colony. In, *The Mathers on Dancing; Including: An Arrow Against Profane and Promiscuous Dancing Drawn out of the Quiver of the Scriptures*, Joseph Marks quotes a sermon by the Reverend Mather:

> Concerning the controversy about Dancing, the Question is not whether all Dancing be in itself sinful. It is granted, that Pyrrhical or Polemical Salutation: i.e. where men vault in their Armour, to shew their strength and activity, may be of use. Nor is the question, whether a sober and grave Dancing of Men with Men, or of Women with Women, be not allowable, we make no doubt of that, where it may be done without offense, in due season, and with moderation. The Prince of Philosophers has observed truly, that Dancing or Leaping, is a natural expression of joy: so that there is no more Sin in it, than in Laughter, or any outward expression of inward Rejoicing.
>   But our question is concerning Gynecandrical Dancing, or that which is commonly called Mixt or Promiscuous Dancing viz. of Men and Women (be they older or younger persons) together: Now this we affirm to be utterly unlawful, and that it cannot be tolerated in such a place as New England, without great Sin. [4]

Continuing in his sermon Mather condemns profane and promiscuous dancing by analyzing the Bible for its anti-dance content. "Grave and sober dancing" was the only form of dance that Mather felt a Christian population might allow its citizens to practice. Certainly dancing for pleasure among mixed company was not to be tolerated, and dance as a performing art was beyond consideration.

In other less conservative colonies of the central and southern Atlantic region, earning one's living by teaching social dance forms, while less socially conflicted as a result of theological discourse, was still at the periphery of acceptable vocations. Still, because ability in social dance was considered an important sign of personal grooming, there was a need for instruction. Dancing Masters toured the estates of the wealthy, teaching the sons and daughters of the social elite lessons in grace and deportment. Dance in performance was also presented in the more populated colonial cities. The romantic ballet for example, was presented fairly regularly in America's larger urban centers throughout the middle decades of the 19th century. [5] Regardless of the social position of the itinerant dance instructor, or the presentation of concert dance performances, dance in America was not regarded or understood as a fine art. Nor was dance considered subject matter of any concern to educators in schools or colleges.

As an example of lingering fear of dance in the late 19th century, consider the following passage from William Cleaver Wilkinson's *The Dance of Modern Society* (1884). Wilkinson's argument against dance is carefully separated from an impassioned plea for propriety. He also separates his thesis from the judgment of God, attempting to clarify his condemnation of dance as a matter or reason. Still, Wilkinson rather disingenuously introduces his "rational" argument via the doors of propriety and religious precedent:

> I do not, it will be seen, affect the candor either of ingenuous inquiry or of judicial neutrality. Much less do I affect the candor of a merely curious unconcern. I appear as an advocate, and I do not expect, as I shall not attempt, to avoid the vehemence of advocacy. I volunteer my office on behalf of several imperiled interests, all of them valuable, and one at least vital. It is the case at once of Health, of Economy, of the Social Nature, of Intellectual Improvement, and of Morality, that I defend. I undertake to implead the Dance in their joint behoof as the common and equal enemy of them all.
> I shall summon the accused to answer, not at the bar of passion, however holy and religious, and not before the tribunal of Scripture, however clear and authoritative, but rather in the wide and open forum of reason, of conscious, and of common sense. If the Dance can escape conviction here, she shall be welcome for me to make her pirouette, and go tilting out of court, free to take her chances of living down, as best she may, the ancient and sacred suspicion against her, which still survives in that one safe sanctuary left for a badgered and brow beaten morality ready to be ashamed of itself - the inviolate bosom of the Christian church. [6]

In conservative Protestant religious communities dance continues to be the subject of consternation and scorn. Marks' text mentioned above concludes with "A Bibliography of Anti-Dance Books (1685-1963)." [7] Ann Wagner (1997), writing in *Adversaries of Dance: From the Puritans to the Present,* presents this caution against the evils of the body and pleasurable movement:

> Yet vestiges of the old notions sometimes appear-as in the small community of Purdy, Missouri, where a legal battle arose not long ago over whether or not the school board could prohibit dancing. In 1987 Hollywood produced *Dirty Dancing,* a film set in the early 1960s about young people who struggled to overcome rules forbidding dancing. [The film's title itself tells us something of popular conceptions of dance]. Some conservative groups still send out anti dance tracts, and some private colleges continue to require students to sign a pledge that they will not dance. [8]

Popular Interest in Antiquity: Resurgent Classic Ideals in a Modern Age; Impact on Physical Education and Dance

For most 19th century Americans professional dance remained a misunderstood activity for society's slackers. In the latter decades of the century changes began to take place in education and in public tastes that would open the door for new ways of considering the expressive use of the human body. In addition to the inclusion of programs for physical education in American schools, by the late 19th century there was a resurgent appetite among adults for the trappings of 'classic' cultures.

Public interest in antiquity had recurring cycles in American popular culture in the years leading up to the end of the 19th century. The images and philosophies of Ancient Rome seemed to fit well with the emerging identity of the young American Republic. In Europe, the French Revolution of the late 18th century, and the Napoleonic excavations of Egyptian and Greek ruins in the first years of the 19th, reinvigorated classical images of antiquity in European education, fashion, the arts, and culture. What was fashionable in Europe sooner or later came to be fashion in the United States. By the end of the 19th century interest in ancient cultures was renewed by further excavations of archeological sites in the middle and far east. Images and stories of "savage," and "lost civilizations" that appeared in the tabloid press were widely popular. In the 1880's for example, New York's newspapers, such as Pulitzer's *World,* and William Randolph Hearst's *Journal,* competed for readers by including stories of exotic, foreign lands. On the more serious side, newly formed academic organizations like the National Geographic Society promoted a more scientific and scholarly understanding of the world through publications meant for middle class audiences. Interest in the 'other,' the 'exotic,' and the 'foreign' had an influence on the American public's conceptions of the body, personal and community health, and education. Descriptions of "lost" civilizations reflected popular notions of European racial superiority and helped fan the American public's increasingly inflated self-image. [9] Comparing themselves with the citizens of ancient Greece or

Imperial Rome, Americans were encouraged to develop their appreciation for the total human being in mind, body, artistic inclinations, and expressive qualities. An important manifestation of the 're-discovery' of the body, and of thought and emotion as expressed through the body, was a new method for training actors and public speakers that was gaining in popularity in American theatrical and liberal educational circles.

Devised by Francois Delsarte, a French music and drama teacher, the Delsarte System was used to develop individual abilities in expression through gesture, posture, and movement. According to Stebbins (1902), "Delsarte welded the whole of his system together with the universal Law of Correspondence." [10] The Law of Correspondence associated humankind with God through the idea of "Trinity." The Christian "Trinity" of God; the Father, the Son, and the Holy Spirit, was reflected in the Mind, Soul, and Life of man. Trinity was also reflected in just about any other triad one might come up with: Mental, Moral, Vital; Love, Wisdom, Power; Attraction, Repulsion, Rest:

> Delsarte's trinity of principles comprehends three distinct states and types of humanity - Intellectual, Emotional, and Vital. In actual practice, the working formula consists of principles which are in themselves impersonal. They are the powers which *individualize the person and lie back of the personality* [authors emphasis]. They consist of the intelligence, or thought-creating spirit, the formative powers, or soul, which is the spirit of life, and the result of their unified action, which we term Emotion....[I]n exact proportion to the strength and range of this trinity within, we are enabled to express the heights and depths of human feeling. [11]

By 1880, an American version of Delsarte's techniques was being pioneered by Steele MacKaye, a well known actor and theatrical talent in the New York dramatic world. [12] In presentations of Delsarte "statue posing and tableaus," the costuming was commonly inspired by Greek and Roman fashions of antiquity. The techniques for expression employed by the American Delsarte Movement reflected the glories of ancient Greek and exotic eastern cultures, imparting to the practitioner a degree of seriousness and refinement that appealed to American audiences. According to Ruyter (1979), Delsartian exercises helped develop an appreciation for personal communication skills, relaxation, emotional

39

expression, body awareness, and 'balance,' ideas that would resurface in the new, art-dance of the early 20th century. [13] Delsarte's system of expression not only attracted actors and others interested in performance, it also appealed to the general population as well; in particular urban women of means. One of MacKaye's students, Miss Genevieve Stebbins, is recognized as the person most responsible for popularizing Delsarte's work with the larger American public. [14] Through her numerous books, public demonstrations, and in lectures at progressive schools Stebbins helped break down many of the social and cultural biases surrounding physical training and expression, especially for women. According to Ruyter:

> Stebbins furthered the Delsarte system in America through extensive work as a teacher, writer, and performer. Most of her teaching was in fashionable seminaries and academies for young ladies - and was apparently sought equally by Protestant, Catholic, and non-sectarian schools. In addition, she taught the Delsarte system and yoga breathing exercises to such adult groups as a philosophy class and a class of middle-aged women studying "nerve-gymnastics" (techniques for relieving nervous tension through correct breathing and exercise). [15]

In addition to being taught at "fashionable seminaries" for young women, elements of American Delsartism were incorporated into programs designed for teacher preparation in physical education. Stebbins' Americanized version of Delsarte's work had a profound effect on the thinking of two young women who were growing up in the 1880's, Ruth Dennis of New Jersey, and Isadora Duncan of California; soon to be recognized as the 'mothers' of a new, American art-dance. Delsarte's ideas appear at the core of the work that Duncan and Dennis (as 'Ruth St. Denis') would later contribute to the professional world of dance, and to dance in education. At the center of Stebbins' work were two central themes - the classical world of antiquity represented the ultimate in man's artistic achievements and that one might commune with the divine through the body. [16]

Another early systematic approach to understanding the nature and elemental structure of expressive human movement was Dalcroze Eurythmics.

Devised by Emile Jacques-Dalcroze in 1898, Eurythmics was a technique for using rhythmic exercises to supplement musical understanding:

> It was Emile Jacques-Dalcroze, the great Swiss music educator, who first realized that musical rhythm depended absolutely on motor consciousness for its fullest expression. His research led him to evolve a system for rhythmic movement designed to develop mastery of musical rhythm...
> ...[B]eginning with the simplest of rhythmic responses and proceeding step by step to the most complicated rhythmic problems, Dalcroze's system of rhythmic training is unique. Eurythmics develops the child's rhythmic potential through the medium of his own body, which becomes, in effect, a "musical instrument."
>
> The study of Eurythmics is based on the following important objectives:
> 1. Utilization of the whole body, involving the larger muscle groups, assures a more vivid realization of rhythmic experience than does the customary use of the extremities, such as hand - clapping and feet - clapping.
> 2. The physical coordination's developed in the well directed rhythm class give the individual the power to control his movements in related activities.
> 3. Bodily movement acts as a reference for the interpretation of the symbols of rhythm. Which become truly significant when learned as the result of vital rhythmic experience.
> 4. Habits of listening are developed by the child in the process of identifying what he hears and what he does.
> 5. Body, mind, and emotion are integrated in rhythmic expression.
> 6. The freedom of expression, which is a cardinal principle of Eurythmics, stimulates the creative impulse in every department of learning.
> 7. Finally, learning becomes joyous and meaningful when it evolves from human needs. The child who has danced his way to music will never turn a deaf ear to music. [17]

Like American Delsartism, Dalcroze Eurythmics contains many of the essential perspectives that would inform and stimulate the thinking of the important "art-dancers" of the early 20th century. These included use of the whole body (as opposed to simply positioning the limbs), tying rhythm to coordination to develop sequential exercises for neuromuscular development, body-mind integration, freedom of expression, and education and learning as evolved from human needs. [18] The Delsarte and Dalcroze agendas fit well with the tenets of Progressive Education. They provided an approach to pedagogy that would soon become the bedrock for curricular attention to the body and its utilitarian and aesthetic potentials.

There were important social issues that also helped shape the focus of early physical education training programs college women. The women's movement for educational-social equality, and interest in matters of women's health and well-being impacted the subsequent development of programs in dance. In the late 19th century, more and more women were attending to issues of health and the needs of the adult female. Practical matters that had a real impact on women's lives included dress reform, personal hygiene, physical fitness, conception, and health in child bearing.

In turn, the health and physical well-being of the increasing numbers of women who were enrolling in coeducational state universities was a growing concern to college administrators. Women's physical education and health had traditionally been attended to at women's seminaries and colleges, but with the creation of state funded, coeducational institutions, a greater number of women could afford to attend college. The greater number of women in college, and the public's interest in women's health, led physical educators to develop classes and programs that would suit the needs of their female students. Administrative interest in the health needs of women led to the rapid development of women's physical education programs in state supported higher education in the last decade of the 19th century. Lee (1983), discusses the historic development of women's physical education programs in higher education:

Vassar was the first college in the United States to offer physical activity classwork for women as part of the school program. This was in 1868. Mt. Holyoke and Rockford colleges had been offering work since 1837 and 1849, respectively, but neither achieved collegiate rating before the 1880's. Wellesley established its departments in 1881. Oberlin college was the first coeducational college to organize a department of physical education for women (1885). A few state universities recognized departments for women before those for men: Indiana, Kansas, Utah, Michigan, Ohio State, and Texas. In three state universities it was the military department that brought about the establishment of a department for women: California (Berkeley), Nebraska, and Wyoming. State University departments for women were founded as follows:

1889 - California (Berkeley)	1894 - Illinois	1894 - Wisconsin
1890 - Indiana	1894 - Michigan	1896 - Iowa
1890 - Washington *	1894 - Nebraska	1896 - Minnesota
1893 - Kansas	1894 - Oregon	1897 - Ohio
1894 - Utah	1894 - Washington*	1900 - Missouri

19

[* Lee does not clarify two references to "Washington." We are left to assume that one refers to the University of Washington, and the other to the Washington State University.]

The 15 years between 1885 to 1900 were a time of swift and rapid fire change in all areas of American life. Politicians, educators, and labor leaders, began to act as they responded to demands for political, social, educational, health, labor, and voting reform. The Age of Progress was a time of technological invention, material excess, and the accumulation of prodigious wealth by some. Cultural and legal barriers that delimited the role of children and women for centuries began to crumble. Legislation intended to reform government, corral big business, improve public welfare, and increase public access to education was passed in swift succession. Liberal educators took bold steps and seized an opportunity that would not be theirs again for many years. The roots of many of their experiments may be traced to American Delsartism and the Dalcroze System and to the Progressive Education Movement that gained in popularity in American culture following the Civil War. [20]

Progressive Education: Origins and Principles

Progressive Education in the United States had its origins in the writings of the English philosopher Herbert Spencer. Spencer's theories reflected an attraction many in science and education had for the work of Charles Darwin. Applying Darwin's concepts on the evolution of the species and natural selection to social existence, individual development, and the education of children, Spencer argues that education should prepare the student for life in contemporary society. In this context, education would involve an active engagement of the student in real life situations. As with natural selection in the wild, Spencer's notion of a social Darwinism had a tough edge; the individual's success in society was a matter of innate attributes coupled with luck. Some where born with a better chance for survival than were others.

43

In his writings Spencer also discussed physical education. Pragmatic to a fault, he felt that the practices science had developed for breeding better farm animals might be adapted and put to use for successful child rearing. Haley (1978) comments:

> Spencer also relies on animal analogies, particularly in his essay "Physical Education," where the comparisons are mainly to the care of livestock and pets. Why is it, he asks at the beginning of his discourse, that most men show an interest in the breeding, training, and raising of animals, but few in the rearing of children? [21]

According to Spencer, physical education should include all aspects of healthy living including regular physical activity, attention to personal hygiene, healthy clothing, and proper diet. His theories encouraged a much broader interpretation of what a progressive and enlightened education might mean. Spencer's influence permitted others to expand on progressive ideals and make the case for physical education and dance as academic subjects.

Ruyter (1979) and Lee (1983), cite G. Stanley Hall as the next important exponent of progressive educational ideals to point out the benefits of physical training, and even dance. [22] Quoting Lawrence Cremin's *The Transformation of the School: Progressivism in American Education 1876-1957,* Ruyter (1979), writes of Hall's contribution as one which "opened the pedagogical floodgates to every manner of activity, trivial as well as useful, that seemed in some way to minister to the needs of children." [23] Hall wrote directly of the value of dance in his text *Educational Problems,* written in 1911.

Hall valued dance as a spontaneous expression of the human spirit that exemplified a harmonious connection between mind and body. Hall's chief interest in dance was as a thoughtful and thought provoking physical activity. Dance fit quite well with Hall's Theory of Recapitulation in which performing and practicing folk and national dances, imitative dances of nature, and dances of love and work provided children with an opportunity to express, to "recapitulate." Through physical activity they would bond more closely with their human potential. Hall didn't advocate the use of theatrical forms of dance. Instead his

44

focus was on using dance to "enlarge the emotional life by making all the combinations of movements that it is mechanically possible for the body to make." [24] Hall's contribution to the eventual inclusion of dance in the college curriculum was in his placement of dance in a progressive context, distancing it from its potential immoral (theatrical) connotation by endorsing the practice of national dances as a tool for individual expression and cultural appreciation. Hall's position as President of Clark University helped lend his arguments academic weight and validity. Certainly his admiration for the dance, and the substance of his persuasive discussion on the merits of dance in education, helped focus and refine subsequent academic initiatives for dance in the curriculum. [25]

Lee (1983), writes that Francis Parker, Superintendent of Schools in Quincy, Massachusetts, was another important early exponent of progressive ideas in education. Lee quotes John Dewey, the man most associated with progressive education, as proclaiming Parker "The Father of Progressive Education." [26] According to Lee, Parker:

> [D]evised a schooling for the children based on observation of life about them, reading of current materials, nature study at first hand, and experiences in doing original writings. With a basis for learning established, he then brought back the use of the textbooks....Before the 1890's his ideas were not widely recognized, but once they were made known through articles in magazines and newspapers, a growing number of educators, unhappy with the old formalism, seized upon his theories, and politicians and reformers, as well as parents and teachers, began pushing for reforms in education. [27]

Following Spencer, and contemporaries of Hall and Parker, were John Dewey and William James. Both were then at Columbia University, and were the next great advocates for a pragmatic, yet progressive, approach to education:

> A psychologist as well as a philosopher, James emphasized the vagaries and the resilience of the mind, and warned against imprisoning intellectual creativity within arbitrary or mechanistic systems. For him the truth of an idea depended on its consequences. Dewey conceived of philosophy as an instrument for guiding action, an instrument he himself used in advocating experimentation in education and government. Tolerance and freedom of belief of expression, Dewey noted, were essential if ideas were to enjoy a competitive chance to prove their merit. [28]

By 1900, reformists in Government, also labeled "Progressives," were beginning to effect change in state politics. The reform movement began in Wisconsin under the political leadership of Governor Robert "Fighting Bob" LaFollette:

> He [La Follette] attracted both a rural and urban following that was essentially middle class in its background and aspiration. Before he became United States senator in 1906, LaFollette made his administration [as Governor of Wisconsin] a model of honesty and efficiency, established a fruitful liaison between the government and the state university, whose distinguished faculty included many valuable advisors on public policy, and overcame the opposition of the Old Guard in the legislature....Wisconsin had become, as Theodore Roosevelt later said, "the laboratory of democracy. [29]

Political "progressives" supported the task of reforming education. By the end of the first decade of the 20th century John Dewey (1859 - 1952), was the acknowledged leader for progressive change in education. Dewey wasn't, as Dworkin (1959) points out, progressivism's singular champion, but, following his work at the University of Chicago, and later at Columbia, Dewey did take on the personification of the progressive educator:

> Dewey's career was the longest among those philosophers for whom there are substantial and verifiable records. The range and quantity of his writings attest not merely his spirited activity until the very end of his life, but the astonishing vigor of the mind that was at work. His first publication, which appeared when he was twenty-two, dealt with problems in metaphysics. The writings of his last fifteen years, which many professional philosophers regard as his weightiest contributions to the continuing philosophic dialogue, were concerned with logic, theory of value, methodology of the behavioral and physical sciences, and theory of knowledge....[B]ut of all his published work, it is his writings on education that have exerted the widest and deepest influences upon life on the United States and other countries. [30]

Dewey's take on a progressive education differed from that of Spencer and Hall in that Dewey believed the student should be much more proactive in learning to prepare for life. Unlike his predecessors, who felt that learning should help the student accept the pre-existing conditions of life and social evolution, Dewey believed that through experience education might in fact shape and direct personal development. [31] Transference of the benefits of educational experience to life and living spoke directly to physical educators looking for rationales and justifications

46

for their work and teaching in higher education. Yet, hitching their wagon to Dewey's star had both its rewards and its drawbacks. While the tenets of progressive education spoke to the educational potential of thoughtful physical experiences, time revealed that an unchallenged progressivism did not support academic rigor, nor did it predict an evolutionary need for physical education and dance to become more professionally oriented and focused. A vigorous turn toward academic professionalism swept the American university in the years following the Second World War and it carried the fields of physical education and dance.

John Dewey's Influence on Programs in Physical Education: Traditional v Progressive Education

At the turn of the 20th century, the ideals and perspectives of progressive education inspired the thinking of educators interested in promoting the value and substance of a "physical" education. However, it was radical at this time to consider that the subject matter associated with physical education might possess enough depth and breadth to be considered an academic discipline in higher education. Without some philosophical perspective to tie it to individual and societal benefit, physical training was essentially just physical activity. The critical question was: Couldn't "physical training" be found in everyday labor? The field's response to this question was one of the reasons the term physical "education" was coined to replace the labels of physical "culture," or physical "training." The point to be made was that a physical education was an education that dealt with healthy living, developed neuromuscular skills, combated the "evils" of a sedentary life, and taught the "standards of sportsmanship." [32] The philosophies of progressive education were used to make significant steps toward refining and defending the idea that structured, invigorating, and culturally relevant movement activities might be beneficial to students.

How did Dewey's writing about the merits of a progressive education fit the academic agenda for physical education and dance? At the center of Dewey's thoughts on the nature of the progressive curriculum was the notion that education should give shape to individual human abilities. Dewey's vision for education encouraged the student to experience events that provoked thought, analysis, and active juxtaposition with other like and unlike events. Dewey advocated the organization of subject matter (curriculum), within experience and his views fit well with the disciplinary goals of physical educators. A brief review of Dewey's thoughts on the nature of progressive education helps clarify the perspectives that many early movement educators adapted to develop their own thinking.

According to Dewey, traditional education consisted of three central perspectives:

1. The subject matter of education consisted of exposing students to bodies of information and to skills that have been worked out in the past; the chief purpose of the school was to transmit these to each new generation,

2. there were standards and rules of conduct; moral training involved forming "habits of action" that were in conformity with such rules and standards, and

3. the patterns of organized education; grades, classrooms, tests, subject matter, the set of relations between students and between students and teachers, constituted the school as a kind of organization quite distinct from other social institutions.

In Dewey's opinion, the rise of progressive education was the result of a discontent with traditional methods and concerns that the precepts of traditional education were not working in a modern age. Progressive education was, in effect, a criticism of modes of education that involved an imposition of ideas and habits from 'above' and from 'outside.' Dewey also thought that traditional modes of education were too adult for children. Learning in these contexts meant a routine acquisition of what was already incorporated in books and in the minds of teachers. Moreover, what was taught in a traditional education was thought of and dealt with in a static manner. The implementation of a progressive curriculum was meant to benefit the modern child in six ways:

1. Imposition of knowledge from above would be replaced with expression and the cultivation of individuality,

2. External discipline would be replaced with free activity,

3. Texts and teachers would be replaced with experiences,

4. The acquisition of isolated skills by drill would be replaced by attaining ends which made direct and vital appeal,

5. Preparation for a remote future would be replaced by making the most of the present, and

6. Static aims and materials would be replaced by acquaintance with the changing world. [33]

Dewey's conviction that there was an intimate and necessary relation between the processes of actual experience and education was the perfect point of .departure for the field of physical education. Advocates for physical education were in need of an overarching rationale for the questions conservative educators asked when they attempted to make the case for a developed and integrative program of physical training in the schools: Why? And to what end? The problem for progressive physical educators was in establishing a context for learning through movement that was in harmony with the principles of learning through experience. Dewey's pragmatic cautions against thinking that all experience could contribute to learning helped frame their task of equating movement experience with cognition:

> Experience and education cannot be directly equated to each other. There are good and bad experiences, experiences that inform and instill and experiences that don't....
> ...[E]verything depends upon the quality of the experience which is had and how that experience is contextualized to benefit the student...
> ...[A] coherent theory of experience, affording positive direction to selection and organization of appropriate educational methods and materials, is required. [34]

John Dewey's philosophies inspired the thinking of early movement educators. From their point of view, the physical self and the sentient, moving body was the perfect medium for experience. Physical educators held the vision their discipline helped students lead an informed and healthy, active life, learn proper hygiene, develop a heightened sense of shared community in democratic living, and experience a deeper connection to racial roots. These were important issues for physical educators at the turn of the century and Dewey's philosophies of experiential learning were congruent with these goals. Dewey's educational philosophy was used to justify sequential, curriculum based learning through movement experience. His contributions to the development and acceptance of physical education and dance in the American university are seminal.

Progressive Education in Retrospect: A Critical Perspective

Not everyone has agreed with Dewey and the other proponents of progressive education. There are many academic historians who feel the principles of progressive education inevitably led to curricula that were lacking in substance and intellectual rigor. Consider one rebuttal of Dewey's influence written well after his time. In *Stability and Experiment in the American Undergraduate Curriculum*, Laurence Vesey (1973), comments on Dewey's influence:

> [Dewey's influence]...reached a peak of prominence in the 1930's. Much of the Dewey rhetoric echoes the utilitarian minded reformers of the late 19th century. Dewey's followers rejected specialized technical training as an appropriate focus of the college curriculum and instead proposed a curriculum based on more universally determined "life needs." These included courses centering on social and family adjustment, on marriage and the home, an indoctrination of Dewey's liberal civic philosophy, and courses dealing abstractly with the problem of choosing a vocation (rather than courses that prepared one specifically for a vocation). Upon reflection the Deweyian model is judged as...the least important of the reform crusades. The colleges which it powerfully affected (such as Bennington, Sarah Lawrence, and Stephens College in Missouri) usually happened to be girls schools or else truly obscure.... [A]dherents of the Dewey persuasion communicated a tone of belligerent sectarian isolation, offering ritual formulas of a low intellectual caliber. [35]

Vesey's criticism reflects his assessment of Dewey's impact on the curriculum as a whole. His comments on the colleges that implemented Dewey's progressive policies (Bennington, Sarah Lawrence, and Stephens College) may be considered sexist and rather harsh, "girls schools or else truly obscure." It is interesting that these colleges were among the first to accept dance as an independent, arts-related, academic discipline separate from physical education.

While Dewey's legacy may no longer permeate whole systems of undergraduate education, his influence helped initiate inclusion of experientially based disciplines that were previously not considered as discreet subjects in the university (i.e. physical education and dance), engaged the professoriate in tying education more closely to real life experience (the development of internships and other educational "field" experiences), and promoted a more receptive academic environment for diverse and non-traditional subject matter. One result of the progressive education movement was the development of policy statements concerned with the value of instructive and socially conscious physical education programs in American schools. In these programs and in the professional societies created to serve physical educators, dance found its first champions in mainstream academia. Turning our attention back to dance and its early connection to physical education, we will see that this relationship, while at first a blessing for the evolution of dance as subject matter within the academy, over time became fraught with complications as the utilitarian nature of physical education clashed with the aesthetic nature of dance.

Anderson, Sargent and Gulick: Three Pioneers for Physical Education and Dance

The American male has never comfortably been associated with dance in American culture and education. Recall the Reverend Increase Mather's sermon on dancing, cited earlier in this chapter, in which Mather contextualizes male participation in dance, "where men vault in their armour, to shew (*sic*) their strength and activity." [36] By the late 19th century "vaulting in armour" had become less of an issue, but the expectation that men would dance only when it demonstrated their strength and activity was still an important aspect of the cultural norm. Male participation in art-dance, the ballet or the pseudo-art-

51

dances of the theatrical spectacles that were popular in the developing vaudeville circuit of the 1890's was highly suspect because aesthetic movement was (and still is), plagued with questions and concerns regarding the masculinity of men who choose to dance in this manner. Folk dances, however, were devoid of theatrical connotation and fit well with the needs of early physical education programs. Hall's Theory of Recapitulation and Dewey's interest in experiential learning provided a positive connotation for folk dance in the physical education curriculum. Interestingly, it was physical educators William G. Anderson, Dudley Sargent, and Luther Gulick who are credited with bringing folk dance into the physical education curriculum. Each contributed a great deal to the development of physical education programs nationally through their writings, organizational activities, and example. And, each could easily be the subject of an extensive biography. In the field of physical education Anderson, Sargent, and Gulick loom large. I reference them only in that their individual interest in folk, aesthetic, and "national" dance helped lend the topic of dance an important degree of academic recognition.

William Anderson was an exceptional physical educator. A native of Michigan, Anderson had his first experiences in physical education training with members of a circus. His formal education included study at Boston's Roxbury Latin School, the University of Wisconsin, and a degree in medicine from the Cleveland Medical College. In 1885 Anderson founded the Brooklyn School of Physical Education, and in 1892 he accepted a position at Yale University as associate director of the gymnasium. He was appointed Director of the Yale Gymnasium in 1903. Anderson remained at Yale until his retirement in 1932. [37] In addition to advocating the inclusion of gymnastics and sports activities in physical education, Anderson traveled extensively in Europe and America studying national, regional, and social dance forms and used these in his classes at the Brooklyn Normal School and at Yale. [38]

Dudley Sargent, a native of Maine, started his training in gymnastics at an early age. Appointed the Director of the Gymnasium at Bowdoin College in

Brunswick, Maine, Sargent began devising his own approach to physical training that predicted the development of natural gymnastics in the early 20th century. [39] In 1887, Sargent founded the Harvard Summer School of Physical Education. Sargent's "Aesthetic Calisthenics", also known as "Aesthetic Dance," was taught by Melvin B. Gilbert at Harvard. According to Ruyter (1979), aesthetic dance was the first established dance system used in American education. [40]

Luther Gulick was born in Hawaii and was the son of missionary parents. As a young man he studied at Oberlin College under Dr. Delphine Hanna, an important early leader in physical education for women. At Oberlin, Gulick roomed with Thomas Wood, who would later develop Natural Gymnastics, an approach to physical training that gained support in American education during the years of the First World War. A prolific organizer, Lee, writes that Gulick was:

> ...[F]ounder of many important movements, such as the establishment of physical education in the YMCA's of America, the Playground Association of America, New York University Summer School of Physical Education, the Department of School Hygiene of the New York Academy of medicine, the position of Secretary of the International Education Committee of YMCA's (he being the first to hold the position), and the Camp Fire Girls....[H]e was one of the founders of the American School Hygiene Association, the Boy Scouts of America, American Folk Dance Association, and American Camping Association. [41]

As a founder of the American Folk Dance Association, Gulick supported the study of folk and national dances in elementary and secondary education. And, as President of the American Physical Education Association (APEA), he chose dance as a central theme of the APEA National Convention held in New York City in 1905. [42]

Benefiting from the influence of many physical educators, but perhaps most importantly from that of Anderson, Gulick, and Sargent, classes in folk and "national" dances became an important part of early physical education curricula.[43]

American Pageantry: Dance for a Democratic Community

The national dances, so appealing to progressive educators like Hall, Anderson, Gulick, and Sargent for their value in replication and reinforcement of what were considered the positive attributes of race, cooperative living, and a Protestant work ethic, found an outlet in community supported art events in the American Pageant Movement of the early 20th century. Introduced from England to America in 1905, civic and educational pageants quickly became an important means of emphasizing the benefits of the healthy, productive activities of work and play, while simultaneously enhancing community based interaction and cohesion. By 1909 pageants were assuming a unique place in American culture as civic expressions of identity, uniqueness, and history. Pageants also made quick inroads into the early physical education curriculum in higher education. The American Pageant Association, formed in 1913, promoted the benefits of pageants as these helped communities deal with the pressing issues of immigrant assimilation, democratic governance, community relatedness and shared history, and social/political reform.

In *American Pageantry: A Movement for Art and Democracy* (1987), author Naima Prevots traces the American pageantry movement during the years that these large scale community endeavors flourished, from 1905 to 1925. In her introductory comments Prevots suggests the kinds and range of pageants produced in America during this period:

> Across the vast open space the pilgrims convoyed forty-eight young women bearing the state flags, as a replica of the Mayflower blazed with light in Plymouth harbor and the chorus sang to words by Robert Frost...In a New York armory women performed a "Dance of Steam" to symbolize modern industry and their role as equal partners in shaping the world...On the sloping banks of a river in North Dakota the Spirit of Prophesy told of the excitement and conflict of extending America's boundaries into the Northwest. Sakakawea, also called Sacagawea and played by a full-blooded Indian, sang in her native language about guiding Lewis and Clark over dangerous mountain ranges...In Boston's Arena, children and adults danced portions of Swedish, Italian, Russian, Hungarian, and other traditional dances. [44]

Figurative retellings of historic and cultural events brought civic and educational communities together in pageant performance. Poetry, dance, storytelling, and dramatic action were supported with visual effects, music, staging, costumes, and props to reinforce local and regional history, community values, and cultural standards. The American Pageantry Movement helped change negative notions of the body and dance in popular culture and the success of community pageants led to the inclusion of course work in pageantry in colleges and universities. Teachers College of Columbia University, an early leader in progressive physical education, was also an early leader in including courses in "pageantry and festivals" in teacher education courses. In researching American Pageantry Prevots found listings for physical education- based classes in pageantry at Teachers College that emphasized dance as an art form with its own unique history. The idea that dance was an art and that there was, in fact, a history of dance to understand was an important conceptual bridge toward considering dance as academically substantive. The American Pageantry Movement helped develop a context for appreciating dance as a historically relevant, democratic, community oriented form of art expression. Many of those who developed and taught educational courses in pageantry at Teachers College were also early leaders in dance education including; Gertrude Colby, Mary Wood Hinman, and Mary Porter Beegle. [45]

World War 1 and the "New" Gymnastics

As has been noted, physical education programs of the 19th century borrowed heavily from the German idea of physical culture and employed German calisthenics and gymnastic systems for training the body. In the early 20th century, the developing political conflict in Europe between Germany and America's traditional cultural and political allies, France and Great Britain, led to an American suspicion of things German. By the time political tensions in Europe led to war in 1914, some in the American press were seriously questioning the patriotism of people who ate sauerkraut. German aggression was condemned not only by the American press and politicians, but also by patriotic elements in the educational community. The German approach to physical training, promoted by members of the Turnvereine, emphasized the use of gymnastic drill and group exercises. In part as a result of the influence of John Dewey, and in part to separate American physical educators from their German counterparts, Thomas D. Wood, of Columbia University, developed a new approach to activity titled Natural Gymnastics designed to replace the old method of response to formal command with a new form that "would embody social and psychological objectives." [46] According to Lee (1983), many physical educators lacked a "realistic understanding" of Dewey's or Wood's philosophy:

> [T]oo many teachers...became involved with class periods in which the pupils had little exercise and attained little in the way of social or psychological objectives and definitely no physiological ones. They had merely wasted their time. This vacuum of attainment most certainly had not been the intention of the originator [Wood], and the leading promoters of the new gymnastics, and these failures led to a division among physical educators. One group would retain the old forms of gymnastics for their own value. Another group would keep the old forms but rob them of their old formal and militaristic aspects. A third group would replace the old forms of gymnastics entirely with Wood's natural gymnastics. A fourth group would have no gymnastics at all in the physical education but would build the program around sports and dance in various forms. [47]

At the same time, in the years leading up to the conflict in Europe, dance was benefiting from the significant progress it had made in academic development as a result of Dewey's and Wood's influence. Natural Gymnastics had its counterpart in Natural Dancing.

In 1913, the first formalized curriculum in dance in higher education was instituted at the Speyer School of Teachers College, Columbia University by Gertrude Colby. The cultural and political atmosphere was right for dance to take such a 'step' at this particular time. In making the case for dance education, early leaders in the field stated that dance was liberal, individually motivated, non-threatening, democratically evolved, and an artistic expression of physical development. Through practice of the "national dances," whose performance reinforced the students connection to "race," and the newly conceived "natural dance," as espoused by Isadora Duncan, the student might artfully express the beauty of the body and appreciation for healthy living. Colby married the "national" and the "natural" together in an ingenious way. We shall see that the

"ColbyIdea for Dance Education" acts as an important bridge between dance as activity and dance as art-based discipline in higher education.

CHAPTER 3

Dance in America, 1895 - 1925: Becoming Art and Business; First Programs in Higher Education

Between 1895 and 1925 there were a number of developments in the professional world of dance that shaped popular conceptions of dance and influenced its future in the American university. Dance artists, Isadora Duncan, Ruth St. Denis, and Ted Shawn broke new ground for dance as art, matured their own vision for dance in education, and paved the way for the American "modern dance" artists and educators who would follow. Like Anderson, Sargent, and Gulick in physical education, Duncan, St. Denis, and Shawn are "giants" in the history of American dance and their lives provide the content of legend. However, unlike the former three, Duncan, St. Denis, and Shawn worked outside the world of the university. Nonetheless, their professional lives had a major impact on developments for dance within the academy.

Isadora Duncan

Isadora Duncan's influences on the evolution of popular, artistic, and academic notions for dance in America were transformative and stemmed from her performance artistry as well as from her writings, pronouncements, and position statements. A native of California, Duncan was the youngest of four children and was born in 1878. Her parents, Mary Grey and Joseph Duncan were "non-conformists." Mary was a disciple of Robert Ingersoll, a popular Irish agnostic with a penchant for life, human kindness, and art. Joseph was a gambler and a poet. Mr. Duncan abandoned his family when Isadora was quite young, leaving Mary Grey to support her children by teaching piano lessons. [1]

As a child, Isadora was exposed to a progressive education; aesthetic exercise, music, folk dance, literature and poetry. Isadora assisted her sister Elizabeth teach dance lessons at Elizabeth's San Francisco studio, and with her other siblings Augustin and Raymond, Isadora entertained neighbors with theatrical productions staged in their backyard. The Duncan children's theatricals became so popular that they toured California's coastal towns performing a "variety" show. In 1895, at age eighteen, Isadora and her mother headed east, for Chicago, Illinoiswhere Isadora found work dancing as a chorus girl. A year later, after a tour of the United States and Britain with Augustin Daly's production of *A Midsummer Night's Dream,* Isadora "retired" from commercial theatre to become a "salon soloist," a performer who brought culture and art into the living rooms of America's wealthy arts patrons. While still in her early 20's, Isadora was making a name for herself as a performer in New York by dancing to poetry, and creating new works of her own to "artistic" music.

In 1900 Isadora left America to go to Europe with her brother Raymond where they found new inspiration in museums and in conversing with European artists and art critics. The Duncan's traveled to France to see the American dance artist, Loie Fuller, and the Japanese dancer-actress, Sada Yacco, at the 1900 Paris Exposition. Fuller's inventive solo performance used drapery and colored lighting to create extraordinary visual illusions with movement and electricity. It was the talk of Paris and the Exposition. Sada Yacco, on the other hand, brought to European audiences the Asian Theatre's detailed attention to gesture and dramatic moment. [2]

Returning to London, Isadora began to reference her thinking on dance to the concepts and ideas she had encountered in attending performances, reading various philosophical tracts, seeing the art of modern painters and sculptors, visiting museum exhibits of renaissance paintings and classical statuary, and frequenting intellectual salons. In short order, Isadora retooled the way she conceived of, and performed, her dances and changed how she made her art. Isadora moved away from the artistic music for dance that was popular for the "salon artist" and instead began to perform her dances to the music of composers such as Chopin, Wagner, Brahams, and Schubert. Duncan also developed a movement technique that was uniquely hers, incorporating the expressive use of the upper body. She "traveled" the stage in movement, developing sequences that were unlike anything anyone had done, or seen, before; running, skipping, leaping with uplifted chest, head thrown back, arms reaching toward heaven.

In time Isadora also began to speak on, and write about her vision for dance. In 1902, or possibly in 1903, around the age of 26, Duncan wrote her famous tract, *The Dance of the Future,* which she gave as a lecture in Berlin. [3] *The Dance of the Future,* is an argument for Duncan's vision of the new dance and the new woman of the 20th century, it is also an argument against the ballet and against the ballet's manifestation of women trapped in the image of "nymph," "fairy," or "coquette":

> The dancer of the future will be one whose body and soul have grown so harmoniously together that the natural language of that soul will have become the movement of the body. She will dance not in the form of nymph, nor fairy, nor coquette, but in the form of woman in her greatest and purest expression. She will realize the mission of woman's body and the holiness of all its parts. She will dance the changing life of nature, showing how each part is transformed into the other. From all parts of her body shall shine a radiant intelligence, bringing to the world the message of the thoughts and aspirations of thousands of women. She shall dance the freedom of women....
> ....[S]he will dance the body emerging again from centuries of civilized forgetfulness, emerging not in the nudity of primitive man, but in a new nakedness, no longer at war with spirituality and intelligence, but joining with them in a glorious harmony. [4]

In later writings and lectures, Isadora contextualized dance in relation to the other arts, and argued for recognition of dance as "high" art. In short order, Duncan discussed the physical and cultural origins of dance, panned the ballet as sterile and lifeless, wrote on the inspiration she received from various philosophical and artistic sources, sought a connection between the body and the spirit through dance, and reinvigorated discourse on an aspect of human expression that had been ignored in western culture for centuries.

Extracting what was needed, in words, ideas, and images from the works of Walt Whitman, Beethoven, Nietzsche, Kant, Chopin, Wagner, of Greek art, or the art of the Italian Renaissance, Isadora redacted these to make her case for a fresh new vision for art-dance. Disciplined and compulsive, Isadora absorbed huge sums of information from readings and ideas that stirred her thinking and passions. In reading the works and philosophies of people like Whitman or Nietzsche, Isadora selected what she chose to remember and reference, taking those ideas that worked for her, and ignored the rest. Duncan found important references to dance, to movement, to education, and strung these together in a series of epistles that had a profound effect on the thinking of other dancers and dance educators. Given to a certain emotionalism in her writing, and prone to sweeping pronouncements and conclusions, Isadora was the first to make the case for dance as an art and educational medium that was co-equal to its sister arts of music, theatre, painting, and sculpture. In many ways Duncan was simply a "force of nature"; larger than life, obsessed with her mission, at times profound, at other times absurd and given to personal excess, which got more and more out of hand as she aged. Still, Duncan was always driven in her advocacy for a new discourse in dance. Duncan was often pedantic, and heavy handed, yet, at the same time she was visionary, inspired, and extremely charismatic.

During her active career Isadora was received by critics and audiences much more favorably in Europe than she was in the United States. Her reputation in America was fraught by real and assumed details of her personal life and her leanings toward the political left. Regardless, Duncan certainly stimulated the thinking of American dance artists, teachers, and progressive educators who read her works, or saw her perform. Gertrude Colby, who established the first curriculum for a creative, art approach to dance in higher education, was greatly inspired by Isadora's writings and artistry, and says as much in her book *Natural Rhythms and Dances*, discussed later in this chapter. [5] Duncan's vision and legacy inspired the spirit of dance as it was re-born at the dawn of the 20th century; in the wake of progressive education, American Delsartism, social and political change, health and clothing reform, revolutions in the visual and performing arts, and unparalleled developments in technology and industry.

Ruth St. Denis and Ted Shawn

Living in the same epoch as Isadora, Ruth St. Denis and Duncan shared similarities in their lives:

> Both were products of American Delsartism. Both studied ballet with Marie Bonfanti in New York. Both launched theatrical careers in the mid - 1890's, and each worked for Augustin Daly....[E]ach abandoned it [a theatrical career] to create her own vision of a great art dance. Both did extensive research in libraries and museums. Gathering material upon which to base their art.... [6]

Both also traveled to Europe and were acclaimed there, both established schools, and both found their first independent success in the parlors of society matrons. Yet they couldn't have been more different in style, in temperament, and in life and living. Duncan was the great trailblazer for a vision of dance as art. St. Denis integrated art and popular culture and prepared the way for the young Americans who would generate a "modern," American dance.

"Ruth St. Denis" was born Ruth Dennis to Thomas and Ruth Emma Dennis in 1879. The eldest of two children, "Ruthie" Dennis grew up on a farm in New Jersey, not far from Manhattan. Ruth Emma was one of the first women medical doctors in America, having received her degree from the University of Michigan in 1872. Mrs. Dennis practiced medicine for one year before the strain of the work overwhelmed her. She apparently suffered a nervous collapse and in the process of attending to her own health, turned her back on the cautious medical advice of her day, and toward physical and metaphysical alternative remedies. At the time of Ruth Emma's illness, the American medical community was divided over the issues that affected women's health. Clothing reform, exercise, health and hygiene, diet and mental stimulation, and domestic science were practical issues important to the nascent women's movement. Ruth Emma, who found her 'cure' in alternative therapies, and remained committed to progressive medicine and education throughout her life. [7]

As a child, Ruthie Dennis was exposed to new practices in education, health, diet, medicine, and religion. Her mother taught Delsarte's principles and allowed her to take lessons in dancing. As Ruthie trained and learned about dance, she expressed to her mother her interest in the theatre and in performance. Tall, and very beautiful, Ruth Dennis' potential was obvious to both mother and daughter. With her mother's help, Ruth found steady work in the developing vaudeville circuit as a "skirt" and "kick" dancer.

Ruth Dennis' first success was in vaudeville, and then in the extravagant theatrical productions of Broadway entrepreneur David Belasco. In Belasco's productions of *The Ballet Girl, Zaza, The Auctioneer,* and *Du Barry*, Ruth traveled across America and Europe, as she acquired a professional sense of the theatrical, polished her performing techniques, and spent a great deal of time pondering what it would take to make her a "star." After taking a fresh look at a poster for Egyptian Deities Cigarettes in Buffalo, New York, Ruth came to her epiphany. A popular brand of the day, advertisements for Egyptian Deities were in most magazines and on many early billboards. Egyptian Deities advertisements featured a "scene" of ancient Egypt, at the center of which usually sat the goddess Isis on a granite throne. One day, one of these ads just happened to be in the right place at the right time and within Ruth's daydreaming field of vision. In the illustration of the Egyptian goddess Isis, Ruth Dennis saw herself reflected and found the image, the context, and the substance of what it was she would bring to the stage. In 1905 Ruth left the Belasco company to set out on her own career, a career like Duncan's, that would revolutionize the way in which dance was presented and understood in American culture.

Ruth was nothing if not aesthetically flexible in the early days of her solo career. After seeing an ersatz "Hindu Village" exhibit at Coney Island, she turned her vision to the culture of the sub-continent of India. In the dances of Hindu culture Ruth felt she could explore the depths of dramatic potential. Ruth's first creation was based on the Indian legend of the maiden *Radha*, who was loved by the God Krishna. Mrs. Orland Rouland, a New York matron of means, saw Ruth perform Rạdha at Proctor's Vaudeville House on 23rd Street. Rouland recognized something special in Ruth's new act and arranged for her to perform for a private audience at the Hudson Theatre. Addressing a trunk of costumes to be forwarded to the Hudson Theatre, Ruth's mother recalled a name David Belasco had given Ruth, "St. Dennis." She altered this by one letter to address the trunk "Ruth St. Denis," and the name stuck. Ruthie Dennis soon assumed the more exotic and pious stage name "Ruth St. Denis" and began to create the dance works that would bring her international fame. [8]

At first, St. Denis's new vision for dance was not primarily theatrical, nor was it commercial. Ruth's initial interest in the dances of India had to do with her desire to combine the spiritual with the theatrical, and to do so she felt her dance must be grounded in 'high ideas' of philosophy, art, and religion, characteristics that Ruth felt were abundant in Hindu culture. Between 1905 and 1906 Ruth created three important works for herself based on Hindu themes; the original work, *Radha*, and then *Incense*, and *The Cobras*. Shortly after embrking on her solo career, Ruth St. Denis left America for Europe in 1906 in search of greater triumphs. While in Europe she added several new dances to her repertoire, including *Nautch*, and *The Yogi*, and in 1909 Ruth St. Denis returned to America an international "star."

St. Denis's "Indian" dances were caught between the realms of the spiritual and the theatrical, and in this netherworld she placed her mark on American art and culture. By combining sex and saintliness, St. Denis found the 'twist' she needed. She crafted a new way for American audiences to simultaneously accept and objectify, both the dancer and the dance. Ruth's was no fairy dancing, no sylphan fluttering, no rhythmic 'to and fro,' St. Denis had created dances of intellectual and cultural substance, dances with character, dynamic changes, storyline, mystic trappings, and perhaps most importantly, dance with recognizable theatrical dimensions.

By 1914 St. Denis had played out much of her initial success as both she and Isadora were being imitated by a large number of less talented performers.

Things on the Vaudeville circuit were changing too, with more and competitive national circuits, more performers on a single billing, and no opportunities for European tours with the continent at War. Finding the financial backing that she felt was necessary to create new work and continue to grow artistically was increasingly difficult. St. Denis turned toward Japanese culture for new inspiration, and found a new dimension in her dancing as she attempted to be more 'authentic.' But the fact of the matter was that regardless of the competition, and the funding problems, the public was growing tired of St. Denis' work.

A few years earlier, in 1911, during a cross-continent tour of America, St. Denis had performed in Denver, Colorado, where a young man named Edwin "Ted" Myers Shawn was in the audience. After seeing Miss Ruth, Ted found himself profoundly moved. He dreamt of her work and hoped that one day he would meet her.

Shawn was born in 1891 and was a native of Kansas City, Missouri. After completing his high school education, he enrolled at the University of Denver to study for the Methodist ministry. In his junior year, Shawn was stricken with diphtheria, loosing control of his legs as a result. Taking up dancing as therapy, Shawn soon talked himself out of his Methodist future and began learning as much about dance as he could. In 1910 Ted made his professional debut in a small Denver nightclub with his teacher, Miss Hazel Wallack. According to newspaper accounts, Wallack and Shawn danced a bit of ballet, some ballroom or 'fancy' dance steps, and threw in a bit of the rage of the day, the dance of *Salome.* [9] Shawn spent the next four years refining his skills and touring as a performer. In 1914, three years after having first seen St. Denis in performance, Shawn traveled to New York and walked into Ruth St. Denis' 89th street studio, just in time to join her small company on a tour of the Southern states and to help rejuvenate her lagging career. By the time St. Denis and company arrived in Los Angeles in late 1914, Ted was Miss Ruth's husband, manager, and performing partner. In the summer of 1915 they opened a professional school for dance, Denishawn, on a hill overlooking downtown Los Angeles. Over the next 16 years,

Denishawn the school, and later Denishawn the touring company, were pre-eminent in professional American dance education and performance.

The creation of Denishawn, was a stroke of business, organizational, and social-artistic savvy. In education, Denishawn blended instruction in dance with a range of related subject matter and by doing so cast the study of dance in a new light. Students at Denishawn learned dance techniques and performance works, while studying culture, history, religion, costuming, accompaniment, social grace, and art. Thus, Denishawn may be viewed as an early, commercialized version of the academic dance department, and an important conceptual "jump" for dance in education. Until Denishawn, dance in America had not been professionally taught in concert with supporting disciplines, and certainly not in context with art history, religion, or literature.

As the first professional school for American dance, Denishawn symbolized dance as institution, dance as entrepreneurial business. A popular slogan of the time affirmed; "the business of America *is* business." [10] Apart from St. Denis and Shawn's contributions toward expanding popular conceptions of dance through their elaborate (and imaginative) presentations of dances from around the world, in many respects it was in their skill in public relations and in conducting the business of dance that may be Ruth and Ted's most important legacy for dance in American culture. One is left to wonder how many children, young women or men, first considered dance after seeing or reading about Denishawn? How many parents permitted their daughters to study dance because of Denishawn's public image; the beauty and extreme visual piety of Miss Ruth, the spiritual pronouncements of Ted Shawn, the Denishawn school as symbol of successful entrepreneurship? According to author Janet Soares (1992); "In a six month period in 1924 Denishawn traveled to 293 cities and performed for over one million viewers." [11] Author Jane Sherman (1979), attributes the following statements to Ruth St. Denis:

A pupil should write down all ideas of technique, of creating, of new gestures, new countries to dance, of dance and health, dance and social poise, dance and business, and dance and art.
...[O]ne should think of dance as art although one may have to do it as business.
12

Together St. Denis and Shawn were adept at connecting dance to popular cultural, and to the religious and educational sentiments of the day. Pious, and yet at the same time progressive, sexy and serious; St. Denis and Shawn made sure their image was solidly grounded in a Christian sensibility; all the while in Egyptian or Aztec head-dress. Their 'Christian' piety only helped accent their interpretive, and imaginative dances of exotic, 'other' cultures. They adeptly manipulated their public and media image; virtuous yet glamorous, worldly, heterosexual, married; husband and wife in a profession still widely viewed as populated by hustlers, "queers," and prostitutes. Their skillful use of the emerging mass media; the magazine, the tabloid photo spread, the newsreel, performances in vaudeville, and the popular cinema, brought their work, and dance, to the attention of millions.

Working outside of the academy, Duncan, St. Denis, and Shawn shaped the thinking of those who were inside its ivied halls. Anderson, Sargent, and Gulick brought the national dances into the curriculum; Duncan, St. Denis, and Shawn shifted attention in the professional world of dance toward the natural and the expressive. Duncan, St. Denis, and Shawn introduced the ideas that dance could be conceptually based, that dance could be tied to the other arts, and that dance reflected the humanities and sciences, both in art and in education.

Dance: First Programs in Higher Education

In the years leading up to the first two decades of the 20th century many influences came together to help dance find its place in American higher education. Changes in the college curriculum reflected the needs and future of a democratic, industrial society. Vocationalism in the university came about in response to economic, social, and geographic expansion. Immigrant academic professionals brought new ideas to higher education. The rapid expansion of eastern and midwestern urban centers, largely due to immigration, led to social, health, and community wellness concerns. The creation of teacher programs in physical education, the American Delsarte Movement, and Dalcroze Eurythmics; each added to the public's new interest in matters of the body. Other influences included; the search for a new spiritualism in response to the rapid and often unsettling advances of science and industry; progressive education; the evolution of mass media and transportation; social mobility; radical change and experimentation in the visual and performing arts; the accumulation of personal and industrial wealth; the creation of a large middle class; the women's education, health, and suffrage movements: all these elements coming together, and playing one off the other; changing, shifting, and evolving.

From events and personalities in the world of professional dance at the turn of the century, and the corresponding changes in American culture, I now turn to the central focus of this text, the story of dance in the American university. We will see that dance evolves in the university in much the same way that the university has evolved in our culture: from the pioneer program or school emerges a network of similar and like minded programs and schools, from the efforts of the early 'giants' in dance art and education, come perspectives and techniques used by many. Over time, dance, like other disciplines in education, became less the province of individual initiation and interpretation, and more the product of group consensus.

Gertrude Colby and Margaret H'Doubler - University Programs in Dance: 1913-1926

The first educational program for a creative, art-dance in American higher education was organized in 1913, in New York City, at the Speyer School, a division of Teachers College of Columbia University, by Gertrude Colby. Colby was a graduate of Dudley Sargent's Boston Normal School of Gymnastics. She had trained in ballet with Louis Chalif, in Aesthetic Dance with Melvin Gilbert, and had studied American Delartism, Dalcroze Eurythmics, and American Pageantry. [13] According to Spiesman (1960), Colby was invited by officials of the Speyer School to establish a physical education program for children which was to be based on three criteria; a program that would be natural and free for children, a program that would permit self-expression, and a program that would harmonize, and be capable of being integrated with, other programs in the Speyer School. [14]

Between 1913 and 1916 Colby worked in the Speyer School developing her ideas and methods of teaching dance for children. However, in 1916, the Speyer School was discontinued. In the next academic year, Colby was invited to transfer her working environment to Teachers College; to develop her courses in rhythmic and "natural" movement into a more substantial teacher training program. In 1918 Colby established her program for dance education at Teachers College, which she labeled "Natural Dancing". Colby outlined her methods for teaching in her text, *Natural Rhythms and Dances*, first published in 1922. [15] Colby remained prominent in dance in higher education until she left Teachers College in 1931. Because the Teachers College dance education program was historically the first in higher education, and *Natural Rhythms and Dances* outlines Colby's philosophy and methodology, Colby's introductory notes to this text provide an interesting starting point for considering the origins of dance as a discreet academic discipline.

Natural Rhythms and Natural Dances: A Beginning for Dance in Higher Education

According to Ruyter (1979), in the course of Colby's career in higher education she trained "hundreds of dance teachers who carried the work to other schools throughout the country." [16] In the introduction to *Natural Rhythms and Dances,* Colbydiscusses her philosophy for dance education, defends dance as appropriate subject matter at all levels of learning, and details her methods for educational dance. The introduction to *Natural Rhythms and Dances* is interesting reading because it clarifies Colby's terms, her approach, and her mission. Colby's

70

introductory comments represent a rationale for dance in higher education as had developed between 1913 and 1922. Viewed from the vantage point of the present, Colby's introduction is essentially a portrait of educational dance in transition. Colby's Natural Dancing was evolutionary because it linked study in the folk and "national" dances, the standard for dance in physical education programs in the latter 19th and early 20th centuries, with the artistic, aesthetic, and "natural" interest in movement that grew out of the work of Isadora Duncan:

The growing recognition of the need in physical education for something less formal and more in harmony with the body with the interests and activities of everyday life has drawn attention to a "new " type of dancing. It is not new, nor is it truly old, for while the dancing of ancient Greece was its inspiration, its development is modern in essence.

When Isadora Duncan gave her great gift to the world it was regarded as a wonderful art; ...here and there over this country various groups recognized its educational possibilities and sought gropingly to open the way for the joy of free rhythmic expression to the rising generation. As a result we have many exponents of Rhythmic Dancing, Greek Dancing, Natural Dancing and many others....

At Teachers College, Columbia University, we have adapted the name Natural Dancing feeling that this term expresses more nearly the thing for which we are working. It is based on such free natural movements as walking, skipping, running, leaping etc. By making ourselves free instruments of expression, rhythmically unified...."We dance ideas, not steps."

For years we have been teaching rhythms and dramatic games in our kindergartens. The singing and dramatic games have led naturally to the folk dances of more or less difficulty for the older boys and girls; but the rhythms have ceased with the primary grades ....[W]ith no thought of the loss to education of their wonderful joy-giving, imagination producing qualities.

Our purpose in developing Natural Dancing has been to carry on the rhythms of childhood to a higher form of the art of dancing - "the only art in which we ourselves are the stuff...."

...The beauty of natural dancing is that it is open to everyone. No skill or background of preparation is necessary, for everyone knows how to walk, and skip and run. And by starting with something known ...we gain confidence and satisfaction in our dancing, lose self consciousness and build new things upon the old....

Our method is to begin with simple primitive rhythms and rhythmic activities in pantomime, such as playing ball, rolling hoops, flying kites and the like....[D]ancing must be based upon rhythm and expression to be worthy of the name. Meanwhile we are listening to music with understanding...

Musicians have complained, and with justice, that most dancers mutilate music to subserve their own ends, changing tempos at will and adding or dropping measures ad libitum. In dancing with a musician's understanding and interpretation of the music, we are learning more than the art of the dance, we are building a real musical appreciation.

The question always arises, "Is there any technic in Natural Dancing?" Yes, but it bears no relation to that of the ballet.

The technique of Natural Dancing is along the line of natural movements with the purpose of developing a greater freedom, a better poise and control - in a word, to make the body a better instrument of expression.

It has been said that technic is the "grammar of dance." Perhaps, but no modern education begins with grammar. Technic - and grammar - should be a means to an end, not an end in itself....When ideals outgrow the power to express, the desire for a more responsive body is felt and the time for technic is ripe.

This technic consists of finding the best way to do a given thing. Of course there must be a standard toward which to work - a "form" as in games and in athletics; but in dancing it is sufficiently flexible to allow for individual variations of physique and temperament. Our standard is based upon art, especially as found in Greek sculpture and vases; upon the laws of line and mass, of balance and opposition. The living embodiment of our standard is, with the exception of a few minor details, in the Isadora Duncan Dancers.

During the last two years there have been constant requests for "material" both from my own students and from those who have seen the work...I have gathered together some studies and dances that have worked out in my classes and present them in this volume....I have tried to be clear in my explanations while preserving the atmosphere in each one as far as is possible on the printed page. The directions are intended as suggestions only and, within the prescribed form, there should be an infinite opportunity for individual expression,

This brings up a point that I feel is an important one. There has been much said of dancing as a means of "self-expression". This may be true according to the layman's understanding of the term. It is true from a psychologist's standpoint only when the dancer expresses in spontaneous rhythm an emotion spontaneously felt. This is rare and is purely an individual, never a group thing. The ideas and emotions in most Natural Dancing are from external stimulus for they are suggested by the music or by the story or idea. In which case it can not truly be called "self-expression." However, once the idea or emotion is stimulated, it becomes a part of the individual and the resulting expression is her own.

The educational value of lyric dancing (an interpretation of music forms, not motivated by an idea) has been questioned. I feel that it can be justified on the ground of training in music appreciation ...It can be compared to the playing of an instrument and, I fear, must be experienced to be appreciated. Often when a group is experimenting with a piece of music there will be such comments as "No, that doesn't FEEL right" or "There, that is good."

Everyone should have an opportunity for creative work...In my classes at Teachers College every senior is required to give one or more original "Children's Rhythms." What a scurrying for music and ideas there is and what an interest when they are presented!...

A word about the method of presentation. We tell first the story or idea that is to be danced and then let the group hear the music and become somewhat familiar with it. With the more difficult music it will be necessary to study it in detail as to phrases, accents, climaxes, and mood as well as rhythm. NEVER teach by counts or measures....Let the music be the inspiration and the guide. In pantomimic action, the music serves as a timer as, for example, in The Dead Bird and The Last Rose. Any effort to reduce it to counts would destroy the spontaneous expression.

....I offer a sample lesson as a suggestion.

BLOWING BUBBLES

Teacher: "You have all blown bubbles, I know. Let me see you do it.
(Class responds by imitating the action)
"What do you do with the bubbles after they are blown?"
Pupil: "Blow them big until they burst."
Pupil: "Throw them up into the air."
Teacher: "Let us sit down on the floor and listen to this music. See if you can tell when it says to throw the bubbles off your pipe."
(Class sits down and listens until someone finds the little accented notes where the bubble is thrown off)
Teacher: "What else can you do with bubbles."
Pupil: "See if you can blow them high up."

Pupil:	"Put your finger through."
Pupil:	"Catch it in your dress." Etc.
Teacher:	"How do you feel when the bubbles burst?"
Pupil:	"Makes your face all wet."
	(One little boy said "It makes you feel all stickery.")
Teacher:	"Where do the bubbles go when they burst?"
Pupil:	"They just go."
Pupil:	"Nowhere."
Teacher:	"Listen to the music again."
	(Music plays while teacher talks.)
	"We will blow the bubbles first. How many are there? Listen! Yes, two. Now we will play with this one - blow it about. It bursts! Oh my face is all wet. Where has it gone?
	(The children follow the action freely while the teacher is speaking.)
Teacher:	"I liked the way Jack got up and moved around when he was playing with his bubble".
Jack:	"I could make it go higher."
Teacher:	"Let us play it again and see how many different ways we can find to blow the bubbles."

In Natural Dancing, from the Children's Rhythms to the highest art form, the idea behind it must be understood and felt before the dance can be given true expression.

Gertrude K. Colby
September 1922 [17]

Colby's text then outlines Free Rhythms, Child Rhythms, Studies, and Natural Dances. A key is given for directions; body facings oriented for the proscenium stage, and a description of "steps," including the waltz, waltz run, accented waltz run, gallop, skip, slide, hop, run and leap, polka, gallop-skip, leap-gallop- gallop, and run-leap-leap. The dances, with titles like *Springtime in Hellas*, *Chariot of Apollo*, and *The Frolic*, are accompanied by appropriate music selected by the author. Each dance is outlined with written movement directions (e.g. " a little girl with her doll in her arms walks slowly forward hushing it to sleep with a gentle swaying motion") followed by the number of measures (in this case 16), expected to complete the directed movement. [18]

And that, in Gertrude Colby 's own words, is what Natural Dancing is all about. Consider what it is that Colby is saying in her introductory comments: first, there is the admission that Natural Dancing is not a new discovery in dance, but rather is a rediscovery of the artistic relevance of natural movement. As Duncan did before her, Colby appeals to her reader to view the broad relevance of dance as a form of human expression rediscovered; like some lost doctrine from the world of antiquity.

Secondly, by tying the practice of natural movements to music, rhythm, and a story line, Colby argues for a dance education that is based on "ideas, not steps." Here Colby frames educational dance as conceptual dance, an educational perspective that was very progressive for its day. Conceptual education in dance is in harmony and is integrative with other programs a school might offer. Additionally, if one dances "ideas, not steps," then dance is not reserved for the physically gifted nor is not limited to imitation of movement, the dance experience is open to all and is at the same time both thoughtful and thought provoking. Colby argues for educational dance that may be of benefit to all; as dance engages the individual physically, intellectually, and creatively.

In addition to the obvious references to the work of Delsarte and Dalcroze, Colby's affirmation that natural movements are inherently rhythmic effectively links dance to another body of knowledge, thereby casting dance in light of its merit as cooperative partner in a liberal education. In order to perform dance/natural movement with clarity and ease, the student must have an understanding of rhythm: dance is intimately related to music, and learning in dance involves acquiring basic knowledge of musical form and structure. Deeper understandings of music are developed as the dancer matures and works with more sophisticated musical forms. Next, Colby connects studies in dance with the humanities through rhythmic movement that leads to the expression of ideas and stories. A theoretical relationship between dance and science is implied in Colby's statement, through the notion that training the body in natural movement also involves learning basic principles in physics and anatomy: the transference of weight in a skip; the spring of a foot, or the straightening of a knee. Developing ideas, "stories," and relating these back to invention in movement, developing "real music appreciation," and developing natural movement skills are clearly a means for couching dance in terms of its merit and worth in cognitive and behavioral learning; dance in a liberal educational context.

74

Colby follows her description of Natural Dancing with an appeal to the reader to consider the potential of dance as it represents the spirit of progressive education. Through references to "lost youth," Colby says that the rhythms of childhood are ignored in education after the primary levels, "with no thought of the loss of education in their wonderful joy-giving, imagination- producing qualities." Colby's purpose in developing natural dancing is " to carry on the rhythms of childhood to a higher form of the art of dancing - the only art in which we ourselves are the stuff." The search for innocence and pure spirit through the natural rhythms and movements of the body is a direct reference to the goals of progressive educators seeking to stimulate the child's learning from within. The point that dance is the only art in which "we ourselves are the stuff," is important because the affective nature of dance, the felt nature of the experience of dance, ties the doer to that which is done. This idea, that in dance education the object (dance) is embodied in the subject (the dancer), coupled with the notion of dancing ·"ideas, not steps," separates Colby's perspectives from those of many of her peers. In this regard Natural Dancing not only acts as an evolutionary form linking the "national" to the "natural" in dance. Natural Dancing bridges the theoretical gap between the aesthetically "natural" and the aesthetically conceptual. Margaret H'Doubler would take this tack as early as 1918 at the University of Wisconsin.

Colby writes that the question of dancing as a means of self-expression is true "according to the layman's understanding of the term," and that "it is true from a psychologist's standpoint only when the dancer expresses in spontaneous rhythm an emotion spontaneously felt." By 1922 Colby seems to have given up on her first charge at the Speyer School, that her program in dance education engage the children in self-expression. To Colby, self- expression in dance is "rare and purely an individual, never a group thing." After her Speyer School experience's, Colby may have learned what to expect if dance in education was turned toward self-expression; coming to realize that children lack the intellectual and psychological wherewithal to generate true self-expression, and that attempts at unhindered self-expression would lead to chaos in the classroom. In stating these opinions, Colby ties dance education to the students preparation for participative, democratic living through group experience. Colby's Natural Dancing was not designed to teach children to express their inner-selves, but was designed to help them work cooperatively, and think creatively, while learning moral values and life lessons that would inform their later participation in a moral and democratic community.

A central weakness in Colby's conceptual framework for Natural Dancing is that once the approach has been worked out it has nowhere to 'go.' Natural dancing for adult learners was not developed beyond the model for children; mature learners would simply pay attention to more complex musical forms, more involved storylines, more elaborate ideas. While story lines, musical forms, and ideas may be expressed through the use of natural movement, these experiences in learning do not generate greater understanding of natural movement itself.

To today's reader Natural Dancing, as a means of dance training, may seem naive and simplistic. One could criticize Colby's method because it doesn't go beyond looking at dance as much more than a form of motion-based storytelling. Natural Dancing isn't so much about movement as it is about using movement to express the ideas and attributes associated with specific musical scores and narratives. While Colby says the teacher should "NEVER teach by counts and measures," the dances in the text are all carefully timed and measured. Ideas for dance do not spring from the consciousness or kinesthetic understanding of the mover, but are derived from and stimulated by external sources; from the nature of a story to be told, the drive of the rhythm, or ebb and flow of the music. Colby's Natural Dancing was not meant for adult learners, it was not about generating personal art ideas, nor was Natural Dancing about a theoretical consideration of natural movement; Natural Dancing was designed and meant for children.

Still, when viewed it in its historical context of 1913-1922 America, Colby's approach was quite radical for its time. This was a time when popular and educational ideas of dance were in a state of beginning and flux. Educational dance was evolving from the "national" to the "natural." The "art" dance of Denishawn, and much of the work of Isadora Duncan, was intriguing yet not educationally framed and still cloaked in the exotic, the libertine, the religious, the political, and the spectacular. Popular notions of dance were wed with the public's fascination for the new music "Ragtime," and the social dances that came out of the "honky-tonks" and "juke joints," or to those made fashionable by the refined gliding of dance personalities Vernon and Irene Castle, who did so much to cast a sheen of glamour on social dancing.

Aside from Isadora and Denishawn, on the theatrical stage in the early 1900's *Salome* was the dancing woman to watch out for, her dancing interpreters invariably clutching a wax head of John the Baptist. As the decade of 1910 - 1920 progressed, dance was captured in images on the cinema's screen as viewed in D.W. Griffith's *Intolerance*, *Babylon* and other dancing orgies. Denishawn dancers were commonly featured in Mr. Griffith's early films. By 1920 the "dancer" was a symbol of a new-found personal, physical, and sexual freedom, particularly for women. However, dance was still largely thought of as sinful and silly, precious and titillating, "fancy," "risqué"; rarely serious. In 1920 America dance was nothing to "really" think about.

The importance of Natural Dancing in the evolution of dance in higher education lies in the fact that Colby couched it as dancing from ideas, not steps. To Colby, dance was an educational medium where object and subject are the same. For dance to be conceptually based was a new and important departure for educational dance. Natural Dancing is also significant transitionally in that it introduced aesthetic notions of dance into the curriculum, thus beginning the process of individuating dance education from its more utilitarian 'sister' activities in physical education, including the folk and national dances. With the addition of art ideas in dance, the content and instruction of dance took on new dimensions that would ultimately lead to its separation from physical education. The idea that the study of dance in higher education was substantive enough to deserve a discipline based approach to its instruction would be the contribution of the other early 'giant' in dance education, Margaret H'Doubler. However, while H'Doubler would define the parameters of the discipline, widespread acceptance of dance as an arts-based discipline in the university would take many years of patient development and negotiation.

Next Steps: Toward a Focus on the Essence of Dance, Human Movement

The teaching of one of Colby's most promising contemporaries, Bird Larson, bridges the work of Gertrude Colby with that of Margaret H'Doubler. In her teaching, Larson began to delve more deeply into the "stuff" of dance itself; human movement. Larson was the first college educator to look at dance movements as separate from any dependency on music and storylines and, according to dance historian Lincoln Kirstein, was the first American dance educator to "turn toward the professional dancer and away from the purely educational field." [19] Kirstein may have meant that Larson's work was geared for adult learning and that her methods in dance education demonstrated her interest in the potential of dance as a mode of self-expression.

Larson had a background in corrective physical education before she began serious study with Gertrude Colby at Teachers College. Studies in anatomy, corrective exercise, and the biological sciences helped Larson conceive of dance as more than just a vehicle for storytelling and musical interpretation. [20] In 1914, Larson began work to develop a dance program at Barnard College, sister college to Columbia University. Although Larson borrowed heavily from Colby's Natural Dancing, she supplemented her teaching with lessons in applied anatomy and physics. Larson believed movement had its origins in control of the torso and paid particular attention to techniques for gaining better control of the body. She developed a system for training called Natural Rhythmic Expression, which included three aspects of instruction; studies in natural body movement, studies in designed body movement, and controlled movement with music to express an idea. [21] Larson's work acts as an important link in the development of a dance curriculum for adult students. Unfortunately she died at a young age in 1927 and did not fulfill her promise as a dance educator. H'Doubler later commented that Larson was someone who "...was seeking too." [22]

CHAPTER 4

In the first years of the 20th century, Wisconsin was a state that exemplified the progressive spirit in its politics and in education. As noted in Chapter Two, Robert "Fighting Bob" LaFollette was Governor of Wisconsin at this time. LaFollette followed the national example set by President Theodore Roosevelt as he squared off against big business and the "Old Guard" Republican political machines of the late 19th century. [1] Progressive action and reform in government and politics supported an activist role for public education. An important result of progressive education was a rethinking of the role of the public university and its service to the community.

The Wisconsin Idea of Education

In 1903, Charles Van Hise was appointed president of the University of Wisconsin. A political and philosophical associate of La Follette's, Van Hise soon began to promote the notion of the "service university"..."where the boundaries of the campus are the boundaries of the state." Van Hise's policy was labeled, The Wisconsin Idea of Education:

> The indefinable Wisconsin Idea, which came into currency during the progressive era, is probably better summarized by some of the popular cliché phrases of the time than by the hyperbole of a "university that runs a state." "The expert on tap, not on top," "the boundaries of the campus are the boundaries of the state," "the service university," "applying the scientific method to legislation," "the democratization of knowledge;" all suggest a congenial interchange between campus and capitol. [2]

In support of the "Wisconsin Idea," the university offered its resources in service to the state and its local communities. Services often included providing the expert skills of university faculty to state and private sectors, community use of facilities, public seminars, access to the arts, sports, and entertainment, and elective curricular offerings. In major and elective curricula, academic departments at the University attended to the relationship between course work and the student's later success in life and as participant in a democratic community.

In 1911, physical education was established as a major in the University's College of Letters and Science for the training of physical education specialists, directors of play and recreation, and coaches of sports and athletics. Independent divisions for men and women were formed and both divisions offered a large slate of non-major courses to the public, faculty, and general student population. The women's physical education division offered leisure, sport, and recreational activities considered appropriate for women, including classes in dance.

In the spring of 1910, a young undergraduate woman by the name of Margaret H'Doubler was completing her major in biology with a minor in philosophy. During her college years, Miss H'Doubler had demonstrated a talent in sports, particularly basketball, and in team coaching. Following graduation, H'Doubler was invited by the women's physical education faculty to stay on as coach of women's basketball and baseball teams. In the fall of 1912 the University hired Blanche Trilling to direct the women's physical education division. Together, the young coach, Margaret H'Doubler, and the administrator, Blanche Trilling, changed the future of dance as education in America.

The Wisconsin Idea of Dance

Margaret H'Doubler was born on April 26, 1889, in Beloit, Kansas. She was the youngest child of Charles and Sarah H'Doubler. Charles H'Doubler was a man of inexhaustible energy and many talents, holding several patents for electrical mechanisms. While still a child, Margaret and family moved to Warren, Illinois. In 1903, when Margaret was 14, the family moved again, this time to Madison,

Wisconsin, Margaret graduated from Madison High School in the spring of 1906. She entered the University of Wisconsin in the fall of 1906 and she expressed an interest in following her brother Frank's lead to become either a medical doctor, or a biologist. [3]

Margaret completed a major in biology with a minor in philosophy in the spring of 1910. In addition to her regular studies in the sciences and the humanities, Margaret had her first regular exposure to physical education at Wisconsin. During her years as an undergraduate H'Doubler participated in many extracurricular sports and excelled in swimming, basketball, and baseball. She studied dance, learning folk, national, and "classical" dancing, taught by an instructor experimenting with the works of Melvin Gilbert and Louis Chalif. Upon completion of her degree, Margaret was invited to become an Assistant Instructor of women's' physical education. During summer sessions in 1911, 1913, and 1914, H'Doubler attended workshops for coaches and physical educators at the Harvard Summer School and the Sargent School for Physical Education in Boston. [4]

Blanche Trilling, a graduate of the Boston School of Gymnastics, directed women's physical education programs at Wisconsin for 34 years; leading the Women's Division from 1912 to 1930, and the independent Department of Physical Education for Women from 1930 until her retirement in 1946. During Trilling's administration dance at Wisconsin evolved from a program of elective study in assorted dance styles, into an academic major, and shortly thereafter, into a graduate degree program. Miss Trilling's political savvy and administrative skill in the academic arena helped shepherd dance in higher education into the 20th century. She is remembered as a persuasive, articulate, and visionary woman committed to the value of all aspects of movement education. [5]

In her first six years on the Wisconsin faculty, 1910 to 1916, H'Doubler enjoyed great success as coach of the women's basketball and baseball teams. She was highly successful in recruiting young women for team sports, and greatly enhanced the public image of the women's basketball program. H'Doubler's success in coaching and her leadership skills did not escape the eye of Blanche Trilling. In the spring of 1916, when H'Doubler requested a leave of absence from her teaching to pursue graduate studies in philosophy at Columbia University in New York, Trilling asked to see her. The following is from H'Doubler's official oral history compiled in 1972, by Professor Mary Alice Brennan at the University of Wisconsin:

After I graduated I was asked to stay in the department and help develop sports. Now have I said to you that I was a biology major and philosophy minor? This is very important to me in my way of thinking, later on....Well I wanted to go out and know more about physical education so the only thing to do was to go to the Harvard Summer School and the Sargent School of Physical Education [the Boston Normal School of Physical Education], you probably heard of that....But I wanted to go on, not so much in that [graduate studies in physical education] as I wanted to go to Columbia for more philosophy. I did go to Sargent's...but I was so disappointed, so disillusioned: it was such a dreadful course. There wasn't (sic) any values - you learned a bone name in anatomy - there was nothing significant about the skeletal structure for movement or anything like that, nothing. Something would have to happen to hold me in this field.

But I was interested in the philosophical side so I went to Columbia, and that was a wonderful experience with the philosophers there at that time....[I] was asked to be the graduate member of the Education Philosophical Club, and so I got a chance to be in on all kinds of discussions of education and their points of view. There was Dewey, and Kilpatrick, and Fitzpatrick [at Columbia]. I got terribly excited about what this human mind, what this human being, really is, the values and all, and it got me very stimulated....I got very interested in doing reading on my own. I became interested in drama and theater. I had access to Matthew's Library...and as I read there and as I would read there I saw what an important part dance had in all civilizations - the older civilizations.

...[B]ut I got very interested in this thing and realized more and more the part that dance had played in the various cultures. From there I commenced to build up and tried to see what could be done in our civilization...And I was taking many courses. I was going to find different ballet studios at the same time. This was 1917.

...[T]here was the fact that I was going to New York to study and Miss Trilling called me in and said "Marge, while you are in New York, I wish you would look into dancing and maybe you could come back and teach dance"....[A]nd she said tears came into my eyes, and I said , "I just couldn't think of that. I don't know anything about dance."

She said, "Well, if you get as many girls dancing as you have girls playing basketball, I don't think you would care." "Miss Trilling, I just can't think of ever giving up basketball." She said, "All right you can keep your basketball."

Well, then I left early in the summer, practically after school was over here [Madison] and went to New York so I could commence to look around to see what was going on in dance before the university opened. I went here and there and was so disappointed. Oh, I was so disappointed. And the ballet I took I thought was very bad, very bad indeed. You were just one of a number. Do this, do that and imitate. I just kept writing back to Miss Trilling "I just can't find anything that I think you would want me to teach or that I care to teach." She would hear of different people that were teaching dance [and send H'Doubler to them]. [6]

As the year went on, and as H'Doubler struggled to complete graduate courses and still pursue the charge Miss Trilling had given her, her frustration increased. The following is from a transcript of a lecture given by Miss H'Doubler to students at the University of Wisconsin in June of 1972, compiled by Carl Gutknecht:

> [T]he more I took of it, the more I disliked dance. Everywhere I went most of what they were teaching was ballet, and I went through that. Of course I didn't get to the work. I stopped before that because I couldn't see where it was going to end. It led to a dead end, and I couldn't find anything that I wanted. And do you know girls, the different places I tried to get people to tell me "what is dance?" Not one of them could tell me. Not any of the teachers that I was taking from. I was working with 7 different studios at the time....I found 2 or 3 different studios that were teaching what they called, I guess, contemporary or modern dance, and they were merely doing a different kind of movement but they were as rigidly taught as the ballet forms were taught. So there, that wasn't it. And then there was Dalcroze, and I thought "Oh, this has a great deal to offer." Again I was disappointed. Constantly writing to Miss Trilling; "I shall never teach dance." [7]

In her interviews and taped comments, H'Doubler never mentions being inspired by the work of Gertrude Colby although she did take classes with Colby at Techers College. Colby had already begun developing her teacher training program for dance educators at Teachers College in 1916, but it wasn't until the 1918 - 1919 academic year (after H'Doubler had returned to Madison), that Colby's curriculum was inaugurated under the rubric Natural Dance. H'Doubler did, however, have an interest in the work of Colby's pupil and contemporary Bird Larson, and mentions Larson in her oral history:

> I don't know whether you have heard the name, Bird Larson. Well, she, I think, would have gone someplace if she had not such an early death. She said "Marge, I don't know where I'm going." But as I watched her teach it was more that she was controlling what the students were doing rather than....but it was freer than anything I had seen.
> ...I just saw her teach once and then she went abroad and I think she was taken ill or died. She was a very attractive person and one I am sure who would have found her way. She was seeking too. [8]

In April of 1917, at the end of H'Doubler's year of graduate study, Trilling wrote and asked that she visit one more teacher. By this time Trilling had scheduled H'Doubler to teach dance during the summer session. Trilling and H'Doubler were both aware that time was running out to develop a course in dance, one that (according to Trilling) would be "something worth a college woman's time."

From the feeling revealed in H'Doubler's statement, "and really the more I took of it, the more I disliked dance," one may assume that H'Doubler took Trilling's charge very seriously. One gets the sense from her oral comments that H'Doubler wasn't interested in teaching dance if it wasn't conducive to a theoretical approach. H'Doubler may have been critical of the dance education she was exposed to for a number of reasons. Certainly her experience in graduate school discussing the tenets of progressive education contextualized her broad goals and thinking in teaching. Her background in the biological sciences encouraged her to think systematically. At this time dance education was anything but systematic. As H'Doubler read, studied, and practiced dance it seems apparent that she intuitively felt there was an undiscovered aspect of dance that would lend itself to substance in a college curriculum.

According to H'Doubler:

[I]n April, she [Miss Trilling] said, "I wish you would look up a woman who does not teach dance but is a music teacher and has her students move in relation to music. Her name is Alys Bentley, if ever you happen to run across such a name." And she was a remarkable creative teacher of music. And you may be interested in this little item - what she did with the children. They sang only their own little songs. She did not teach them other songs or melodies, they made their own and she was interested - I told her what my problem was - and she was interested enough to take me. She had a group of 5 - 7 girls and one of them was Ruth David...a lovely mover - and I think her group was called a group of "dancers," though they did not give programs, I don't believe. Movement, as such, was not taught. She [Miss Bentley], would say "Now you do what Ruth is doing, that's what I want." But here's the thing I feel so beholden to her for. That is that she got us down on the floor and had us do some rotations and work with flexions and extensions - as we would say - but not talking or telling us why or anything about it. But then it came to me like a flash; of course, get on the floor where we're away from the pull of gravity and then work out what really are the structural changes of position of the body when it can move freely. And then I commenced to get quite excited. I talked to her again about it and she said "Stay here in New York and develop this because you never can do it in a university. Whoever heard of anything artistic coming out of a college?" [9]

On the floor of a studio in Carnegie Hall, Margaret H'Doubler had the revelation that would help her make dance "something worth a college woman's time." H'Doubler's epiphany seems to have come to her quickly. The essence of her inspiration was that studies in dance must be grounded in knowledge of the moving body itself. This revelation led H'Doubler toward an approach to dance that she could associate with substance and it led her toward a science of dance. Attention to the scientific underpinnings of dance must have made perfect sense to H'Doubler. She was educated in the biological sciences and in the philosophies of progressive education. H'Doubler came to dance with experience teaching in physical education where rules, strategies, and measurements dominate the disciplines approach toward instruction. After H'Doubler's experience with Alys Bentley, an intellectual "door" had been opened. H'Doubler felt she could begin to explore her role in conceptualizing and teaching educational dance:

> I wasn't interested [in staying in New York] - I wanted to teach. Well, I commenced to talk to others about what I thought could be done, nobody could see it....I thought I should talk to Dr. Karl Schroder and Dr. Sargent. They'll know what I am talking about. No, they just didn't know that anything like this could exist, like this that I had in mind. **10**

H'Doubler returned to Madison in the early summer of 1917 with little to go on other than an intuition that what she had in mind could and would work:

> So...I came back to teach in summer school I didn't have a thing but an idea...fortunately the summer group that came to study was a marvelous group, and they, too, were dissatisfied with this kind of dancing [styles of dance that had previously been taught at the university]. We all had to teach it, and the students who had to take it took all year to teach a sequence of a dance called the *White Rose Mazurka*, and the students didn't like it, and that was why Miss Trilling thought there could be some other kind of dance that would have some vital meaning and could qualify as an art experience, and an educational experience for the students. **11**

The statement quoted above sheds additional light on the intentions of H'Doubler and Trilling. They were interested in a kind of dance with vital meaning, dance as art experience, and dance as an educational experience. Trusting that H'Doubler needed time to develop her approach further, Trilling allowed her to teach dance during the 1917 – 1918 academic year. At the conclusion of the spring 1918 term, H'Doubler's class was scheduled to present their work to the campus community. Throughout the year Miss Trilling had stopped in to observe classes on occasion but always arrived at the beginning of class, and only saw the girls working on the floor. H'Doubler became convinced that Trilling had serious reservations about her work and the educational benefits that might stem from it. H'Doubler offered to resign her position if the presentation they had planned that spring was not up to Miss Trilling's standards. Following her presentation, Trilling told H'Doubler that what she had done was remarkable in its uniqueness, educational value, and artistic promise. [12]

While there are no records of exactly what went on in the studio during H'Doubler's first year of teaching, her 1921 text, *A Manual of Dancing*, was begun in the forms of notes during this period and acts as an important reference for understanding her original methods. [13] H'Doubler approached instruction in dance procedurally; beginning classwork with the introduction of a motor activity for rhythmic, kinesthetic, and scientific exploration. [14] The daily lesson might involve investigating a specific joint action (rotation, or flexion and extension), natural movements of the body (such as a crawl, or rising from a lying position to standing), or a rhythmic step (skipping, galloping). These kinds of motor activities she labeled "fundamental." Exercises in the *Manual* include "folding and unfolding," "the prancing step," and "rolls." After movement activities had been experienced they were analyzed kinesiologically and rhythmically. Attention to analysis brought the experience into conscious awareness and promoted intellectual understanding.

H'Doubler's ideas for dance in the summer of 1917 were just that, ideas. During the summer session she began to refine these and put some to use in her teaching. In the next academic year, she continued her investigations of other avenues of thinking for their use in the dance classroom. At this point in the development of her methodology, H'Doubler began to actively seek out ideas and information from other sources to help her refine her vision.

Besides Miss Trilling, who had inspired H'Doubler to seek dance that would be vital, artistic, and educational, H'Doubler gleaned her original inspiration from her experience in Alys Bentley's studio. H'Doubler's interaction with

Bentley framed her reference for a starting point in dance education, prompting her to first consider the mechanical and rhythmic principles of movement. Following her return to Wisconsin in 1917, H'Doubler discussed her ideas with Gertrude Johnson, her roommate and a member of the theater faculty at Wisconsin. Johnson encouraged H'Doubler to consider the role of human emotions as source material for movement. Her suggestion led H'Doubler toward study of the organization of the brain in search of links between feeling and moving states. Ruth Glassow, a colleague of H'Doubler's in physical education, and a pioneer in the field of kinesiology, recalls Johnson's influence on H'Doubler's thinking and early teaching in dance in her oral history:

> She did not really get anything that developed her ideas but somehow an inspiration came to her of what rhythmic movement could mean to the individual in development. It was that she began to get into, and I think she was very much influenced by a friend of hers who was in dramatics here at the University of Wisconsin [Gertrude Johnson]. In dramatics, there is a good bit of your bodily movements conveying the emotions....I'm sure she had a lot of influence and was able to stimulate the thinking of Margaret H'Doubler in connection with this. They were very good friends. [15]

Pursuing the link between emotion and movement, H'Doubler credits Dr. Frances Hellebrandt, a faculty member in neuro-physiology at Wisconsin, with helping her understand the nervous system, motor learning, and the physiology of the brain. [16] From these studies H'Doubler began to use the idea of the kinesthetic sense in her teaching. The kinesthetic sense, the subjective-sensory feedback received from proprioceptors (nerve endings), located in the inner ear, and in muscle and connective tissues, informs the mover of joint position and pressure, the body's relation to the horizontal, and its velocity. [17] It had first been described by H.C. Bastian in his book, *The Brain as an Organ of Mind*, published in 1885: [18]

> [I] knew my anatomy and I knew movement. Oh, but I did read like crazy on the nervous system....I discovered for myself, the feedback and relay stations of the thalamus....I checked it with Dr. Hellebrandt....I went to her because of this. I got so excited about it and she herself, really hadn't realized that there was that connection in the thalamus and the cerebral cortex. [19]

H'Doubler referenced the kinesthetic sense as the subject's appreciation of the objective experience. As she developed her methods, the concept of the "objective-subjective" evolved as a central concept in H'Doubler's teaching. In 1948 she clarified this apparent dichotomy in a position paper titled "A Way of Thinking."

> Through the kinesthetic sense we are not only made aware of body positions and of moving parts, but also of the particular organization of time and stress factors of any particular movement. That is, our sensations of rhythm, and its organization is dependent on the movement sense. We base our judgment of force and duration of movement upon these sensations, and these judgments are the basis for further general judgments of effort, resistance, and weight. Our sensations of space, as well as of time, are also associated with the movement sense....This objective - subjective relation between the "knowing subject" and the "object known" forms the structure essential to a vital learning experience in any field, for the subjective phase of experience can act creatively only as it is interactive with the stimulating forces. [20]

H'Doubler's attention to the kinesthetic sense was unique to her method in teaching: referenced to develop the student's cognitive understanding of the nature of subjective sensation, the inherent rhythmic structure of movement, and the mechanical parameters of motor response.

Understanding the physiology of movement supported H'Doubler's developing interest in rhythm and how practice in rhythmic movement could then lead to a deeper awareness of the kinesthetic sense. H'Doubler references "Dr. Dawson" (a colleague in Physiology of Exercise), whose research in electromyography allowed her to see a visual manifestation of rhythm. After observing the electromyographic apparatus H'Doubler remembers "getting the idea of what rhythm really is":

> Well, it was an isolated muscle that was put up [attached to the electromyographic device]; and there was a marker on a rotating drum with smoked paper; and then the muscle was stimulated and it made this kind of thing [a graphic representation of neuromuscular activity]. Well there's your whole story. He didn't tell it to me but I got it from there just the same. You never heard the word rhythm used - why you could just see it! [21]

Even with her initial success in teaching dance, H'Doubler was reluctant to be too open about her methods and techniques. According to Remley:

Miss H'Doubler was not satisfied that her theories were either sound or perfected. Ideas were still in the budding stage, various teaching techniques were being tried at various levels of student development, and a philosophy of dance was just beginning to evolve. [22]

Yet H'Doubler was less reticent in thinking of new applications for her budding theories. Observing individual differences in her student's skills and needs, H'Doubler began experimenting with the idea that her "fundamentals" might have an application in the form of "corrective" dancing. According to Remley, H'Doubler altered her fundamentals to "meet the requirements of postural and lateral conditions." [23] Physical examinations were required for all women students entering the physical education program. Students were assessed for posture (posture tracing's were taken of all women students starting in 1920), physical fitness, coordination, and athletic skill. Students who failed to meet base requirements were referred to the Women's Physical Education Correctives Program, managed by Louisa Lippit. Miss Lippit allowed H'Doubler to offer a corrective class in dance in 1921. [24] Corrective Program classes in posture, relaxation, dance, and corrective exercise led to the eventual development of a program in Physical Therapy (1929), and later in Dance Therapy (1949). [25]

At the center of H'Doubler's "budding" methodology was the importance of first developing a sound and scientifically based approach to learning in human movement. She began with analysis and practice of fundamental principles of movement. After these concepts had been investigated and control of the body obtained, student explorations in class then focused on rhythmic possibilities in movement, and finally on the expressive creations in dance that might subsequently evolve.

Besides being inspired by Bentley to use the floor for the purpose of getting away from the effects of gravity in exploring movement, H'Doubler also acknowledges the importance of Bentley's creative method on the subsequent development of her own method:

> I must say at this point her [Bentley's] main interest and her biggest work was with children and she was simply marvelous with them. She did not teach them songs or melodies, she had them create their own. She was a highly creative person, the first one that I had contacted. [26]
>
> [A]nd you may be interested in this little item - what she did with the children. They sang only their own little songs. She did not teach them other songs or melodies, they made their own. [27]

H'Doubler's interest in Bentley's approach to the music-dance relationship seems to have been that Bentley didn't teach her students "songs and melodies," but that she had them make their own. A cross-over of this idea appears in H'Doubler's later method of having students generate and understand their own solutions to creative problems presented in class.

What is particularly interesting about the development of H'Doubler's methodology in dance education is that she seems to have generated her approach quite independently. All indicators point to a remarkable, and independent, conceptual development on H'Doubler's part in a very short period of time. The data collected from H'Doubler's oral histories, texts, recollections, position statements, teaching syllabi, and writings, do not suggest any substantial ties to the work of her contemporaries in dance education. H'Doubler herself makes no reference to being conceptually, behaviorally, or methodologically influenced by others in the small circle of nationally recognized dance educators working in the same time period; Mary Wood Hinman, Mary Porter Beegle, Ruth St. Denis, Ted Shawn, Lucile and Agnes Marsh, Helen Norman Smith, or Gertrude Colby. Nor, for that matter does H'Doubler reference her work in relation to that of her contemporaries in Germany; Rudolf Laban, Mary Wigman, or Harald Kreutzberg.

In H'Doubler's oral history, Mary Alice Brennan asks pointed questions about stimulating influences, both educational and artistic, and H'Doubler's responses concern the individuals identified above; Trilling, Larson, Bentley, Johnson, Dawson, and Hellebrandt. Wisconsin colleagues; Otto and Koffka

(Professors of Philosophy), Hagen (Professor of Art History), and Meiklejohn (Professor of Education), are other important influences and while not mentioned in her oral histories, they do turn up in H'Doubler's writings and in other scholarly works on H'Doubler. [28] At one point in the interview Brennan questions the possibility of influences from other dance educators, directly referencing Mary Wigman; "Did you find any other teachers who might have been teaching along this line? And the students, did they come from other people who may have been teaching in this way? Did you find any, say, from Mary Wigman?" To which H'Doubler's reply is, "Well, Mary Wigman didn't teach this way." [29] While this may be interpreted as an ambiguous answer, it clearly suggests that she wasn't "finding teachers who might be teaching along this line." Mary Lou Remley (1975), addresses the matter of influences in a footnote to her article The Wisconsin Idea of Dance: A Decade of Progress 1917 - 1926:

> Gertrude Colby, Bird Larson, Isadora Duncan and others have been variously credited with stimulating H'Doubler and her theories of dance education, and Miss H'Doubler credits her development and refinement of the idea to a composite of many sources. After study of Alys E. Bentley's early writings, further discussion with Miss H'Doubler, and perusal of her writings, this writer is convinced that the main impetus for Miss H'Doubler's idea of dance was a direct result of her contact and brief study with Miss Bentley. [30]

By 1921 H'Doubler felt more confident in discussing her methods and in allowing students the opportunity to present their work on a more regular basis. In that year a studio devoted exclusively to dance was opened in Lathrop Hall. [31] A student group was also formed so that student's would have an organized activity outside of class time and a venue for their creative work. Miss H'Doubler offered her group the name Orchesis, after a Greek term she had uncovered in her reading which she translated as "the science of movement in action and repose." [32] Students elected to use her term and the first Orchesis was formed. The Orchesis idea was later transplanted to colleges and universities across the country and today Orchesis groups still exist in many dance departments. A large number of

93

current dance major programs can trace their evolution back to an Orchesis group founded on their campus after 1921.

A Manual of Dancing

In 1921 H'Doubler's first text, *A Manual of Dancing* , was published. This is a short volume of only 103 pages, many of which are left blank for "memorandums," pages for notes on the use of the text by the reader. The text is divided into 5 sections: (1) "Teaching Interpretive Dancing as an Educational Activity." (2) "Exercises for Fundamental Motor Control: "Upper Part of the Body," "Lower Part of the Body," "Coordinating all Parts of the Body," and "Drawing of Fundamental Exercises," (3)"Realization and Appreciation of Music through Movement ," (4)"Plan of Lessons," and (5), an annotated Bibliography.

The creation of *A Manual of Dancing* is extraordinary because it came so quickly in H'Doubler's development as a dance educator. Just five years earlier she had burst into tears when Trilling asked that she look into dance while on leave in New York. H'Doubler evolved quickly, yet did so with a very mature sensibility. In the introduction to the *Manual* H'Doubler carefully states that her aim in writing this book is to: "evolve a scheme of training (in dance) worthy of a place in an educational curriculum." *A Manual of Dancing* was written: "not to create argument or to question the definitions of others, but...to clarify her procedure in teaching dancing as an educational activity." [33] In opening comments H'Doubler states:

> Dancing is self-expression through the medium of bodily movement; a revealing of mental and emotional states, stimulated or regulated, or both, usually by music. I say usually by music for we have long been accustomed to associate dancing only with music. [34]

H'Doubler alludes to rhythm as the more powerful driving force in dancing and references poetry as another form of accompaniment to dance because of its rhythmic nature. Dance is; "an art form since the chief characteristic of all art is self-expression and like all expressive art forms it (dance) takes deep root in human experience, feelings and emotions." [35] She then turns her attention to means of expression and brings forward the idea that at the root of dancing lies movement and that an understanding of the fundamental nature of human movement is necessary to prepare the dancer to move with feeling and conviction:

> Plainly the body is our instrument, our medium of expression. If the body then is to communicate our ideas, thoughts and feelings, our first task is to render it capable of being sensitive and responsive to the demands placed on it. This means the physical mechanism must be studied, the function of various parts understood and their relationship to the whole appreciated. [36]

That dance should be understood from the perspective of the science of the moving body, in part and wholly related, was progressive thinking for the time. H'Doubler's scientific approach was a new paradigm for the consideration of an approach to educating through dance. To achieve control of the body H'Doubler defines what she feels are; "fundamental exercises that are basic and necessary for all further work in dance." [37] Here we have the beginnings of the H'Doubler technique for dance. "Fundamentals" are meant to:

> ...[E]stablish habits of muscular guidance and control in order that the student may have full use of the physical mechanism free from inhibitions. Always the laws of natural movement, namely, movement according to the joint-muscular mechanism are applied. The source of the movement made clear and then allowed to "follow through."
> By "follow through" is meant, that any movement when initiated in the body, or in any of its parts, shall continue to the climax, without obstruction, constriction, or inhibition at any point. [38]

The idea of identifying movement fundamentals was another of H'Doubler's departures from the work of previous dance educators. In this regard H'Doubler's analysis of movement in dance went much deeper than that of her peers. H'Doubler's reinterpretation of natural movement is also interesting. Having taken, classes with Gertrude Colby at Columbia, H'Doubler was aware of the use of the term "natural" in reference to Colby's teaching, where natural meant that which seemed innate. But H'Doubler's purpose was not just to analyze the gross aspects of natural locomotor movements such as walking, running, skipping, and hopping. She meant to analyze the body structures that permit such movements; the movements of flexion, extension, or abduction, which occur at the hip, the shoulder, or spine. H'Doubler's use of the idea of "follow through" is also worth considering. Today we know that this is an important aspect of training in professional dance technique because the dancer must be able to fulfill and project their movement in performance. For H'Doubler, the idea of follow through was individually important for students to fully feel each movement, receive kinesthetic feedback, and to acquire the ability to move with confidence. "Follow through" may have been a creative adaptation of her teaching in sports where the idea is commonly used to effectively manipulate external objects such as basketballs and baseballs.

H'Doubler defines her fundamental exercises as:

> [A] series of movements which in themselves demand fundamental coordination's, most of them beginning in the spine and extending in a well ordered progression to all the smaller muscle groups of the extremities. Because of the muscular activity involved in the upright position, many of the fundamentals are executed lying on the floor, thus relieving the body of the pull of gravity. A chief function of the first exercises then is to prepare for the upright position. When the fundamental principles of movement upon the floor have been mastered, the next step is to carry these principles over into the upright position, adding the coordination of the muscles which support us in the standing position.
> At first every movement has to be under conscious control, and is the object of attention, otherwise the correct reflexes or habits would not be established. Later we can trust to our impulses and no longer need to think out every movement.
> Because of the very nature of the kinesthetic sense and its value it is of the utmost importance that it should be well developed. This the fundamentals also aim to accomplish. All this is of course, not dancing; it is merely getting at the things which make dancing possible. [39]

In these statements H'Doubler reveals the nature of her scientific approach to dance. For the first time dance is clearly equated with its origins in the fundamental aspects of human movement: individual joint actions and restrictions, reflexive movements, and development of the individual's kinesthetic sense. H'Doubler recognized that it is only through increased understanding and skill in both non-locomotor and locomotor movements that art dance becomes possible. After discussing the necessity of training in movement fundamentals (the non-locomotor), H'Doubler goes on to analyze locomotor movements accompanied by music. She understood locomotor movements as "elements of construction for dance steps." And, she considers music structures and their influence on time as an important element in moving. Still, however, H'Doubler says:

> So, this part of our study may be called the appreciation and realization of music through movement [note that she does not say "movement through music"]. Still this is not dancing". This process is a building of movement vocabulary with which the student is meant to "later express herself...,

In preparing to dance H'Doubler felt that:

> [T]he student should be so taught that she may give expression to her own reactions, and not those of another. Here, it seems, is where much of the dancing taught, fails almost entirely as an educational activity. It is at best an imitative process, a type of work which does not grow from any creative germ. It is destructive to any stimulus for originality. It is mechanical, an application, not a creation. There should be no imitation or memory, as far as set movements and gestures are concerned. How can there be if we adhere to our definition of dancing - self-expression through movement. **40**

This perspective would stay with H'Doubler throughout her professional teaching career. First and foremost H'Doubler was an educator, thoroughly committed to the development of the individual, and the potential of creative and expressive movement in that development. H'Doubler's ideas on dance and dance education were liberally and individually based. Her philosophy and approach were neither vocationally or professionally oriented. H'Doubler's educational idealism is summed up in the closing paragraph of her introductory statement for *A Manual of Dancing*:

> It is perhaps needless to say that if dancing is to hold a place of importance in an educational curriculum those who teach it must have as broad a background as possible. The better the background the better the teacher. Those teaching this activity should believe in its values, not as performance, but as an educational influence of the finest type. Considering the aim of modern education, namely, development of the individual, I sincerely believe that the type of dancing I have attempted to suggest hold values we have been too slow to appreciate, and is as important a factor in physical or any other education as any subject in the curriculum. **41**

Creating a Major in Dancing: 1926

Throughout the 1920's H'Doubler continued to work on her ideas; developing her fundamental exercises, defining relationships between rhythm and dance, and expanding the body of knowledge of educational dance. As time went by, and as students took her ideas into the field, H'Doubler's model was increasingly referenced by college educators developing dance programs on their own campuses. In response to increased interest in her approach, H'Doubler and students crafted a lecture-demonstration on educational dance. Lecture-demonstrations began with fundamentals and progressed to expressive aspects, finishing with a review of the materials used to teach and train in dance. The format and focus of the lecture-demonstration helped promote H'Doubler's idea that educational dance was first and foremost a learning activity and was not meant for professional entertainment.

Based on the positive reception to H'Doubler's lecture-demonstrations and her text, requests also began to come in for H'Doubler trained teachers. Remley (1975) notes that:

> Long before the establishment of the dance major, alumnae from 1919, 1920, 1921 and 1922, were teaching "Miss H'Doubler's Dancing" at Northwestern University, the University of Washington, Michigan State Normal School, the University of Texas, Illinois State Normal University, North Carolina College for Women, and Wellesley College. [42]

By 1923 the increase in requests for teachers trained in "Miss H'Doubler's Dancing" had led to the development a minor in dancing for women. The minor consisted of 12 credits distributed in physical education and course work in speech, philosophy, music, and psychology. The dance minor prompted H'Doubler toward making the case for dance as a major discipline. Miss Trilling didn't think a major in dancing would have much chance being passed by the University faculty. H'Doubler agreed that her chances were slim but went ahead anyway thinking, "if not this year, then next":

> Pretty soon we commenced to receive requests for teachers in dance. I went to MissTrilling, oh so excited about it. And she said, "My Lord, Marge can you see this faculty, this University ever consenting to a dance major course"? And I said, "No Miss Trilling, I can't. But let me make a course of study and I'll present it and they will refuse me the first year. And then I will present it the second year and I'll be refused. And the third year they will accept it to be rid of me." She said. "All right, go ahead." [43]

In 1925 H'Doubler published her second text, *The Place of Dance in Education*, as a philosophical preamble to her efforts. *The Place of Dance in Education* is the first in a series of philosophical treatises, position papers, and policy statements that H'Doubler generated over her long career meant to clarify her liberal, humanist educational perspective. [44]

On June 8, 1926, H'Doubler submitted a curriculum for a specialized major in dancing within the course in Physical Education for Women to the Faculty of the College of Letters and Science. Assisting her in the process of crafting the curriculum design were Miss Trilling, and John Sellery, Dean of the College of Letters and Science at Wisconsin. On October 13, 1926, the School of Education, Department of Physical Education Women's Division, (after approving the curricular design for dancing at their October 11 meeting), submitted the course outline for the specialized Major in Dancing to the faculty of the College of Letters and Science for final approval. The curriculum was approved and the first university major in dance began accepting students in the spring semester of 1927. Later that year the curriculum in Dancing was expanded to include the M.A. in Physical Education with a specialized major in Dancing. [45]

Margaret H'Doubler's contributions to dance in the American university were seminal. Perhaps the most important of these was her work in developing the substance of dance as an academic discipline. H'Doubler promoted the notion that the study of dance should involve a variety of conceptual approaches, and that different aspects of dance should be learned in their specific context. H'Doubler's legacy is in the idea that dance, as a field of study, included course work in the science of movement, (kinesiology), practice in developing fundamental movement skills (technique), understanding historical perspectives (dance history), manipulating movement creatively (composition), understanding the relation of movement to rhythm (rhythmic analysis), how to teach the body to move (teaching methods), and developing an understanding of classic and contemporary thinking on the moving body (dance philosophy).

The other great contribution of Margaret H'Doubler, one that she took several steps further than her colleague Gertrude Colby, was that dance in education was liberal in nature and that its purpose was to inspire individual kinesthetic awareness, intellectual understanding, and individual creativity. H'Doubler believed that the function of dance in education was to enable students to discover themselves, physically, mentally, and creatively, through expressive human movement. After the creation of the major in dancing, H'Doubler spent her remaining years in academia reiterating this point over and over. Yet, while core elements of H'Doubler's philosophy on dance in education have had a lasting impact on dance in the university (among these the idea that dance must be taught conceptually and that the individual learns best through structured experience), her argument against professionalism in the dance curriculum was overcome by the evolution of the discipline and the necessity for dance to define its role in higher education through association with the other fine arts. With the definition of dance as a fine and performing art, the influence of the professional dance world made quick inroads into the curriculum.

Dance, arguably the first of the arts, was the last to enter the realm of structured learning, and it did so through the door provided for by its association with physical education. A shared focus on the benefits of practice in human movement was, at first, the mutual reference point in education for physical education and dance. Over time however, the subjective, aesthetic nature of dance found itself at odds with the utilitarian, objective desires of physical education. Both turned away, one from the other, toward allied areas of study in the face of external questions and doubts raised about each as an academic discipline.

In the space of ten years 1917 - 1927, dance had been propelled out of obscurity toward academic substance and definition. The university was now a place for dance to define and understand itself. Margaret H'Doubler's contributions toward that end were transforming for dance education. Regardless of her position against bringing vocational attitudes and professional standards into the dance curriculum, Margaret H'Doubler's gift to dance in education was

100

extraordinary: to revolutionize dance in education, to develop a body of knowledge for dance, and define for dance a meaningful place in the American university.

The next great leap forward for dance in the American university would be toward melding educational goals with professional standards. And the 'giant' in dance in the American university who would spark this was a young academic with a gift for organization and an unerring commitment to the dance artist: Martha Hill.

CHAPTER 5

Establishing An American Modern Dance: 1926 - 1940

In a striking coincidence, just as dance was coming to recognition as a major area of study at the University of Wisconsin in April of 1926 modern dance appeared as an emergent art form on a concert stage in New York City. Over time modern dance would become the most pervasive stylistic influence on dance in the American university. In the 1930's, the term "modern dance" was used to label a highly stylized and expressive dance form, an art-dance, that was conceptually based on similar trends in the areas of theatre, music, and the visual arts. Modern dance emerged out of the studios of a small group of New York concert dancers. In its educational manifestation, modern dance blended rigorous training in technique with conceptual studies in dance composition, rhythm and music for dance, the history of dance, and aesthetics. In higher education, modern dance made significant inroads in replacing the more liberally based "interpretive" perspective that had dominated dance in the university over the previous two decades.

Not all dance educators were able, or willing, to go to the lengths that Colby, Larson, or H'Doubler had to develop their own conceptual framework for educational dance. Most were trained as physical educators, where a game's rules and strategies were defined and easily accessible in a manual. The most intellectually taxing thing the uninspired educator had to do was to understand and adhere to matters of boundaries, kinds of "plays," the rules of offense and defense, and records keeping. Those who gravitated toward dance found modern art dance hugely attractive. Its conceptual underpinnings were qualitative; its description metaphorical. The modern dance could be imitated. Replicating it lent a certain artistic credibility to the vision and intentions of physical educators who were interested in an arts-based dance experience for their students. At the same time, by the abstract, qualitative, art conscious nature of its presentation, modern dance alienated many others in physical education. These were people who were either not comfortable with the notion that dance was, or could be, more than just another "activity," or who where suspicious of the pedagogical implications of allowing artists so much influence in the form that this educational dance took.

As interested educators in the field were exposed to the dynamic, individual, and artistic approach of modern dance, revelation stimulated their desire for academic independence for dance. Some began to call for dance to break away from physical education and to align with the other fine and performing arts. Throughout the 1930's, educational discourse that emerged out of the debate over dance was found primarily within academic journals devoted to health, physical education, and recreation. A few major urban newspapers included the writings and commentary of a resident dance critic, and some texts were produced. As a program within physical education, modern dance faced a skeptical audience. This troubling new kind of dance, that some educators seemed so ready to accept, was of great concern to educators who still looked at dance as a movement activity. The struggle for academic parity, and mutual respect between physical education and dance, began in earnest in the 1930's, and, in many ways, continues to this day.

The future of dance as an arts-based discipline was shaped by a cadre of " the leaders of modern dance," at Bennington College, a small, liberal arts college that was organized in the town of Bennington, Vermont in 1932. A model of progressive education in action, Bennington was conceived at the height of the "Roaring Twenties" and came into being during the darkest days of the Great Depression. From Bennington, the seeds of the modern dance were dispersed to educational programs in colleges and universities across America. Led by dance educator Martha Hill and her administrative colleague Mary Josephine Shelly; dance artists, Martha Graham, Doris Humphrey, Charles Weidman, Hanya Holm, composer Louis Horst, and dance critic John Martin, were the core faculty who helped reshape the academic world of dance with their new vision for dance in art and in education.

The Pioneers of an American Modern Dance: Martha Graham, Louis Horst, "Tamiris" Doris Humphrey, Charles Weidman, Hanya Holm, and John Martin

As noted earlier in Chapter Three, between 1915 and 1925 the Denishawn company and school had been the nexus of professional training and concert dance in America. Denishawn toured internationally and featured "star" performers in addition to Ruth St. Denis and Ted Shawn. Out of Denishawn came new artists who developed their own approach to dance, eventually classified as modern. Unlike the dance performances inspired by exotic or ancient cultures which were a hallmark of the Denishawn company, the modern dance as a concert form was labeled expressional, and like modern art, reflected the contemporary concerns and experiences of the choreographer and performer. [1]

Martha Graham and Louis Horst; "Tamiris"

The woman who ultimately became the living symbol of modern dance for the American public, and the first to leave Denishawn in 1923, was Martha Graham. After quitting Denishawn, Graham enjoyed an active career as a performer, teacher, and choreographer that spanned 7 decades (1923 - 1991).

The daughter of an early, pre-Freudian, psychiatrist, or "alienist," Martha was born in Allegheny, Pennsylvania in 1894; the eldest child of George and Jane, "Jennie," Graham. In 1908 the Graham family moved to Santa Barbara, California where Martha and her sisters Mary and Georgia, "Geordie," lived a comfortable, upper middle-class life. In 1912, Martha was taken by her father to see a performance by Ruth St. Denis in nearby Los Angeles. The event proved important to Graham, stirring within her a latent desire to dance. [2]

Following graduation from Santa Barbara High School in 1913, Martha registered to attend the Cumnock School of Expression in Los Angeles. The Cumnock School was a progressive institution, with an educational mission based on the belief that art and life were inseparable. While still a student at Cumnock, Martha enrolled in a summer course at Denishawn in 1916. At 23 years of age Graham completed her course work at the Cumnock School in 1917 and immediately enrolled as a full time student at Denishawn.

There was little in Martha's early character and dancing to indicate that here was a great artist in the making. St. Denis felt Martha was far too shy and timid a personality; too small, dark, and troubled looking for a career in dance. But, being a full-time and paying student, Martha was gingerly placed in Ted's care and he took an interest in her development. Graham worked diligently and Shawn began to cast her in roles. In 1920 he created a ballet for himself and for Martha titled, *Xochitl*, a melodramatic spectacle based on Shawn's imaginative readings of Aztec culture. *Xochitl* proved a great success and Martha began to bloom as a star performer.

Graham left Denishawn in 1923 after receiving an offer for a regular position with John Murray Anderson's Greenwich Village Follies, a fashionable dance review in New York City. Martha performed with the Follies for two years as the "art" dancer in the show. In 1925 Graham accepted Anderson's offer to teach dance at a new school he was forming for performing artists in New York. She also accepted a teaching position in the Dance and Dramatic Arts Division of the Eastman School of Music in Rochester, New York. For the next two years Graham commuted between jobs. It was during this period that Graham began to form her own thinking on dance, perhaps all that time on the train provided a regular environment for contemplation. Regular teaching in a formal setting seems to have prompted Martha to develop a philosophy regarding new ways to use the expressive body in generating art.

In May of 1925 Louis Horst left Denishawn. Horst had come to Ruth and Ted in his mid-thirties, after years of playing piano for silent movies. Like Ted Shawn, Louis was a native of Kansas City. Horst had developed a mentoring relationship with Graham during their time together at Denishawn. Some of Graham's biographers have concluded that Graham and Horst's ties were artistic and romantic. Regardless, the product of their relationship was the evolution of modern dance. Upon leaving Denishawn Horst traveled to Vienna to further his studies in music composition. Louis didn't find Vienna fulfilling and was in regular communication with Graham. In October of 1925 Horst returned to New York. On April 18, 1926, Graham, with Horst accompanying, presented what is generally accepted as the first concert of modern dance at the 48th Street Theatre in New York City. [3]

Within a year of Graham's foray into the field, other names were starting to crop up in the small circle of modern dancers. In 1927, Helen Becker, who assumed the stage name "Tamiris," presented her own concert of modern choreography. Doris Humphrey and Charles Weidman, former Denishawn dancers and were contemporaries of Graham and Horst, followed Tamiris in 1928. In New York City, these modern dancers began experimenting with new approaches to dance teaching, performance, and composition. Concert activity in the new professional world of modern dance at this time has been described as prolific. According to dance historian Marcia Siegel (1987), the 1928 - 1929 season was;

> ...unprecedented in its dance activity. The writers who were given the most space to cover dance, John Martin at the New York Times and Mary F. Watkins at the New York *Herald Tribune*, toted up 129 concert dance events for the season. [4]

Doris Humphrey and Charles Weidman

From the fertile breeding ground of Denishawn came most of the dancers responsible for beginning the modern dance. Graham, Horst, and Tamiris were joined by Doris Humphrey and Charles Weidman when the Humprey-Weidman partnership presented their first concert of original choreography in the spring of 1928. The break from Denishawn was not as clean for Humphrey and Weidman as it had been for Martha Graham. Humphrey and Weidman prolonged their affiliation with St. Denis and Shawn throughout 1927 and into the summer of 1928. But, by August of 1928, Humphrey and Weidman had completed all contractual agreements with Denishawn and they were on their own. Like Graham, Humprey and Weidman attracted the talents of a Denishawn musician, Pauline Laurence. Laurence was musician, publicist, costumer, and booking agent for the Humphrey-Weidman Company until the group disbanded in 1944. [5]

In Denishawn, Doris Humphrey had been Miss Ruth's chosen protégé. A lithe and agile performer, Humphrey grew up in Chicago, studying with an assortment of ballet teachers and with Mary Wood Hinman, an early teacher of folk and national dances. Hinman, an instructor at John Dewey's experimental school at the University of Chicago, had an important influence on Humphrey. Dance historian Marcia Siegel comments, "Hinman represented the most enlightened approach to dance education, a pioneering spirit who never ceased searching for new materials and modes of teaching." [6] Through her study with Hinman, Doris may have framed many of her own future teaching perspectives. Seigel writes that Humphrey was "ambivalent about Mary Wood, as she was about all the powerful women in her life." [7] However, as a teacher Miss Hinman was very much in sync with the progressive education policies of John Dewey, and progressive teaching methods were a hallmark of Humphrey's later pedagogy. In June of 1917, Mary Wood sent Doris a brochure for the Denishawn School in Los Angeles. Seigel quotes a note from Hinman to Humphrey about Denishawn, "It is so full of what one wants, I feel that she (Ruth St. Denis) is in your line and she could make a lot out of you - she is of tomorrow." [8]

Charles Weidman came to Denishawn from Lincoln, Nebraska. His first teacher there was Doris Humphrey. Over the next several years Humphrey and Weidman established a working relationship and by 1926 when Denishawn was struggling to survive were making preliminary plans to establish their own school and company.

Like Graham and Horst, Humphrey and Weidman contributed a great deal to the development of modern dance in America. The Humphrey-Weidman School offered winter and summer sessions for teachers that were very popular with dance educators in the colleges. [9] According to Margaret Lloyd (1949), dance historian and author of the *Borzoi Book of Modern Dance:*

> In the late twenties, as news of the new dance got around, dance-minded gym teachers from all over the country began taking vacation courses at the New York studios of Doris Humphrey and Charles Weidman and of Martha Graham. The techniques were different, and it must be added, more easily adaptable in the Humphrey-Weidman studio. Although rhythmic and artistic, the work was, in the teacher-students' estimation, fundamentally and functionally gymnastic, utilitarian. [10]

Teacher training sessions at the Humprey-Weidman and Graham studios helped generate a client base for the Bennington Summer School of the Dance in the late 1920's and early 1930's.

Hanya Holm

In the decade prior to the beginnings of modern dance in New York City, a contemporary dance movement was also gaining momentum in Germany. The German version of modern dance, as developed by Rudolf Von Laban, Harald Kreutzberg, Mary Wigman, and Kurt Joos, had emerged in the years leading up to the First World War with distinct characteristics of its own. Following the War, the German dancers had regrouped and reclaimed their place in developing this new kind of art-dance. In 1929 the "German dance" was introduced to American audiences in a concert tour by Harald Kreutzberg, and was reintroduced in 1930-31 through a series of concerts dates by Mary Wigman and her dance company. Following the success of her first American tour, Wigman returned to Germany. Before leaving America however, Wigman saw that a school was established in her name in New York City. Wigman's school was left to operate under the direction of her assistant and principal dancer, Hanya Holm. [11] Holm stayed in America, and while not immediately establishing herself as a choreographer, was quickly recognized as an important teacher of the German dance. The German influence would play an important role in dance in American higher education, adding an intellectual component to dance studies in dance accompaniment, improvisation, and pedagogy.

John Martin

The other significant figure in the early years of modern dance in America was dance critic John Martin. Martin came to the *New York Times* in 1927 from a career as an actor and theatrical director. He had been recommended for a part time position as dance critic to Times editor Olin Downes by Elsa Findlay, a teacher of Dalcroze Eurythmics. Martin's original plan was to work at the paper for a few months, until further work in the theater became available. However, Martin was at the right place at the right time and understood and could write intelligently about the new dance movement still in its formative stages. Martin joined the Times staff in October of 1928 as the nation's first full-time dance critic for a daily newspaper. From 1927 until his invitation to join the Bennington faculty in 1934, through his column in the Times, and in lectures on art and dance that he organized at the New School for Social Research beginning in 1931, Martin clarified the meaning of a modern approach to art-dance. He promoted the work of American and foreign modern dance artists (prominently among these both Harald Kreutzberg and Mary Wigman), and helped define the academic realms of dance history and criticism. [12] By 1930, the recognized artists of American modern dance were all based in New York and Martin was reviewing their work.

Modern Dance 1930 - 1933: Organized Activity, Dance Repertory Theatre

The first years of the 1930's were not easy ones for most Americans, let alone performing artists in dance. The Stock Market Crash of October 1929 was devastating to many financially. To survive and prosper to the degree that they might expect to, the small group of recognized choreographers organized under the leadership of Tamiris to create the Dance Repertory Theatre. [13] Dancers with a thirst for a national reputation wanted to show their work on Broadway, because it was only through performances in Broadway theaters that substantial recognition from the press was likely. The Dance Repertory Theatre was designed to be a cooperative effort in producing dance concerts, to attract the greatest audience, and resolve scheduling conflicts. Unfortunately Dance Repertory Theatre only lasted two seasons before artistic temperaments, and a repeal of the legal prohibition on Sunday evening concerts, caused it to go under. Before the creation of Dance Repertory Theatre options were limited since most theaters were booked throughout the week and closed on Sunday evenings. With the repeal of the Blue Law for theaters, Sunday evening concerts became the standard for modern dancers. One of Martha Graham's dancers participating in Dance Repertory Theatre productions was Martha Hill. Author Sali Ann Kriegsman (1981), speculates that the failure of Dance Repertory Theatre may have had a lasting impression on Hill as she would later use great skill in keeping most of these artists working in close proximity to one another at Bennington College. [14]

Symposia on Modern Dance 1930 - 1933

By 1930 modern dance was beginning to be widely known in academic circles. Martha Hill (New York University), and her colleague Mary P. O'Donnell (Teachers College), were members of the American Physical Education Association (APEA), and through the APEA's Eastern District were active in promoting the modern dancers in academic circles. Members of the APEA, including H'Doubler, Hill, and O'Donnell were beginning to organize on a national level. In 1931 they successfully petitioned the APEA to create a National Section on Dancing (the history of the National Section on Dancing is covered in Chapter 7). Academic Journals (i.e. *Health and Physical Education* and the *Journal of Physical Education*), and popular magazines (i.e. *American Dance* and *Dance Magazine*), included features on the new dancers and their modern perspectives on

111

dance as art and in education. John Martin's lecture series on modern dance at the New School in New York City was a great success, stimulating scholarly discourse on the nature and potential of dance as art. Martin asked dancers, composers, artists, and educators to participate in an open forum of demonstration, which was then followed by discussion and debate. Audience members were often quite eager to question the motives and substance of the modern dancers work because, from its beginnings, modern dance had a popular reputation as very serious and self-indulgent. Through the demonstrations, followed by the question and answer format, dancers honed their extemporaneous speaking skills while defending their points of view, and educated audience members about the discreet differences and similarities of modern dance.

To supplement their meager incomes and to survive between performance seasons, Graham, Humphrey, Tamiris, and later Holm, taught regular classes in their respective studios in Manhattan. Teacher training sessions during winter and summer breaks in the academic calendar were increasingly popular with collegiate dance educators. In 1932 and 1933 symposia for college dance professionals were held at Barnard College. They attracted instructors and directors of dance programs in women's physical education from prestigious Eastern colleges and universities. Participants discussed the methods, aims, and principles of the modern dance. According to Soares (1997), representatives from New York University, Mt. Holyoke, Vassar, Russell Sage, Smith, Sarah Lawrence, and Wellesley colleges attended the 1932 symposium. [15] Sessions at the American Physical Education Association conferences, meetings at other professional societies, articles in magazines and journals, and educators who visited the New York studios and schools all helped disseminate the news about the modern dance.

"Out of One Happening:" Martha Hill and Bennington College

Into this evolutionary mix stepped Robert Leigh, the first President of Bennington College. According to dance historian Sali Ann Kriegsman, writing in *Modern Dance in America: The Bennington Years* (1981):

Bennington College had been ten years in the planning when it opened on 6 September 1932 to its first class of 87 women. The college was conceived in the Jazz Age, but its proponents met with one setback after another, capped by the stock market crash of 1929, which almost scuttled the project. When the original campus site in Old Bennington was withdrawn, the Trustees gratefully accepted Mrs. Frederic B. Jennings' offer to donate 140 acres of her North Bennington Farm....

...[T]he college faculty were themselves practitioners in their fields, honoring the progressive philosophy that doing is a potent means of learning. (John Dewey was among a raft of eminent advisors in the college's planning, and William Heard Kilpatrick of Teachers College, Columbia University, was an ardent advocate.) [16]

Leigh and Bennington's other early academic managers wanted a comprehensive arts curriculum that would be on par with the college's other academic programs. Leigh's wife thought up the idea of an arts based "exercise program" because the construction of a gymnasium was outside the college's meager budget.

Leigh approached Martha Graham for a possible recommendation for the position of Director of Dance, and Graham referred him to Martha Hill, introducing the two at the 1932 Annual Dance Symposium at Barnard College. [17] Hill declined Leigh's offer to become either full-time director of dance or of physical education but did agree to devote two days a week to Bennington while maintaining her position directing the dance program in physical education at New York University (NYU). Hill commuted between positions until 1951, when she was appointed Chair of the newly formed Dance Department within the Juilliard School of Music. Soares, quotes Hill in a 1993 interview:

..."I was young and inexperienced," Martha Hill admitted, but she believed in Leigh's ideas. Leigh was "...in the business of way-breaking' in his call for 'high intellectual standards freed from the dry and stuffy aspects that had been the pattern at women's colleges." Hill had found her modus operandi... "From the beginning I imported the best dance to the university setting." [18]

Martha Hill and Mary Josephine Shelly

Martha Hill was born in 1901 in Palestine, Ohio. As a young woman she attended the Normal School of Physical Education, later known as the Kellogg School for Physical Education, in Battle Creek, Michigan. After graduating from the Kellogg School in 1920, Hill accepted a vast array of teaching assignments that would keep her on the move until 1932.

Following her graduation from the Kellogg School, Hill was retained as an assistant to Marietta Lane, supervisor of the School's dance curriculum. Hill taught courses in pageantry, ballet, athletics, and kinesiology during her first year and replaced Lane as Dance Director at the Kellogg School in 1922. In the fall of 1923, Hill left Michigan to take a position in physical education at Fort Hays State Teachers College, in Fort Hays, Kansas, where she was Director of Dance in Physical Education, teaching classes in ballet and gymnastics. While at Fort Hays State Hill demonstrated her talent for organization by working with music faculty in the production of elaborate spring festivals for music and dance. Hill directed the dance component of the festival with costumes and scenery rented from New York City. [19] Summer sessions in 1924 and 1925 were spent at the Perry-Mansfield Dance Camp in Steamboat Springs, Colorado.

In the spring of 1926, Hill moved to New York City to begin the undergraduate program in physical education at Teachers College. Hill saw Martha Graham's second independent concert at the Klaw Theatre in New York City on November 28, 1926: "When I first saw Graham I was bowled over. It was an instant conversion. I immediately went to study with her at the John Murray Anderson-Robert Milton School of the Theater." [20] Because of the strength of Graham's vision for dance, Hill studied with her through the fall and winter of 1926 - 1927, while simultaneously working on her degree requirements at Teachers College. In the summer of 1927 Hill traveled to Wisconsin and enrolled in Margaret H'Doubler's summer teaching course: "That summer confirmed my belief in Martha Graham. At Wisconsin, they never used anything below their waists. Everything was arms. No torso. That would be too erotic." [21] The marked difference in the approach Hill and H'Doubler each took toward the teaching of dance in higher education was soon apparent. Kriegsman quotes Barbara Page (1981), a former student of H'Doubler's, as saying:

Martha (Hill) was offered a job at the University of Oregon in the Physical Education Department and went out and developed this wonderful kind of dance in education that she expanded so beautifully later at New York University and Bennington. (The H'Doubler inspired teacher) wore costumes of chiffon and did little things on the order of Duncan, all "inspired", and here came Martha in a leotard and nothing else. [22]

Page's recollection portrays a stark image. Following her exposure to Graham, Martha Hill was on to something else in her teaching, something more dramatic and focused, akin to the early images of the modern dance that have entered the popular consciousness; dance that was streamlined, percussive, anxious to express, and art conscious. From 1927 to 1929 Hill continued to teach and develop her ideas on dance in education at the University of Oregon. The summer of 1928 was spent teaching at the University of Chicago. In 1929 Hill returned to New York to complete her B.S. at Teachers College. Back in New York, Hill renewed contact with Mary Josephine Shelly, an instructor of women's physical education at New College, a satellite curriculum of Teachers College. A fellow graduate of the Kellogg School, Shelly had known Martha Hill professionally for several years and had recommended Hill for the teaching positions at the University of Chicago, and the University of Oregon. [23] Soares (1997) writes:

[I]n 1929 she [Hill] returned to New York City anxious to enter the professional dance world. "These were exciting times. Thrilling....We were avid to learn anything in art....We went to concerts and galleries. I was designed by my experiences." She completed her undergraduate degree at Teachers College while rehearsing and performing with Martha Graham. She appeared on stage as Martha Todd, sensing that her 'white-gloved' professors disapproved of the wicked ways of the village artists with whom she conspired. [24]

Between 1929 and 1931, as Hill was finishing her undergraduate degree, Shelly was completing the Master's degree in physical education at Teachers College. Soares reports that at this time:

Hill and Shelly began co-authoring a book on dance theory. "At the time John Martin was defining modern dance. We thought it was terrible that he wanted to call it the modern dance. We wanted to write our own definition." The working title for their manuscript was *Sources and Characteristics of the New Dance.* [25]

In the winter of 1932, after meeting Bennington President Robert D. Leigh, Hill and Shelly came back to Leigh with a plan to hold a six-week summer workshop in the modern dance at the College. Leigh accepted their proposal and submitted it to the Bennington College Trustees. Following approval of the Trustees, plans were made to begin the project in the summer of 1934.

Hill and Shelly: Architects of "The Bennington Experience"

As the principal organizers of the Bennington Summer School of the Dance, Martha Hill and Mary Jo Shelly are central to this chapter in the story of dance and the American university. While Hill and Shelly may not have anticipated the effect Bennington would have on dance in higher education at the time they established their summer program, it was the "Bennington Experience" that was largely responsible for introducing professional dance artistry and standards into the university dance curriculum. Through Bennington the professional and academic worlds of dance intersected and reoriented the nature and focus of college dance from the liberally based model that had evolved under Gertrude Colby and Margaret H'Doubler, toward a more vocational and professionally focused one. With Graham, Horst, Humphrey, Weidman, Holm, and Martin, Martha Hill and Mary Jo Shelly revolutionized dance in higher education in terms of teaching, performance, technique, composition, production, pedagogy, and criticism.

During the summer months between 1934 and 1942, hundreds of dance educators and young professionals worked side by side with the modern dance artists and educators Hill chose to represent the field, in the studio, on the stage, and in the classroom. As a result of their exposure to the Bennington Experience, dance educators in America's universities began to ask important questions regarding the nature of their discipline: Was college instruction in dance about developing dance artists, which then would necessitate the inclusion of professional standards in the curriculum? Or was the promise of dance as a non-professional mode of self-expression and exploration? Could it possibly be both?

116

The first Bennington session promoted the following as a statement of mission and philosophy. According to Sorrell (1969):

> Under the auspices of a college which includes all the arts as an essential part of its curriculum, the Bennington School is designed to bring together leaders and students interested in an impartial analysis of the important trends in the dance. The modern dance, in connection with the other arts of this period, is a diversified rather than a single style. At the same time it possesses certain identifying characteristics which are common to all of its significant forms. The most advantageous plan of study is, therefore, one which reflects this diversification and, by affording comparisons, aims to reveal the essentials of modernism in the dance. The Bennington School presented contrasting approaches to technique and composition and, by giving a larger place to the related aspects of the dance, such as music, undertakes an integrated analysis of the whole structure of the art. Under this plan the student of the dance has access to the experience necessary to the formation of a well-rounded point of view. [26]

In the first sessions held at Bennington, 1934 - 1936, the majority of students were college dance educators from physical education departments who had come to expand their professional understanding and development. Dance historian Margaret Lloyd (1949) writes:

> Their [physical education students] training in the Normal Schools of physical education had included the theories of Delsarte and Dalcroze, modified ballet, folk forms, and the free, pre-modern interpretive dancing stemming from Isadora. That is, what was done in bare feet was interpretive, what in ballet shoes, aesthetic. They knew little of choreography, but did ready made dances such as "At Dawn," "The Brook," "To a Wild Rose," and endless Scarf Dances [the Colby model], until slowly through the twenties a new type of program developed, which offered the pupils opportunity to compose dances of mood and emotion for themselves [the H'Doubler model]. The dances were romantic, loose to form, and led to considerable rhythmized emoting around the campuses.
>   This was the background of the majority of physical education teachers, who taught dance along with field hockey and basketball, and other sports, exercises, and athletics of the full course, when they began to look into modern dance. They appropriated it as advanced calisthenics, as a logical successor to the interpretive dance, and because it was more assimiable and practicable for educative purposes than ballet, modified or classic. In the early days of modern dance infiltration in the colleges, the point of view was preponderantly that of evolved gymnastics, and choreography was mainly a combination of movement techniques with little or no imagination in the use of space, and without expression. But it was a time of ferment and change. [27]

Courses in teaching methods were an important part of the Bennington curriculum during the first two years of the program; 1934 and 1935. After 1936 classes in teaching methods were dropped. [28] The changing composition of the student body was one reason for the shift away from teaching at Bennington, after

1936 there was a greater mix of students, educators, and aspiring young professionals. Another reason courses in teaching methods were dropped was that it soon became clear to Hill and her colleagues that the college teachers who had come to study with the leaders of the modern dance movement were taking what they had learned back to their programs and using these methods and perspectives indiscriminately, and often inappropriately. Their attempt to infuse a garbled collection of ideas and methods into their own teaching was of serious concern to the Bennington faculty.

In his biography of Martha Graham, author Don McDonagh mentions the problem of whom Bennington was serving during the first years of the summer sessions:

> What no one among the organizing group quite realized at first was that the students, for the most part, were never going to be professional dancers. Only three or four years later did younger students come to Bennington in sufficient numbers, these then to be recruited for the various companies....Through them (the first students; college educators) and the others who came in subsequent years, modern dance was to enter college curriculums, through the gymnasium in most cases, and later through the performing arts departments. [29]

Sali Ann Kriegsman (1981) writes:

> The School of the Dance granted no degree (although credits could be applied toward a degree elsewhere) and offered no certificate or grades. Nonetheless because Bennington was the first coherent representation of the modern dance as a movement, it became something of a "Good Housekeeping Seal" for those who were affiliated with it; those who weren't were left out. Moreover Bennington and "the modern dance" had become synonymous, so that in a sense Bennington did promulgate a "method" or "approach" - that which was taught at Bennington. Given the school's concentrated authority and success and the geometric expansion of its influence through students, this was perhaps inevitable. Bennington's curriculum, its methods, and its approach to training and composition, were widely imitated.
> Technique was confined to the three major schools represented within the Bennington hierarchy - Graham, Humphrey-Weidman, and Holm - and to basic modern dance technique taught by Martha Hill and Bessie Schönberg, principally to teachers.
> The curriculum was designed not only to foster greater technical proficiency but to get students to pay more attention to form and structure in dance making. Louis Horst introduced notions of discipline and historical model. He insisted that to dance meaningfully one must first learn the craft of choreography. Horst's theories, based on musical form, and his teaching methods were powerful correctives to amorphous self expression. But soon, in lieu of the dances he disparagingly called "collegiate plastique," pale replicas of pre-classic and modern forms (course titles for Horst's approach to composition) began to crop up across the landscape. Simultaneously, the techniques of the Big Four [a name for the group: Graham, Humphrey-Weidman and Holm], absorbed

118

by students during a summer's intensive orientation, were taught in turn to their students. The modern dance was, for the first time, in double jeopardy of becoming academized through repetitious formulas and diluted through the well meaning (but not always accurate) efforts of students who came, saw, and returned to their classrooms to teach after the briefest of encounters with the Big Four.

Kriegsman concludes: "These problems were to become more serious as the interval between originators and disciples increased. Perhaps Bennington accelerated the process of dilution by precipitating a dispersion of the modern dance." [30]

The impact of professional standards on dance in the university might have been a passing issue of concern had not the success of the Bennington sessions also acted to stir up demand for visits by modern dance artists to college campuses. Upon returning to their programs educators who had their "eyes" opened at Bennington pressured their college administrators to bring modern dance to their campus. In the throws of the Great Depression, the possibility of college performing dates, and the accompanying stipends, was very attractive to Graham, Humphrey-Weidman, and Holm. By 1935 a modern dance-based touring schedule, the "Gymnasium Circuit," was beginning to take shape. It was labeled the Gymnasium Circuit because most activities were organized and conducted through college physical education programs, and dance performances more often than not were held in the college gymnasium. The circuit remained an important means for survival for modern dance companies well into the 1960's. In many cases the professional standards in technique and composition alluded to by dance educators returning from Bennington were reintroduced by the artists themselves during their visits. While the Gymnasium Circuit helped bring professionalism in dance to college programs across the country, and lent credence to the efforts of dance educators who had studied at Bennington, it also aggravated a growing perception by faculty in physical education that modern dance was suspect as source material for educational dance. In the opinion of the physical educators familiar with the dance pedagogy of Margaret H'Doubler, the modern dance was ugly, distorted, and possibly harmful to students who practiced its techniques.

119

The debate over the place of modern dance in the physical education program sparked by Bennington and the Gymnasium Circuit helped set the stage for the eventual shift of studies in dance from their traditional academic home in programs of physical education to alliance with programs in the fine and performing arts.

The legacy of Bennington for dance in higher education is multifaceted. One important aspect of this legacy is that the Bennington Experience empowered dance as arts education, shifting the nature of studies in dance from a recreational and liberal creative focus to a fine arts perspective. In this context modern dance placed emphasis on the individuals participation in, and contribution to, art-dance. Sequential training in topics that spanned the breadth of the curriculum was necessary to enable the student to generate and perform in contemporary dance at an advanced level. The modern focus for dance in the colleges was educational, but as an approach to dance in education it set a high standard for participation in its advanced study. This was attractive to dance educators who where looking for two things - a definition for dance that would distinguish their work from recreation and physical education, and an educational paradigm that would permit them to offer a comprehensive and sequential curriculum in dance as fine art.

The Bennington Experience: A Legacy for Dance in Higher Education

Bennington offered the first department model for dance in higher education - a place where different experts in the same field come together to teach a variety of topics within a single discipline. H'Doubler had identified the many aspects of higher learning in dance. Hill and Shelly sorted them out and assigned their instruction to specialists. Within the curricular model offered at Bennington, particular attention was paid to learning in the new techniques for dance performance as developed by the Big Four. Their training techniques were becoming more conceptually based and sequential in their instruction, leading toward a new formalism in developing the movement skills necessary for the practice of concert dance. Each artist was developing her or his own unique approach to training the body for dance. Doris Humphrey, who began to fully develop her teaching methods at Bennington, based her approach to technique on the notion that dance was essentially "the arc between two deaths," a metaphor for her belief that dance was the play between balance and movement away from balance. Over time Humphrey developed a series of training studies and exercises that led the student toward more complex neuromuscular patterning and a more professional level of dance technique. Yet Humphrey's work in this area remained largely an approach, and not a system for turning students into little versions of herself. There was considerable room for self-initiation and individual interpretation within Humphrey's technique. This aspect of Humphrey's work in technique connected it to the original rationale for dance in education as that had been articulated by Colby and H'Doubler: within the approach was latitude for individual learning, experience, and personal adaptation. [31]

Dance composition also took on a new formalism at Bennington. Under the guidance of Louis Horst, students were discouraged from making the dances that Horst had termed "collegiate plastique." Composition courses were crafted to introduce the student to ideas of form and the intelligent use of structural device. Horst examined compositional forms and devices found in music, the visual arts, and in dances he labeled "pre-classic" and "modern forms" to inspire the art of choreography. Horst is remembered as a harsh critic and task master. He was unrelenting in his drive toward making sure students understood and referenced basic forms and devices in dance making. Author Marcia Siegel (1987) writes:

> For years (following Bennington) there wasn't a modern dancer who did not know how to make an Air Primitive study, an ABA form, or a Pavane as a result of Horst's classes and their many successors in dance departments throughout the country. [32]

In *Louis Horst: Musician in Dancer's World* (1992), author Janet Soares quotes Alwin Nikolais, himself an internationally known figure in modern dance artistry and a Bennington student, as saying:

> Louis was the one that changed my life. It wasn't Martha. It wasn't Hanya. It was Louis....He trained my eye. I place him as one of the great enforcers of my career. It was success with Louis that made me decide to give up music and become a dancer. His

terseness appealed to me and his exactness.... You couldn't get away with anything. After you finished a dance, he'd say, "You know in the sixth measure on the fourth beat, you did this. Why?" he required precise aesthetic reasoning of you. [33]

Contributions to the legacy of Bennington also came from the artists themselves. During their summer residencies, Graham, Humphrey, Weidman, and Holm had the opportunity to choreograph some of the masterworks of 20th century concert dance. Humphrey's *New Dance*, Weidman's *Quest*, Graham's *Letter to the World*, and Holm's *Trend*, are just a few of the works created at Bennington that stand out as extraordinary examples of modern choreography. These and many other choreographies created at Bennington came to represent the 'literature" of dance and helped establish legitimacy for modern dance both as fine art and fine arts discipline.

Dance analysis and criticism, and dance history, were subjects developed by John Martin at Bennington. Martin had strong views on what principles constituted a modern approach to dance. By the time he joined the Bennington faculty Martin had published the first of his many books on modernism and dance. Martin thought that the best way to eliminate the possibility of modern dance collapsing into a set of rival art approaches was to offer study with all the "legitimate" artists simultaneously. This idea helped structure the way in which Bennington was organized during its sessions. The opportunity to study with the leading figures in dance at the same location called on the administrative and scheduling skills of Hill and Shelly. There was, and had been, a smoldering animosity among the modern dance artists who dominated the Bennington program. Stories of artistic and professional sabotage and backbiting color the school's anecdotal history. In some cases students found themselves caught between their loyalty to the artists and their own professional development as they sought exposure to each.

Besides classes in dance technique and composition, history and criticism, studies in music for dance and dance production were an important part of the Bennington curriculum. Music and accompaniment were taught by Ruth and

Norman Lloyd and Louis Horst. Dance production and design was brought to new levels of sophistication by Arch Lauterer. The breadth of study available to students at Bennington had a great effect on the subsequent development of dance curricula nationwide. In the years following Bennington, dance curricula slowly began to become more organized in comprehensive programs, and then into departments, outside and beyond its traditional placement in the curriculum of physical education. The trend toward separate, arts related dance departments began first in women's liberal arts colleges, especially those with a strong tradition in John Dewey's educational philosophies; Sarah Lawrence College 1935, and Adelphi College, 1938, in New York; Bennington in 1940; and Mills College of California, in 1941.

Ballet, as a dance art, also made positive inroads into the mainstream of the academic world at Bennington. In the early decades of the 20th century ballet was panned by many in the arts and in education to be sterile and lifeless. The rejection of ballet as a viable form of educational dance had its origins in the writings and teachings of Isadora Duncan. H'Doubler was also an adamant foe of use of the ballet as a means of dance education. In fact, all the early modern dancers were fairly unanimous in their opposition to ballet, as art and as educational medium. Hill and Shelly, however, invited recognized figures in the ballet, led by Lincoln Kirstein, to Bennington in 1937. [34] This was considered an important symbol of an end to the strict separation of dance arts that had been a matter of fact for many years. The study of ballet in higher education was facilitated by the inclusion of classical dance in the Bennington lecture and performance series.

The Bennington Experience ended on that campus in 1942. Martha Hill reinvigorated summer sessions in dance in 1948 with the organization of the Connecticut College Summer Dance Program. Hill, with assistance from faculty member Ruth Bloomer and President Rosemary Park, developed the summer sessions with Louis Horst, Martha Graham, Doris Humphrey and Humphrey's protégé, José Limón as faculty. The Summer Dance program at Connecticut was

123

quite successful and over time evolved into its present manifestation as the American Dance Festival. The American Dance Festival stayed at Connecticut until 1978 when the Festival moved to Duke University in Durham, North Carolina, where it continues today. [35]

The Federal Theatre Project: Works Progress Administration

The Federal Theatre Project of the Works Progress Administration was a product of Franklin Roosevelt's New Deal. The Project's contribution to public awareness about modern dance was important to the development of dance in the colleges. In America's major cities Federal Theatre Projects supported dancers and dance performances in the darkest hours of the Great Depression.

Economic relief for America's citizens in the first years of the Great Depression (1929 - 1931), was slow in coming and hard to access under the Herbert Hoover administration. Upon defeating Hoover in the Presidential election of 1932, Franklin Roosevelt proposed a range of federally sponsored programs to alleviate the people's suffering and hardship that were collectively labeled the "New Deal." A part of the legislation of the New Deal was the creation of the Works Progress Administration (WPA), a federal agency designed to help people get back to work. The WPA was created in part to manage public works and to provide improvements to the nation's infrastructure. In 1935 the WPA expanded its relief roles to include project employment for performing artists; creating a Federal Theatre Project. The Federal Theatre Project branched into a related Federal Dance Project in January of 1936. Between 1936 and 1939, the WPA's Federal Dance Project produced a number of small and large scale dance productions in New York, and in other urban centers like Philadelphia, Chicago, and San Francisco. Choreographers, performers, and other dance professionals were considered in one of four Dance Theater project categories: modern dance, ballet, vaudeville (entertainment in public institutions), and service (for educational projects). [36]

The Federal Dance Project was hastily put together and suffered greatly in its translation to real activity. From the start Project administrator's found themselves conflicted by their responsibility to "select." When one is faced with excruciating economic hardship, the idea of anything but the most fairly constructed selection process takes on a menace and threat that can be hard to transcend. Project administrators were quickly accused of conflicts in interest, graft, and artistic nepotism. Problems also surfaced in scheduling works and in managing the delivery of services to help mount productions. Regardless of the ups and downs of selection, scheduling, or timely assistance, the benefits of the WPA's Federal Theatre and Dance Projects were real: the larger Project itself represented the first time the federal government took an initiative in funding the arts and artists, the Dance Projects exposed thousands of citizens to dance for the first time, and helped generate new visions for dance outside the Bennington laboratory. The Federal Dance Project supported important new works of social relevance by Helen Tamiris, funded Katherine Dunham's explorations of African-Caribbean themes, and sponsored the work of American ballet choreographers like Ruth Page. Federal funding for the arts also stimulated organized advocacy for dance. One important group to emerge out of the New York project was the American Dance Association (ADA), which remained an active voice in American dance until 1941.

According to Heymann (1975):

The stimulus given to native cultural expression by the relief programs was of crucial importance to the arts in this country. American dance triumphed, no longer viewed as a shabby substitute for European ballet. It had proved able to celebrate American themes with a freshness and vitality lacking in the worn and decadent traditions of romantic dance. In this, the Dance Theatre shared with the other arts projects a new-found pride in the American heritage....Statistics support the fact that unprecedented numbers of Americans were able, for the first time, to see live performances of music, dance, and drama and to partake in free instruction in the arts. It promoted a general cultural enrichment of localities all across the country, and helped create a new concern for the fate of the artistic community. Many in congress were so impressed with the accomplishments...that they moved to establish a Bureau of Fine Arts in 1937 and 1938. Unfortunately, the political climate was too heated in those years for the controversial Coffee Bill, or any form of permanent federal sponsorship of the arts, to be legislated in Washington. [37]

Elizabeth Cooper, writes that the "heat" referred to by Heymann was fanned by two Republican Congressmen sitting on the newly created House Un-American Activities Committee; Martin Dies and J. Parnell Thomas:

> Dies claimed the "WPA was the greatest financial boon which ever came to the Communists in the United States," and that "Stalin could not have done better by his American friends and agents..." According to Thomas, the Federal Theatre Project was "infested with radicals from top to bottom...a hotbed for Communists...not only serving as a branch of the communistic organization but also one more link in the vast and unparalled New Deal propaganda machine." [38]

Although caught between culture and politics, a liberal New Deal and a growing fear of communism, government support for dance in the brief three year period of the Federal Dance Theater helped dance acquire a more refined and nuanced cultural and educational relevance. Funding for dance and dancers in performance, in service, and in research was helpful in expanding notions of what dance was, and what it could mean. The WPA's Federal Dance Theatre supported not only main stream choreographers, but also those who, for any number of reasons, had traditionally been marginalized. The work and creativity of dancers of African heritage were among these.

The Hampton Institute Creative Dance Group

Another college program in dance developed during the 1930's deserves attention, the Hampton Institute Creative Dance Group, located in Hampton, Virginia. Until federal legislation was passed in the 1960's, American education, reflecting the broader social context, involved issues of segregation. Barriers of race existed and were accepted in the arts, but it was also in the arts that barriers of race first began to erode and crumble. Some of the early modern dancers of European heritage like Helen Tamiris and Lester Horton were willing to confront racism. Tamiris deserves recognition for bringing issues and influences from African-American life and living into focus in her concert work of the 1920's and 1930's. Similarly, Horton's work with Native-American themes and with dancers of color, was groundbreaking in the 1930's and 1940's. But the fact remains that throughout the first half of the 20th century, separation of the races was common in American higher education. African-American students enrolled in traditionally "black" colleges for advanced learning. In *Black Dance in America: A History Through its People* (1990), author James Haskins discusses the importance of the Hampton Institute in bringing the African-American perspective to dance in higher education. Haskins also makes an important reference to Bennington as a place where one African-American dance educator refined his skills in dance:

> By the 1920's most if its [the Hampton Institute's] students were middle class, but because there were so few career opportunities open to blacks, Hampton, like other black schools emphasized practical training courses, especially teacher training, over liberal arts courses. By the middle 1920's students at Hampton and other black colleges were complaining that the schools should upgrade their curricula so that graduates could compete on an equal footing with white college graduates. The unrest led to student strikes on many black campuses, including Hampton.
>
> This unrest on the part of the students may have spurred Charles H. Williams, Director of Physical Education at Hampton to seek administration approval to form a creative dance group at the Institute. Williams was interested in movement, and especially in dance. He had read widely on the subject of dance, and believed that African and African-American dances were marvelous examples of pure bodily expression of emotion. He felt that the students would benefit greatly from a dance program, not only because it would help them with their physical coordination but also because it would give them a new pride in their heritage. With the help of Charlotte Moton Kennedy, an instructor of physical education at the Institute who was also interested in dance, he founded the Creative Dance Group for Hampton students....
>
> ...What made the programs of the Hampton Creative Dance Group so innovative was the choice of material presented. The programs covered the range of African-American dance, from the "Juba" and the "Cakewalk," to the "Buck and Wing," and popular dances of the day. But they also included African dances based on demonstrations by African students attending the Institute.
>
> Some of the more memorable were "Mamah Parah," which was danced on stilts, and "The Fangai Man," which was about magical customs....
>
> Charles Williams also choreographed dances that told the stories from black American history, like "Middle Passage," which dealt with the slave trade and included dance renditions of black spirituals and folklore.
>
> The Hampton Institute Creative Dance Group made its first appearance outside the Hampton campus in Richmond, Virginia, in 1935, and from then on it was in considerable demand locally. [39] Meanwhile, Williams began to spend portions of his summers developing his skills in choreography at Bennington College, a white girls school in Vermont, which sponsored an annual Bennington Festival of the Dance....
>
> ...Not only did the group bring to the public a wider appreciation of African and African-American dance as an art form - not merely an entertainment form - it also helped the image of the Hampton Institute....[T]here is no question that the Institute was proud of its dance group and eager to exploit its popularity for the benefit of the college. The Hampton group spawned similar groups at other black colleges, including Spellman in Atlanta, Fisk in Nashville, and Howard in Washington, D.C. [40]

Williams developed a successful dance program at the Hampton Institute. The Institute's touring company contributed toward breaking down popular notions of racial stereotyping. Besides acting as a model for other college programs, the Hampton Institute's Creative Dance Group was an inspiration for community based dance programs in America's urban centers. In an article appearing in *Dance Observer* in 1937, Williams writes:

> The two motivating influences in developing the interest [in modern dance] are, first: The recognition that the dance will always have an important place in the recreational life of young people; and, second, the existence in abundance of great native capacity among Negro youth. We believe at Hampton that if this capacity is developed in a way to make the students think creatively, it will have unlimited possibilities for inspiring and enriching life; and will aid in developing a feeling of pride and genuine appreciation for a great racial heritage....
>
> ...[T]he African Dances [as part of the Hampton Group's repertory], are designed to give something of the tribal life and customs of the native Africans and the great abandon with which they dance. The aim is to present these dances in a serious authentic form. Due to the fact that African students are members of the Creative Dance Group, it has been much easier for our regular students to grasp the genuine African spirit in which the dances are done from those who not only have seen them, but have taken part in them in their native land. [41]

In perspective, Williams remarks may be readily interpreted as addressed to a "white" audience. He is to be commended for educating and informing both "black" and "white" audiences about the substance and nature of African dance and its centrality in African culture. The Hampton Institute Creative Dance Group was an important catalyst for expanding the conception of what dance "was", in the academy and to the public.

CHAPTER 6

Discourse on Dance 1930 - 1940

The most important legacy of Bennington and its successor programs was the grafting of professional art standards with academic goals in the dance curriculum. A result of dance educators accepting the Bennington model for dance was an intense focusing of the discourse on academic alignment for dance with either physical education or the other fine arts. The idea that dance education was arts education, and that professional artists might be involved with teaching dance in higher education, was foreign and uncomfortable territory for many physical educators. Issues surrounding these matters were discussed and debated in professional journals such as *Health and Physical Education (HPE)*, and the *Journal of Health and Physical Education (JOHPE)*. A representative selection of these articles are reviewed and commented on in this chapter. Such topics were, however, not the exclusive venue of scholarly journals. The popular press had its own influence on matters of dance in the universities.

In February 1934, Louis Horst introduced *Dance Observer*, a journal for contemporary dance. From the start Horst's magazine took on the role of champion for the modern dance. In *Dance Observer* columns and articles, the events of the day were detailed and, to some extent, analyzed. Throughout the 1930's a column on dance programs in the schools and colleges was included, as were regular features on company activities, east and west coast seasons, government/political activities in the arts, individual biographies, individual programs like the Hampton Institute Creative Dance Group, and Bennington news. Featured columns usually listed activities, dates, places; who did what and what they planned to do in the future. Articles focused on practical matters such as music-dance relationships, or costuming, and reviewing concert work. However, in its first decade *Dance Observer* rarely engaged in any critical analysis of educational programs or policy. Criticism and commentary in *Dance Observer* was reserved for the politics, choreography, and performance of dance. The editorial focus on performance-related criticism, and the forthright nature of the promotion of modern dance, had its own impact on dance in higher education. *Dance Observer* became an important literary symbol of the dynamic new dance and it taught its readership to use a more refined language of dance. *Dance Observer* remained in print until Horst's death in January of 1964. [1]

John Martin had a regular feature for the *New York Times* titled *The Dance* and, on occasion, Martin would address a topic related to dance in education. Martin's more significant contribution to matters of education are found in his lectures to audiences at the New School and in books like *The Modern Dance* (1933), and *Introduction to the Dance*, written in 1939. An analysis of this latter text is included in this chapter. Walter Terry's 1940 article titled "Collegiate Dance" is also considered here. Terry was dance critic for the *New York Herald Tribune*. Finally, in looking at the tone and substance of the debate on professionalism in dance in higher education, I return to the writings of the woman who did so much to establish a place for aesthetic movement in the academy by including consideration of Margaret H'Doubler's 1940 text, *Dance: A Creative Art Experience.*

This representative sampling of articles, chapters, and texts illustrates the range and tone of the discussion on dance in higher education during the 1930's. It was of growing concern to scholars and educators in both fields to define the unique educational nature of dance or recognize common ground for dance and physical education. A closer look at the evolution of this debate contextualizes the issues surrounding dance in physical education during this period. The discussion acts as an important ground against which the subsequent development of dance in the American university in the 1950's may be viewed. For the emerging discipline of dance, the 1940's was a decade in education for the most part lost to the social, political, and military circumstances of World War II.

Ruth St. Denis

In 1932, Ruth St. Denis and William H. Bridge wrote an early position paper on dance in academia. Following the breakup of Denishawn in 1931, St. Denis attempted to reclaim a place in the professional and educational fields of dance through solo concerts, lecture-demonstrations, and by writing articles. In an article for the January 1932 issue of *JOHPE*, titled *The Dance in Physical Education*, St. Denis and Bridge argue that dance should not be equated with athletics or the utility of games because dance is "a method of human development superior to all other inventions." [2] Unlike art-dance, popular dance trends of the times ("toe," "tap," "soft-shoe," "jazz," etc.,"), athletics, and games did not stimulate the emotional or artistic sensibilities of the student nor did popular or athletic dance engage the expressive capabilities of the self through the instrument of the body. St. Denis and Bridge separate activity-based dance from what they felt was the more noble pursuit of educating through movement that is expressive and communicative; and that is found in art-dance.

Lucile Marsh

Lucile Marsh was a student of Gertrude's. Following her studies at Teachers College, Marsh went on to become a faculty member at Smith College. She co-authored an early text for dance, "The Dance in Education", with her sister Agnes in 1924. In October, 1932 Lucile addressed dance as a fine art in an paper titled *The New Dance Era* written for *JOHPE*. Her title is listed as "Director, the Dancer's Club New York City." In the introduction to her article Marsh writes:

> Today, the dance is accepted as a fine art on a par with music, painting, sculpture, and literature. Physical education teachers can feel proud that they have been most influential in bringing this most human of the arts back into life today. Beginning, as they did,

with folk dancing, then adding rhythmics, and finally organizing a whole dance program in the schools, physical educators built up a general acceptance of dancing that paved the way for the great modern movement that is now sweeping the country. But there is always danger that the pioneers of one generation may become the conservatives of the next. Physical educators must guard against just that. It would be tragic indeed if they were guilty of standing in the way of the future progress of dance, after they had done so much to bring it to its present eminence. We must all realize before it is too late that a new era of the dance is here and we must all qualify ourselves anew if we are to retain leadership in the field. [3]

Marsh's article encourages a flexibility and progressive thinking in teaching dance that many physical educators may have had a difficult time accepting. Certainly for most physical educators in 1932, the idea that dance was a fine art did not drive their thinking, nor did it shape their teaching. However, in this article Marsh opens with "Today the dance is accepted as a fine art...." Marsh warns the liberal pioneer against turning into the over-cautious conservative. She wants her reader to know that dance is a fine art, that physical educators are, at least in part, responsible for this and cautions her colleagues not to stand in the way of this development.

In developing her article, Marsh defends the idea that dance education, like education in the other fine arts, should go beyond attention to craft and its associated recreational stages, and toward education in dance as art expression. She follows this with an outline for a dance curriculum in primary and secondary education that is centered on "interpretive" dancing and the relation of dancing to other subjects in the curriculum. The use of the term "interpretive" in this context may have confused some of her readers; "interpretive dance" was generally used to describe the approach to dance that Colby's and H'Doubler's disciples were teaching. In the physical education parlance of the day, "interpretive" and "modern" dance were coming to be known as two very different things. Marsh's reference to dance and its relation to other subjects in the curriculum was a fairly progressive point of view for a dance educator writing in the early 1930's. Her perspective that dance is "a finer form of physical education because it is a fine art," [4] and that physical educators must master dance as an art and teach it as such, predicts and articulates a central, and thorny, point in the literature for dance education for the next 30 years.

Following the establishment of the Bennington School of the Dance in the summer of 1934, the subject of dance and its place in education shifts much more fully toward defining, understanding, and accepting the role of modern dance in education. The "modern movement sweeping the country" mentioned by Lucile Marsh, reached significance nationally as more dance educators and their colleagues attended the Bennington summer sessions. Gradually, the term "modern dance" replaces the more generic term "dance" in subsequent writings.

George Beiswanger

In April of 1936, George Beiswanger, Professor of Philosophy and Dean of Instruction at Monticello College, Godfrey, Illinois, presented a paper to the "Dance Section" of the American Physical Education Association at the St. Louis Convention. Titled, "Physical Education and the Emergence of the Modern Dance", (*JOHPE*, 1936), Beiswanger asks a set of questions about "modern" dance. First he defines the term "modern" as:

> [A] convenient tag. Every art is modern in its own day, *if it is alive* " [author's emphasis]. The author uses the term "modern" because it serves to remind one of the truth just stated, and also because there is at the present time no more satisfactory term.
> 5

Following his definition of modern art, Beiswanger asks:

> [I]s the modern dance an expression of the basic values and ideals of physical education, or is it fad, a passing reaction against older and more solid forms of dance? Are its physically demanding techniques fundamentally sound? Are they within the range of the average college and high school girl or do they strain the body beyond the precepts of a sane kinesiology? To what extent can the reaction of the average audience against the modern dance be discounted as a natural response to a new art form, destined in time to be changed into enthusiastic appreciation as the art becomes more familiar? What bonds of relationship are there between the aims of physical education and the purpose of the modern dance which justify the promissory note that the director of physical education gives when she engages an instructor to teach it and extends her cooperation and support?
> 6

After this introductory set of questions, Beiswanger states that modern dance:

> ...is the kind of dance which results when the goals of physical education are clarified and communicated on a conscious and artistic plane. The modern dance puts into art form the meanings and the philosophy of life for which physical education stands. It is physical education's own dance, its own art. [7]

In many respects, with this last comment, Beiswanger addresses and answers most of his own questions. Beiswanger's article is an insightful and intelligent defense of modern dance as the art expression in physical education. He looks at the transformation of physical education and dance from their common origins in romantic sensibilities of spontaneous, emotionally charged movement. Physical education and dance were first generated without an extended consideration of the educational goals of each, or the development of a scientific (or in the case of dance, what Beiswanger references as a 'mature') approach to technique, to a point where both are considered mature products - one in the field of education, the other in the field of art. Here we have a fine defense for the modern dance, or art-dance, as mature, art expression. Beiswanger's paper, as it was delivered to members of the Section on Dancing of the APEA (an organization that will be discussed in the next chapter), it seems clear from today's perspective, was an attempt to lend credence to an art approach to dance, and in doing so empower the dance educator in a department of physical education. This was an attempt to bridge what Beiswanger felt was a growing gap between dance and physical educators, exacerbated by misunderstanding, a lack of historical perspective, and perhaps through the phenomenon of Bennington. But through his articulate perspective on modern dance as a "free medium of art," and his erudite discussion of the merits of the modern dance, Beiswanger's article may have added weight to the scale of decision for dance educators as they considered the necessity of recognizing their discipline as something more than activity, as more than recreation, as more than "physical education."

Mary Josephine Shelly

Mary Jo Shelly, Administrative Director of the Bennington Summer School of the Dance, was also invited to address the "Section on Dancing" at the 1936 APEA Convention. Her paper titled "Art and Physical Education - An Educational Alliance", was published in *JOHPE* in October of that year. In this article Shelly looks "...over the fence at the area of art education, which appears to lie no more than a stone's throw away from our own area of physical education." [8]

Shelly was an insightful and politically astute writer and thinker. As both an important member of the APEA and co-founder of Bennington, she was in a unique position to comment on the growing friction between physical education and art-dance as they sought to share common ground, common space, and common resources in education. In her paper Shelly points out that while the dramatic growth of modern dance as a part of physical education has "provoked the greatest agitation since the merits of formal gymnastics split the ranks of the profession," [9] the real issues for dance and physical education to consider come not from their apparent differences, but from their inherent similarity and from outside the field. Addressing the latter issue Shelly writes:

> On the side of common adversity, that point of view toward life and learning which regards play as non-essential may be depended on to see art in the same light. In this view the school theater and school gymnasium are manifestations of the same frivolous generosity, and it requires an equal tolerance to spend the tax payers money on paints and music or on hockey sticks and baseball....[W]e in physical education and our contemporaries in art must in all common sense range ourselves on the same side. It therefore behooves us to find and strengthen any reasonable alliance between us. [10]

To make the case internally, as these branches of the field relate one to the other, Shelly argues that dance as art, and physical education as play, both spring from a human urge to give outward form to internal impulse. While play and art may find different expressions in the urge to give form to each, their tangent has a common origin, and it is this that Shelly thinks members in both fields should remember.

Shelly's argument has great merit, in its unfolding and clarity, and in its synthesis and application to issues in art and physical education. But it also implicitly reminds us that there is in fact "a fence," and that while art and play may spring from a common urge, it is how the urge is manifested, the form taken, that counts. Asking an audience of dance educators to "look over the fence" from physical to art education isn't too much of a stretch, that is really where most of them would like to "go." But asking physical educators to do the same is another story entirely. By this point in time, as a field, physical education was ever more closely aligned with athletics and sport. The practical was superseding the aesthetic in value and orientation; bases were made, balls were hit, points were accumulated; and for the physical educator, measurement was all. The practitioners of physical education were those who were (and are) attracted to utilitarian aspects of movement. The practitioners of dance were those who were attracted to movement's aesthetic, expressive potential. While Shelly's call for those involved in the arts and sciences of human movement to look at the big picture is laudable, it was doomed by the momentum in both movement art and movement science that was accumulating at that time. In retrospect, we must view Shelly as the exception to the rule, as one who could clearly see the art of play and the play in art. Shelly's is a liberal perspective, grounded in interdisciplinarity. At this time however, forces in the university, and in the professions, were steadily moving disciplines toward increased academic specificity. The result in the case of dance and physical education was that the arts of movement as expressed through movement invention and aesthetic inquiry gravitated toward other arts disciplines, while the science of movement, as expressed through the understanding of biological systems and the practice of sport, settled ever more comfortably on its own side of the fence.

Ruth Murray

Ruth Murray, a dance educator in the Department of Physical Education for Women at Wayne University in Detroit, Michigan, and an important early organizer of the "Dancing Section," added her perspective to the growing controversy between dance and physical education in an article titled "The Dance in Physical Education" written for *JOHPE* in January of 1937. [11] Addressing the concerns of her more conservative colleagues, Murray states:

> In the field of physical education, at the present time, there exists no area of activity which has excited as much confusion as that of dance. It is comparable to that historic period in our educational development when certain courageous, far seeing souls proposed a program of natural activities to replace the systems of formal gymnastics that were in place everywhere. We looked upon these people with suspicion and ridicule. Children were dangerous when they were allowed to get out of a line or circle....That is ancient history now. But another formidable foe of tradition, a disturber of complacency, is looming on our horizon. We view it with questioning and alarm. What is this new dance? What is it doing in physical education? [12]

Following this introduction, Murray reviews the basic canon of dance history in western culture as that was commonly cited in the 1930's. Dance is the most ancient of arts and the Catholic Church's attitude toward the body caused dance to be condemned as an invention of the devil during the Middle Ages. Folk dance forms evolved into highly structured court dances and court dances led to the rise of the ballet. The essentially static nature of ballet and its 19th century trappings were the reason for ballet's lack of innovation in the 20th century. This history ends with Duncan's contribution to "the modern school." Murray feels Duncan was misinterpreted by many dance educators with the result that art-dance was commonly perceived as a "silly, devitalized, and pseudo-artistic pursuit no red-blooded person could possibly enjoy." [13] Following this overview, meant to contextualize the rest of her paper for the reader, Murray defines "modern dance" as a term used to equate developments in dance with changes in other art forms in the 20th century. Here, the important theme of her article is fully articulated: that modern dance is art-dance. Art-dance, according to Murray, is concerned with forms, with demanding techniques, with contributions to human expression; art-dance stands alone and is not dependent on other art forms for support.

After making this point Murray returns to the historical record and looks at the development of dance in American education. She outlines this brief history commenting that dance found its first manifestation in education through folk forms and that the practice of folk dances "became the beginning and end of the dance program." [14] Murray comments that folk dances were laundered in education, coming out of the wash as limp, devitalized, "pretty, graceful little affairs." Soon, tap dance followed as the preferred form of dance instruction in public education, due to popular demand, with folk dance gradually replaced by tap and contemporary social dancing.

Returning to the developing sense of educational dance as art-dance, Murray outlines what she feels are the important areas in dance education that may emerge out of the influence of modern dance. Murray melds ideas previously articulated by H'Doubler with perspectives emerging out of Bennington. In Murray's opinion, a new approach to teaching dance as an art demands consideration of rhythmic fundamentals (learning and responding to the relation between movement and accompaniment, analysis of rhythms, tempos, dynamics, and accents); movement fundamentals (experience in the fundamental movements of locomotion, understanding concepts like direction, level, shape and intent); dance composition (the crafting of movement into conscious form, following ideas for art generation and working with structural devices), and exposure to practice and performance of formal dances, where the student ties all her previous experiences into the act of "doing" the dance; but now she "does" the dance with knowledge and personal understanding.

Murray's article sets another stone in the bridge that dance educators were building toward the idea of dance education as art education. While the article is titled "The Dance in Physical Education" in retrospect it may have been more aptly titled "The Dance in Art Education" because Murray outlines an approach to teaching art-dance.

Eugene C. Howe

Eugene C. Howe, Professor in the Department of Hygiene and Physical Education at Wellesley College, wades into the debate in "What Business Has Modern Dance in Physical Education?" written for *JOHPE* in 1937. Here, Howe discusses the error in the common assumption of the day that there is a natural or mutually beneficial relationship between modern dance and physical education. [15] Howe states that the idea of dance as art first found its way into the curriculum through the door opened by Margaret H'Doubler when she argued for inclusion of dance as a creative art expression for educational purposes. Howe goes on to say that modern art dance found its application in physical education programs through the activities of educators influenced by their experiences at Bennington. Howe's point is that the conflict bred by injecting art standards into physical education programs was creating situations where faculties became divided and students ultimately were not being served.

An interesting aspect of Howe's article is his strong rejection of ballet (and by rejecting ballet he surreptitiously presents an implied case for rejecting modern dance) as a dance form of merit or of worth in education:

> The dance in physical education has always followed the dance of the stage. From the point of view of physical education there are two questions regarding this relationship which need clarification: first, the conditions under which teachers of the dance in education achieve their training; second, the justification of any given phase of the dance as part of physical education....
> ...With regard to the dark ages of modified ballet in the schools we can agree that the first question has become a dead issue. As to the second also, there now appears to have been no reason why the various ballet entertainment troupes which have toured the country from time to time should have ever strengthened the position of the dance as a form of art vital to us or as a part of physical education in the schools and colleges....Its growth has been that of a crystal; beautiful after a fashion, sharp edged, smooth-faceted, and self limited. Nothing in its origins, its artifices, its snobbery, and its ballet-hoo allies it with democratic education, and the numerous reasons for its unsuitability as a part of physical training are too well known to need enumeration. In education it remains only in a few finishing schools as an "extra" on a par with American French and drawing. [16]

Following this onslaught on the ballet, "American French, and drawing," Howe returns to the subject of modern dance. He comments on the work of Margaret H'Doubler in training many of the dance educators who were, as a result of H'Doubler's vision, " prepared to integrate it [dance] with other aspects of physical training, physical education, and education as a whole." Interestingly, Howe comments on the "unauthorized bathos" into which the H'Doubler inspired work sometimes fell.

Howe then turns his attention to Bennington and identifies it as the source of the:

> ....[R]ecent adoption by the profession of the leading concert dancers, critics, and counselors as *professors extraordinaire* ....The dance of the 1920's in physical education, though the seed came from the work of the art, grew up in and for physical education; the dance of the '30's in physical education is for and by the concert artists in that he now virtually heads up the activity in a field foreign to his primary interests and about the nature of whose objectives he may, quite naturally and justifiably, be assumed to have no detailed and comprehensive understanding. The situation obviously has possibilities for both good and ill. In the opinion of the writer, the former far outweighs the latter. But it is a situation that calls for comment and the most surprising thing about it is that little from the point of view of physical education has as yet appeared. [17]

Howe's perspective is clearly that of the physical educator and he may be commended on his ability to think "out of the box" when he writes that "Intuition whispers that it [dance] is as ill at home as an etching in a machine shop" in questioning the place of art dance in a physical education program. To relieve this situation Howe asks that his fellow physical educators submit to "some enlightenment and make certain compromises." Howe admits that he and others in physical education have an "increasing delight in quantity as compared to quality, in records as compared with the perfection of movement." [18] Here he identifies the struggle in physical education as it met dance: the desire to be objective while playing host to subjectivity. Like Shelly, Howe recognizes the similarities that exist between the art of play and the play in art, but he also recognizes the different nature of art and play as they are brought to action.

While Howe acknowledges the error of physical education's pursuit of the measurable, he does not take this to task to the degree he does of art-dance as it continues down a path in pursuit of professional standards. We are left to ask, aren't these manifestations of the same desire, the desire to bring any endeavor toward some identifiable end? In the case of physical education an identifiable end was increasingly wrapped up in the demonstration of sport, in dance it was wrapped up in the demonstration of technically challenging, creative movement invention. How different are these desires? Is one more educationally viable than the other?

Howe concludes his article by articulating a concern of physical educator's that dance educators have never really fully addressed: if the dance teacher's interests are in the end result of dance performance, don't they have an obligation in an educational environment to carefully consider (scientifically investigate) the implications their methods of training have on bodies as they push students towards a professional level of skill? This is a constructive criticism that still has merit, particularly in modern dance techniques. In Howe's view, art-dance loses its place in physical education when it neglects to recognize its commitment to understanding its essential nature as physical endeavor. [19]

Mary Josephine Shelly

The last of the scholarly articles considered here is another written by Mary Jo Shelly and delivered as a paper at the APEA Convention in San Francisco, in April of 1939. Shelly's paper was later published under the title "Facts and Fancies About the Dance in Education" in the journal *Health and Physical Education,* in January of 1940. Here, Shelly reports on a study undertaken by the Bennington staff to assess the present status of studies in modern dance in higher education. Shelly writes:

> Concerning the dance in colleges and universities, the study yields a wealth of information...[T]hese facts come from over three hundred institutions and an equal number of individual teachers representing a complete cross section of types, locations and sizes of public and private colleges and universities. [20]

The statistics cited show that in 1939 most colleges offered some courses in dance and approximately two thirds of the courses were in modern dance. In 98% of all cases dance was offered through physical education. A few institutions offered a dance major and a moderate demand for a separate major existed in "a considerably larger number." Approximately 27,000 women and 300 men students were enrolled in dance classes. Only 78 of 300 institutions polled made dance classes available to men. Shelly notes that dance clubs on college campuses served dance in the same manner that intramural athletics served women's sport.

Most dance clubs in this sample were organized through Women's Intramural Athletics programs which limited male participation in dance studies.

When asked if dance educators felt there was adequate undergraduate preparation for teaching in dance, the response was overwhelmingly negative. Shelly concludes her remarks on the results of the survey by stating, "the present, and so far as one can see ahead, the future fate of dance in education rests in the hands of physical education." [21]

After reviewing the data in her article Shelly rhetorically asks, "where do we go from here?" She recognizes the debate on the issue of dance in physical education that had unfolded over the previous decade, and paraphrases the common sentiment among physical educators with a dislike for modern dance:

> ...[M]odern dance, which seems to be assuming more importance than any other kind of dancing, is ugly, morbid, and unchildlike. Look at the professional dancers, what do they know about education? And again, is the modern dance not a lop-sided development in physical education because only the women are interested in it? [22]

Shelly answers these questions from the perspective of one who has experienced her singular position as physical educator and administrator of the most successful symbol of the dynamic of modern art-dance. In Shelly's response to the questions posed the reader detects a tiredness and frustration with the sameness of the complaint, the lack of evolution in thinking, and the lack of resolution. As it reads today, we sense the challenge the field of dance faced in the days leading up to World War II. The future of dance rested in the hands of colleagues who didn't particularly like what modern dance was about and who were struggling for academic recognition for their own perspective in athletics and sport, for measurement for bases made and balls hit. What were they to do about an art located in a corner of their gymnasiums that seemed to confront all their conservative sensibilities, that refused to be pinned down long enough to be measured, and that expressed the feminine in a world in love with the masculine?

John Martin

In his text, *Introduction to the Dance*, John Martin includes a chapter on "Dance in Education." After citing the benefits of dance in the curriculum in light of its merits as part of a progressive education, Martin raises the question of dance as art or exercise rhetorically asking; "Is it exercise, then, or art?... If it is exercise, what is it doing with emotion? If it is art, what is it doing in the gymnasium?" [23] Martin asks these questions and then proceeds to answer by saying; "...it is both these things and at the same time neither of them." [24] He then presents a progressive, liberal justification for considering dance as both exercise and art, and for teaching it in both contexts. In the dance education program, Martin considers the dual nature of dance a part of its attractiveness in education.

Following this part of his chapter, Martin turns to a discussion on the growing influence of professionalism in college dance. While Martin was no apologist for the inclusion of dance in physical education programs, he does write:

> In the meantime that [in the physical education program] is where dance has found itself placed, and there is no reason to disturb it until it can ultimately be made an independent activity around which education in general centers. There is however, every reason to advocate its better treatment. There can be no doubt that the majority of physical educators are unqualified to teach it!... [25]

Regarding this latter phenomenon, Martin blames the physical educators reticence on the fact that dance has become patterned on 'the systems of the professional dancers":

> This is a perfectly natural thing to do, to be sure, for in a subject so comparatively new as the expressional dance, with no tradition whatever within the field of education itself, where is one to turn to for guidance except those few artists who best exemplify its principles? The mistake lies not in the sources that have been turned to but in the application of what has been found there to the purposes of education. It is a common experience to find classes of youngsters being taught exercises taken directly from the studio of some celebrated concert dancer, or perhaps even several sets of exercises from several different studios. [26]

Martin's point is sound: a substantial part of the problem of perception by physical educators was based on the dance educators imitation of the professional and lack of educationally sound, scientifically studied, movement experiences in dance. The blatant imitation of concert dancers irritated the physical educators as much as did the professional artists presence in the gymnasium. That the dance educators were so ready to imitate was coming from within their field, not from outside. Blaming physical educators for not "understanding" dance or for not "treating it better" could, in part, be laid at the doorstep of a thoughtless imitation. Martin suggests that the relationship between the professional dancers and the educator be reversed; that the professional come to the educator to learn to teach. "But such a result is not likely to be even within the bounds of possibility until the educator quits going to the professional dancer for routines." [27]

In retrospect, Martin's writing on the issues peculiar to dance education in *Introduction to the Dance* is pretty much on the mark - dance will remain a part of its parent discipline until it establishes its own educational center. Dance educators had to build their own educational foundation. They had to stop blaming physical educators for not understanding them and stop imitating their glamorous cousins in the professional world.

Margaret H'Doubler

The success of Bennington's influence, and the subsequent turn of some dance educators toward professional attitudes and standards in college programs was not lost on Margaret H'Doubler. H'Doubler viewed an encroaching professionalism with concern. The consummate educator, H'Doubler responded to change in the field in her third, and perhaps most widely referenced tract, *Dance: A Creative Art Experience* published by the University of Wisconsin Press in 1940.

H'Doubler's preface to this volume clearly raises her concerns and situates her perspective on the substance, value, and future for dance education and the dance educator:

> In essence, *Dance: A Creative Art Experience* is a discussion of the basic aspects and enduring qualities of dance, which are within the reach of everyone. Its main purpose is to set forth a theory and philosophy that will help us to see dance scientifically as well as

artistically....[I]t parallels certain phases of my earlier book, *Dance and Its Place in Education*....[M]aterial from the earlier book has been included here in an expanded form. But the purposes of the two are different.

...[T]his book is designed to show that dance is available to all if they desire it and that it is an activity in which some degree of enjoyment and aesthetic satisfaction for all may be found. If we can think, feel, and move, we can dance. In presenting dance from this point of view I have made an attempt to show its nature and conditions. From a knowledge of these conditions the reader may evaluate for himself the trends in contemporary dance; he may distinguish according to his own understanding between those phases that are evanescent and those that are lasting.

If dance is to be brought into universal use, if it is to help in the development of a more general appreciation of human art values, it must be considered educationally. The future of dance as a democratic art activity rests with our educational system. Not everyone can avail himself of studio training, and even those who can afford such training will find that few studios are interested in this aspect of dance. One of the ways dance can reach everyone is through the schools. If every child in every school from his entrance until his graduation from high school or college were given the opportunity to experience dance as a creative art, and if his dancing kept pace with his developing physical, mental, and spiritual needs, the enrichment of his adult life might reach beyond any results we can now contemplate.

Dance considered from this standpoint can be of great social value, but to achieve these results we must bring it within the reach of the laity. It must be a vitalizing experience to them. Dance's power of civilization has always been felt whenever it has been experienced as a control over life in giving artistic form to its expression. Only when dance is communally conceived can it exert a cultural influence.

...[A]s a growing and struggling art, dance needs above all the philosopher-scientist-artist, and in turn he needs a sympathetic public informed on the value and meaning of art. [28]

H'Doubler's comments are clearly aimed at proposing a compromise to the issue many of her colleagues were dealing with throughout the 1930's. Like Martin, H'Doubler's perspective supports a need for education *between* activity influenced physical education and professionally influenced art-dance. The philosopher-scientist-artist must instill in students a life-long interest in the creative, expressive body. H'Doubler clearly qualifies the dance educator as the "philosopher-scientist-artist." In this sequence the educator's grounded perspective (philosophy), is of foremost importance followed by understanding a rigorous conceptual framework (science), and then by creative vision and interest (art). *Dance: A Creative Art Experience* goes on to develop H'Doubler's argument in subsequent chapters.

In *Dance: A Creative Art Experience*, not only does H'Doubler cover territory she addressed earlier in *Dance and Its Place in Education* , making the case for her centrist educational philosophy and approach, she also reaches toward the art side of the issue by presenting her practical theories on the subject of training the dance artist. Here we have H'Doubler's opinions on developing the student's "technique"; the pursuit of physical expressiveness and virtuosity, and composition; rules for using dance as a medium for art expression. One of the more important points H'Doubler makes is a call for attention to the intellectual-physical relationships that must be recognized and activated in developing the motor and creative skills necessary to art express through dance. H'Doubler's idea of the "knowing subject and the object known," in retrospect, is uniquely her own. It seems to have challenged, and in turn been confronted by, both generally accepted notions of dance, and the foibles of human nature.

H'Doubler asks her readers - educators, students, and public alike - to intellectualize dance in a scientific manner. While the work and product of the modern dancers who, for the lack of a better term, had come to represent H'Doubler's "pedagogical competition," was conceptually inspired, they were not inclined toward scientifically deconstructing the expressive act, nor the expressive body. For instance, consider the work of Doris Humphrey. Humphrey settled on the idea of exploring the dynamic of movement as this was reflected in the individual's struggle with gravity and balance. Establishing and moving away from balance was metaphorically referenced by Humphrey as "the arc between two deaths." Humphrey established this point of view and explored its ramifications in designing technical exercises and choreographic statements, but did not seek to establish empirical, scientific truths about the neuro-physiological apparatus necessary to achieve and perceive balance, nor did she go to great lengths to understand the relationship between the rhythm of movements and balance. Had H'Doubler used the same metaphor as an educational reference for dance her inclination would have been to analyze the phenomenon of balance scientifically and then use her understandings to begin to work creatively. Such an approach demands a consistent discipline of mind and conceptual creativity in designing an individual approach toward using such information educationally.

However, and perhaps unfortunately, most dance educators were not as intellectually disciplined or as scientifically curious as H'Doubler. H'Doubler was altruistic in her expectations that others were of like mind, or even similarly adept at philosophically contextualizing and scientifically deconstructing the corporeal-creative act. And, as a result of her interest in approaching dance education in this manner, H'Doubler's writing had become "thick" with nuance and implication. Extraction of H'Doubler's meaning and implication for the ideas presented in *Dance: A Creative Art Experience* demands a rigorous intellectual focus and patience from her reader. There is a metaphysical quality to this work. H'Doubler's attempt at range, density, and depth demands constant attention and interpretation. But, H'Doubler was not always successful in communicating the substance of her thinking in a clear manner. Consider, for instance, the following short passage on "technique':

> Although the will is of importance in the expressive act, it can never be a substitute for the impulse for expression. The will is ever present, but blended with the intellectual, emotional, and spiritual actions in a perfect unity. This blend of mental forces results in a kind of super intelligence that knows the effect before it starts the cause. This co-operation with the other mental faculties is one of the secrets of success. The will can control and guide, but never can supply the impulse to expression except as it serves mental concentration. In this capacity it holds the mind to the idea in hand, directing and restraining impulses until they become diffused through the whole organism. It collects a scatterbrain and makes an artist of the artisan. [29]

What is H'Doubler saying here? She is talking about the disciplined use of "will" in support of educational-artistic growth. While "will" cannot replace inspiration in developing a more sophisticated and nuanced artist - one cannot will an impulse toward expression, intellectually forcing inspiration - when will is at ease with that which inspires it(i.e. the emotions, the spirit) then will, coupled with inspiration, and in harmony with critical awareness leads toward a sort of prescient reversal in the traditional concept of the linear 'cause and effect' continuum in thought and creation. The super-intellect, represented by a marshaled will and inspiration rises above the plodding wondering of "what might happen if I do this" to anticipate effect. The use of will as a sort of supervisor for a sustained-conscious-intellectually managed-inspiration "collects the scatterbrain and makes an artist of the artisan." Yet this understanding is not immediately apparent in H'Doubler's passage. One has to think and use "will" to focus understanding in reading her writings. Unfortunately dancers in this culture have suffered, and yet fancied themselves; resisted, and yet often bought into the notion of being "scatterbrained." Dancers have sometimes cast themselves in this light: inspired, yet intuitive; savants of the body, in touch with what is felt, resistant to intellectualizing the responsive body through "over analysis." Resistance to analysis is not without practical merit in the experience of dancers, athletes, and others desiring control of the body. Any teacher of physical activity will tell you; think too much *in action* and you'll get in your own way. This maxim takes effect at different points for different students. Some are able to simultaneously think and 'do,' while others start to think or analyze and motor skill is impaired. An unfortunate result of a caution with analyzing while in motion may be a spill over effect of caution into other realms of a considered practice in dance-art making. Thus, a cultural reluctance among dancers (and many dance educators), to readily engage in theorizing, a certain anti-intellectualism, has traditionally shaped the thinking of many in the field.

And so, while H'Doubler's treatise was considered an important text for those who would champion dance in the academy, its diffusement into the "trenches" occupied by the majority of faculty and students, and its substantial application in the field was limited. Because *Dance: A Creative Art Experience* is so analytic, and its application demands a longitudinal discipline of mind, its substance wasn't easy to access. H'Doubler's writing makes for difficult reading, and because H'Doubler remains the liberalist and never establishes a style; everything remains conceptually referenced and beyond the imprint of individual taste. Culling meaning and reference from H'Doubler's text necessitates the individual reader's personal investment in understanding, contextualizing, and activating what H'Doubler is saying. The reader has to personally engage the text's message through individualized commitment. H'Doubler does not 'tell'

148

anyone how to 'do' anything; only what must be considered. To a population used to being told what to do and how to do it, and fearing an intellectual approach to their dancing, the message of H'Doubler's text was, for the most part, lost to a wide audience. H'Doubler's writing has a certain tautological nature that causes its message and substance to flatten out and become circuitous, repetitive, and numbing; sometimes incomprehensible. Yet, strewn among the amorphous, ethereal wanderings, and pseudo-philosophical justifications, are adages that attest to her great revelations as an educator:

Man fashions as he knows.

Technique transforms experience into the form of its expression.

We are our own laboratory, textbook, and teacher.

Science certainly cannot make art, but it can contribute to a truthful art. [30]

Even though the substance of H'Doubler's message may not have been widely and regularly referenced, H'Doubler's contribution to the literature through *Dance: A Creative Art Experience* was reaffirming and important at this time. Dance in higher education was still the province of women's physical education and H'Doubler's conceptual "voice" was a welcome addition to the troubling trends and discourse of the decade, as perceived by the wary physical educators familiar with her message and critical of a 'carte blanche' acceptance of modern dance in their programs.

Walter Terry

The last article considered in this chapter is one written by an important dance advocate and concert critic of the day; Walter Terry. *I Was There*, is a compilation of articles and editorials authored by Terry during his professional career as dance critic for the *Boston Herald* (1936 - 1939); *New York Herald Tribune* (1939 - 1967); and the *Saturday Review* (1967 - 1976). Terry would sometimes take a look at the variety of issues for dance in and outside the

149

academy. He addresses matters related to dance in higher education in *Collegiate Dance*, an article published for the *New York Herald Tribune* on June 9, 1940. Here, Terry critiques the (then) current state of dance in American higher education. This article provides us with a sense of what the tone of discourse on dance was outside of the university at the beginning of the new decade, and after the impression of Bennington had been firmly felt.

Terry's article is an interesting place to end this chapter because, unlike the academics commenting on the growing rift between dance and physical education, Terry isn't quite as politic in his message, shooting "straight from the hip," and not pretending to disguise his bias. In doing so he illustrates the intellectual, even emotional, gap that existed between academic advocates for dance and those who were either unimpressed with dance, or were at odds with its independent, and (they may have felt), often self-aggrandizing nature. Those who counted themselves among dance's champions, of whom Terry is certainly one, framed its study and practice as a foundation for healthy living, a positive "mold" for character development, and as a conduit to a better humanity and even a higher consciousness:

Collegiate Dance
June 9, 1940.
You'll find the word dance in the catalogues of almost every major American college. And what does that word suggest to you? One person will summon memories of the exquisite and unreal Pavlowa, another will think of the strong and sometimes ferocious qualities of the modern dance, some will remember the exotic motions of an Oriental St. Denis or the unhampered sensuousness of a Duncan, others will find that the joyous physical gusto of the folk dance comes to mind. There are, also, a great many people who assume that "dance" means social dancing or, on a plane of great skill, tap.
The diversity of approach is reflected in the collegiate dance to such a degree that a plea for recognized standards of dance education would probably be tossed aside as the ravings of a dance faddist. During the last few years I have frequently discussed the evils which mark the educational dance, pointing out that one college grudgingly offers the dance because of student demand, another because it is a good substitute for calisthenics and still another (and this rarely) because its directors recognize the power of the dance as a molder of character as well as a valid mode for artistic, physical and emotional expression. [31]

Following this introduction, Terry outlines the results of a survey of "120 American colleges and universities asking a few simple and direct questions about dance courses offered in each of the institutions." [32] In his survey Terry asks 5 questions and provides a place to add additional comments. Paraphrased, they are:

1. Is the dance a credit course?

2. What techniques are offered?

3. Are classes offered in Physical Education, Drama, or in a dance department?

4. Is dance offered because its directors believe in its benefits, student demand, or a combination of both?

5. What do you believe are the benefits of dance training? Is it focused toward preparation for a professional career? Physical development? Better health? Cultural growth? Do you believe dance molds character?

6. Additional comments.

Terry's survey is a thinly disguised attempt to prove what he suspects is wrong, yet true, about how dance education is viewed by many academics. "Statistics may be dull, so I shall make mine as brief as possible...Only half the letters were answered, and it is natural to assume that silence meant the lack of any dance courses."

Of respondents:

Fifty three colleges offered the modern dance, forty seven colleges gave folk dancing, thirty four colleges presented ballroom, thirty two taught tap, three presented Denishawn, two offered ballet, two gave Dalcroze Eurythmics, five taught clog and several offered courses entitled "basic rhythms." All these courses overlapped, with some institutions presenting several techniques while others presented only one.

In fifty seven of the colleges the dance came under the direction of the department of physical education, at Colorado College it was directed by the music department and at Adelphi College it boasted its own department. Benefits resulting from dance training were extremely varied. Physical development, health, cultural growth, recreation, dance appreciation and character molding all had their adherents. Some institutions stated that calisthenics could take care of physical development and health, and that cultural growth was the goal of dance. Others snapped their professional fingers at culture and upheld the recreation aspect.

Here are a few of the examples of diversities of opinion, not healthy variances, but completely opposed dance viewpoints. Mabel Lee, director of dance at the University

151

of Nebraska, says: "I certainly would not say that the dance molds character. That is absurd. Just as absurd as to say that football molds character." Lehigh University finds that the dance fosters "facility in the amenities of social intercourse." Only ballroom is available there, of course. But at Connecticut College for Women Elizabeth Hartshorn, dance director, finds that the contemporary dance stimulates desire for activity, integrates the body and the mind, leads to appreciation and acquisition of beauty in human movement, increases sensitivity to environment, develops interest in the other arts as well as the dance, develops poise and self assurance and accuracy.... [33]

With regard to the comments attributed to Hartshorn, when read today, had Terry added "...and does not promote tooth decay," to the list of the benefits of dance Hartshorn suggests, her reported response to the question of the benefits of dance would have taken on a bit of the 'tongue in cheek' a skeptic may feel such claims merit. The bias here is unmistakable, and its tone was not an uncommon trait in newspaper accounts of the time. However, the strident advocate's role in support of 'cause' is not as common in today's journalism: "increases sensitivity to environment,... develops poise and self assurance and accuracy?" One is left to wonder exactly what these phrases mean. The tendency to couch the benefits of dance in glowing and universal terms is not uncommon among dance's advocates. Such praise may, however, speak differently to skeptics and suggest a discipline unsure of its real value in education. We may suspect that the student benefits from study in dance to the degree suggested, but what proof have we, then or now? Regardless, Terry's comments and tone encapsulate the subtext and general tenor of discourse between two camps circa 1940: "either for dance or against dance, 'and ne'er the twain shall meet.' "

Interestingly, Terry mentions professional preparation as a outcome of dance education-training. Overt attention to that idea, while in some circumstances attended to, was still years away from large scale acceptance and was not yet central to the mission of most dance programs in 1940. He may have recognized an implicit new goal of dance education at that time, especially the kind of program that followed the influence of Bennington. Terry also anticipates another future issue at the front end of this article, couching this request as the ravings of a faddist, he mentions the need for "standards." Programmatic standards for dance education were increasingly in need of clarification, but this

152

would not be dealt with in a substantive manner for another 35 years. Finally, as an interesting aside, Terry quotes Mabel Lee (whose comments on the history of physical education and dance were referenced in Chapters One and Two), an early leader in the organizational history of dance in higher education (discussed in the next chapter). Lee's important role in the history of dance in higher education cause her remarks, as quoted above, to ring with a certain degree of irony.

The debate over the evolution of dance from what physical educators felt was the non-confrontational, educational dance of the 1920's to the modern, provocative, and often perplexing, art-dance of the 1930's, in large part sparked by the Bennington Experience, fed scholarly discourse in the field of physical education throughout the 1930's and into the early years of the 1940's. At one point or another most every perspective and point of view had its day in print. Very little was resolved but the stage was set for the academic struggle that would consume dance educators for the next several decades as they continued to search for an identity for dance in American culture and in the American university. But, because the middle years of the 1940's were dominated by the social and political issues of war, this discourse was put on hold until the 1950's.

To understand the evolution of dance in the American university in the years following World War II, we must not only consider the points of view of individuals but also the beginnings of organized activity for progress in dance education. From the 1930's to the 1980's the history of dance in the American university, reflecting changes in American educational and business circles, becomes much more influenced by the efforts and activities of organized groups of like minded individuals. Organization leads to pressures for specificity and standardization: the organization serves a certain clientele, and gravitates toward standardized practices. Standard practice may be in shared opinion, in the creation of a product, or in an approach to problem solving. The slow struggle toward standards for educational dance, called for by Walter Terry, began in the discussions and sessions of the first national, professional organization for dance educators, the National Section on Dancing of the American Physical Education

Association (NSD of APEA); formed in the dark winter of the first years of the great depression, and in the face of great internal resistance, by some very persistent women dance educators in 1930 - 1931.

CHAPTER 7

The National Section on Dancing: 1930 - 1950

As the American university recognized a greater range of disciplines and became more diverse in its educational offerings, programming was balanced by standardization in the disciplines of higher education. Academic programs of similar nature were organized in specific colleges, and appointment, promotion, and tenure processes became more related to discipline based criteria. Issues of academic specialization and standards, the boundaries of disciplines, and peer review of teaching, research, and service for promotion, led to the establishment of professional standards of excellence. Professional associations were formed to serve the needs of the growing number of teachers in higher education. Like other programs, physical education was a discipline in need of service organizations.

The first national organization for physical educators was formed in 1885 as the American Association for the Advancement for Physical Education (AAAPE). By the turn of the century the AAAPE had changed its name to the American Physical Education Association (APEA):

> The national organization promoting the development of health and physical education is the American Physical Education Association. The Association is one of the oldest national societies. It was founded in 1885 as the American Association for the Advancement of Physical Education. Its sponsors were a group of physicians, educators, and specialists in bodily development.
> ...The present Association has a membership of approximately 7000. It is divided into six districts: Eastern, Southern, Mid West, Central, Northwest, and Southwest.[1]

APEA Districts were comprised of representatives from states in a geographic region. Other organizations shared affiliate status with the APEA and worked with its members towards common goals. In 1930 APEA Sections were formed to serve the needs of specific populations within the field. The creation of Sections permitted independent affiliate groups to come under the APEA umbrella. [2]

The story of how a National Section on Dancing (NSD) was created is the focus of this chapter in the history of dance in American higher education. The National Section on Dancing was the first national organization for dance educators in the schools and colleges. For many years the NSD was the primary organization for dance educators in higher education, providing a much needed forum for determining the focus and substance of educational programs in dance. Over time the National Section on Dancing evolved into the Dance Division of the American Association for Health, Physical Education and Recreation (1963), and then into the National Dance Association of the American Alliance for Health, Physical Education, Recreation and Dance (1974). The NSD's founding is important to the history of dance in the American university. Through the NSD, university dance educators found their "voice" and prepared the way for the eventual development of dance as an academic discipline.

To begin this part of the story of dance in the American university, we have to backtrack a bit to the years 1930 - 1932. The starting place is an annual meeting for an affiliate group, the Middle West Society of Women Physical Educators (MWSWPE). [3]

The MWSWPE was comprised of women physical educators teaching in higher education and in the public schools. Many MWSWPE members were also members of the APEA and the National Association of Directors of Physical Education for College Women. In March of 1930, the MWSWPE held its annual meeting in Milwaukee, Wisconsin. Conference participants were provided with a dance demonstration by Margaret H'Doubler and students from the nearby University of Wisconsin-Madison . After H'Doubler's demonstration, MWSWPE members met to discuss dance and its educational potential. A decision was made to submit a proposal for a program on issues related to dance education to the APEA for their next convention scheduled for April 1931 in Detroit, Michigan.

The program proposed by the MWSWPE was not the first on dance to be sanctioned by the APEA. Programs for dance had been presented at national and regional APEA conferences for many years. Folk and national dance were central themes at the 1905 APEA National conference in New York City, and Gertrude Dudley of the University of Chicago organized a dance demonstration at the 1917 APEA Chicago Convention. [4] But the MWSWPE proposal was not meant to be another demonstration of dance styles. The program was focused on establishing standards and identifying issues in educational dance. The dance sessions proposed by the women of the MWSWPE acted as a catalyst for a subsequent request to create an official organizational appendage to the APEA, a National Section on Dancing.

The APEA had been governed and managed by its male members since its inception. [5] In the winter of 1930, the APEA Legislative Council approved a new constitution designed to open the organization up to different constituencies. Changes to the constitution allowed for new organizational structures and for women to hold leadership positions within the APEA. Following the 1930 national convention, Mabel Lee, a physical educator from the University of Nebraska, was elected to the APEA Board of Directors as APEA Vice President. [6] APEA rules enacted after the 1931 convention permitted Section status for constituent groups, provided these groups submitted a petition for recognition signed by twenty five active APEA members at least thirty days prior to a scheduled annual convention. With APEA approval, Sections could organize regular meetings at conventions and petition the APEA Legislature for funding. A Section for dance was a real possibility following the 1931 Detroit convention. With Mabel Lee assuming the Presidency of the APEA in 1931, APEA members with an interest in dance felt the time was right for action.

Within weeks of their Milwaukee conference, the women of the MWSWPE met again at the April 1930 APEA conference in Boston. H'Doubler restaged her demonstration on dance and MWSWPE/APEA members reaffirmed their plans for the 1931 conference. APEA President F.W. Maroney appointed

Dorothy LaSalle to prepare and chair the program on dance for the Detroit meetings. [7]

The appointment of LaSalle was later confused with an earlier recommendation by MWSWPE members that Ruth Murray chair the 1931 APEA dance sessions. The question of whom would chair the dance program was resolved by President Maroney and Vice President Lee. They recommended that LaSalle direct the part of the program on dance in the elementary schools, and that Ruth Murray manage the rest. LaSalle recalled her version of the events surrounding the program and subsequent creation of the National Section on Dancing (NSD) in a 1969 letter to National Section on Dance Past-President Gladys Fleming:

> At the 1930 convention in Boston of the National Society of Directors of Physical Education for Women, Margaret H'Doubler, University of Wisconsin, presented a demonstration of dance for college women. Following the demonstration an extensive discussion ensued regarding how to develop interest of college women in dance. Their lack of skill was one factor in their disinterest. D.LaS [Dorothy LaSalle] (who was, at that time, Secretary for the Committee on the School Child of the White House Conference on Child Health and Protection), made a plea for greater interest and attention by college directors to dance in the elementary schools....
>
> Blanche Trilling, Director of Physical Education for Women at Wisconsin, moved that D.LaS be appointed chairman of a committee to develop a report on dance in the elementary schools....[I]was agreed that the report should be ready for the APEA convention the following year....[A]mong the items the report discussed were: objectives, methods, curriculum, dance for boys, and teacher preparation. The committee emphasized the need for more scientific study of objectives, child interests, further experimentation with dance for boys, teacher preparation, standardized terminology, and bibliography.
>
> The report was presented at the APEA convention in Detroit in 1931 at a meeting of the Midwest Section on Dance (Midwest, at that time was independent of, but affiliated with APEA). It was the largest meeting on dance associated with APEA to that date and was chaired by Ruth L. Murray, chairman of the dance section. Dorothy LaSalle made the presentation. The report was well received and subsequently published in The Research Quarterly for December 1931.
>
> At the Detroit convention the decision was made by a group of interested persons to petition the APEA Board of Directors to permit the organization of a dance section. Leaders of this group were: Martha Hill, Dorothy LaSalle, Ruth Murray, Mary O'Donnell, and Mary Jo Shelly. Section status was not approved by the Board of Directors because the group was not organized with elected officers and had not conducted business for a year on a probationary basis (as required by the APEA constitution). Other factors which undoubtedly influenced the rejection were the unfamiliarity with dance by the Board which was composed of all men (women were not permitted to hold office), and the feeling that dance was not a legitimate part of physical education.
>
> ...[T] group immediately organized and elected Mary P. O'Donnell as chairman. To her fell the responsibility of guiding the new section through the academic year 1931 - 1932....

> At the 1932 convention of the APEA in Philadelphia, Miss O'Donnell requested the Board to grant official section status. Members of the Board questioned the desirability of and need for such a section and considerable discussion followed. In the end, however, chiefly because of Mary O'Donnell's excellent presentation and argument, the request was approved.
>
> Under Miss O'Donnell's leadership, A.S. Barnes and Company agreed to publish the refined report. In March 1933 it came off the press as "Dancing in the Elementary Schools." This was the first publication of the Dance Section (now Division).
>
> At the 1933 convention Margaret H'Doubler was elected chairman of the Dance Section but was unable to serve. The President of APEA Jesse F. Williams, subsequently appointed Helen N. Smith, University of Cincinnati, as chairman. [8]

LaSalle's recollection of events contains some inaccuracies. By 1931 women were allowed to hold office, as Mabel Lee was then President of the Association. And, although official recognition for a Section on Dancing was withheld, the Section was authorized to conduct business during the year and to reapply for Section status in 1932. In the official petition to the APEA for recognition of the Section on Dancing, dated March 9, 1932, Mary P. O'Donnell states that the April 1, 1931 dance meeting at the Detroit APEA convention was attended by "more than one thousand individuals." [9]

Mabel Lee had her own recollection of events surrounding the beginnings of the section. On January 1, 1931, Lee assumed the office of President of the APEA. At the encouragement of dance educators belonging to the APEA, Lee took the original idea of the upcoming convention program on dance several steps further and began to make the case for creating a National Section on Dancing as an official unit of the APEA. In a letter to Dorothy LaSalle and Ruth Murray dated January 9, 1931, Lee clarified her instructions and articulated her goals in developing a National Section on Dance:

> As I recall the situation, Miss LaSalle was asked at the close of the Boston meeting by Dr. Maroney President of the APEA, to prepare a report on dancing in elementary schools for the Detroit convention....[S]he was asked at the College Women's Section meeting in Boston to be chairman of the committee to plan a program on Dancing in the Elementary Schools to be presented at the dancing section at the Detroit convention. Previous to this, Miss Murray was asked at the Mid West convention at Milwaukee in March by a group of people interested in dancing to head up a committee to prepare a program of practical work and discussion for the Detroit meeting. This, of course causes over-lapping.

As the newly elected President of the American Physical Education Association, I am going to ask that the two of you undertake the work for the Detroit program as follows:

Miss Murray, will you please, as the Detroit representative of a Mid West group already organized in the interest of dancing, prepare a discussion demonstration program to take place for the convention at that time....Will you please on your program give a place for Miss LaSalle's report on Dancing in Elementary Schools or a place for her program on dancing, whichever she desires to make it...At the close of your demonstration save time for a business meeting of all delegates to the convention who are interested in organizing the permanent dancing section. I would suggest that you reserve at least a whole half hour for this.

Now I am asking you Miss LaSalle, to act as temporary chairman of the dancing group to be planning a permanent organization and Miss Murray, will you please act as temporary secretary of this group?

APEA has adopted a new constitution to go into effect immediately at the close of the Detroit convention. According to the new constitution, any group interested in any phase of physical education may organize a section in that activity, provided that they submit to the council a petition for recognition. This petition is to be presented thirty days prior to convention and signed by twenty five members of the APEA who are interested in the organization of such a section. The petition should be accompanied by organization plans and the name of the duly selected national chairman of the group. I suggest that if interested you get your petition of twenty five signatures to me by March 1st, that will give you a right to attention in council meetings at Detroit which will be held immediately after the convention. Then you can be working on your tentative organization plans and present them at the close of the business meeting of the dancing demonstration. Also, at that time, you can elect your permanent chairman for the coming year. Your plans and chairman name can then be submitted to me at the close of your meeting and before Saturday, April 4th.

Your organization should not be too highly organized and too formal....Each section should have committees at work throughout the year on the problems of their own interest and the convention program should be in culmination of the years work with recommendations for future undertakings. In that way the Dancing Section of APEA should, in a few years growth, be the recognized authority on dancing problems.

Once the dancing section is organized and officially recognized by APEA, your chairman will be a member of the National Council and your group will always be given a place on the program as well as demonstration programs and APEA will look upon the Dancing section as its final authority on dancing matters. [10]

La Salle deferred her organizing responsibilities for the 1931 APEA meetings to Mary P. O'Donnell, instructor of Physical Education at Teachers College, Columbia University.

In February of 1931, Ruth Murray submitted a petition to the Council of the APEA for recognition of a Section on Dancing with the requisite twenty five signatures. [11] At the April 1931 Council meeting, several influential male members adamantly opposed any new section for women. They felt that because the APEA had already accepted a section for women's athletics and allowed women to hold office in the organization, women had gained enough in the APEA.

[12] Despite some resistance, the Council voted to allow the Section to function unofficially through 1931, and formally accepted the National Section on Dancing at their 1932 convention. Dance education now had a national professional organization. For many years the National Section on Dancing was the premier organization for America's dance educators. Throughout the 1930's, in paper presentations, conference sessions, and articles printed in the *Journal of Health and Physical Education*, the Section's activities attest to the range of thinking on the subject of dance in higher education.

The key players who worked to form the National Section on Dancing included Margaret H'Doubler, Martha Hill, and Mary Jo Shelly. H'Doubler was a member of the Section's first Executive Committee but declined her election as National Section Chair in April 1933. Her inability to assume the chairmanship of the National Section is not revealed in the letters, notes, and minutes from the archival material reviewed. Martha Hill assumed leadership roles for dance in the . Eastern District of APEA, organizing conferences and meetings such as the 1932 Dance Symposium at Barnard College.

By the late 1930's the Section's leadership was beginning to show signs of a growing dissatisfaction with being so closely aligned with physical education. Meeting at Mary P. O'Donnell's Manhattan home, Section leaders debated moving the Dancing Section from its place within the Physical Education Division to the Recreation Division. APEA President Hernlund made a personal appeal to the Section's executive committee to stay with physical education. [13]

From 1932 into the late 1950's, the work of the National Section on Dancing was steady and largely concerned with developing criteria for implementing dance programs at all levels of education. Between 1941 and 1945, during the active years of America's involvement in the Second World War, the Section's function was curtailed as meetings were canceled and work put on hold due to military rationing and travel restrictions.

Following World War II, events began to unfold that would have a profound effect on both the National Section on Dancing and dance in the university. The consequences of America's post-war military obligations and American economic domination of world markets, Congressional enactment of the GI Bill to help subsidize returning military personnel in job training and education, a corresponding expansion of higher education, and technological developments in transportation and media, all had dramatic effects on education and dance. For dance educators in the university, the implications of the profound societal changes that followed America's involvement in World War II were not immediately apparent in the late 1940's. In 1950 few people could guess what was about to happen in higher education, culture, or dance. There was one young woman, however, who was exploring the issues that had not been resolved in the discourse of the 1930's; Alma Hawkins.[14]

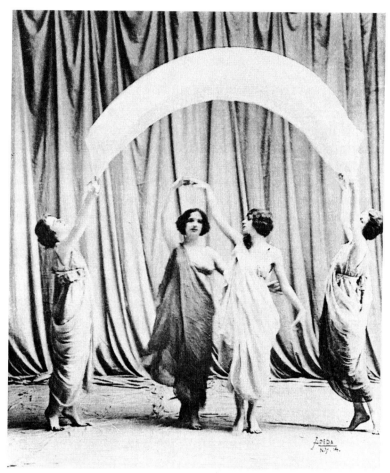

Figure 1 Isadora Duncan Dancers, circa 1915
Photograph by ADEA, courtesy of Irma Duncan Collection
Dance Division
The New York Public Library for the Performing Arts
Astor, Lennox and Tilden Foundations.

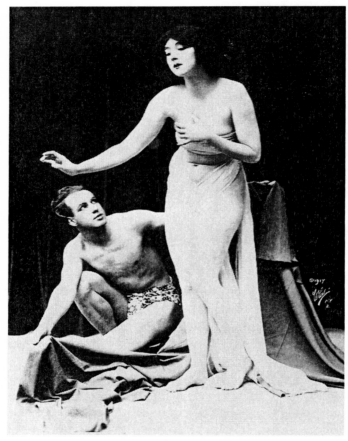

Figure 2 Ruth St. Denis and Ted Shawn in "Greek" attire, circa 1917
Photograph by White Studio, courtesy of Denishawn Collection
Dance Division
The New York Public Library for the Performing Arts
Astor, Lennox and Tilden Foundations.

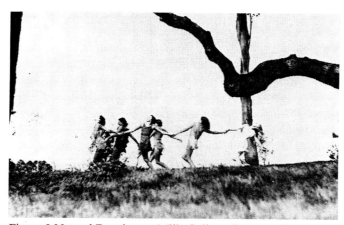

Figure 3 Natural Dancing on Mills College Campus, circa 1929
Photograph, courtesy of F.W. Olin Library
Mills College, Oakland, CA.

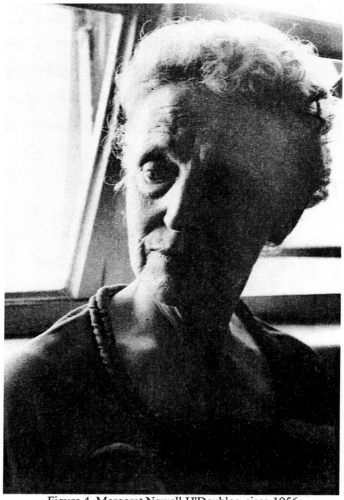

Figure 4 Margaret Newell H'Doubler, circa 1956
Photograph by Adger Cowens of Ajax, courtesy of Dance Division
The New York Public Library for the Performing Arts
Astor, Lennox and Tilden Foundations.

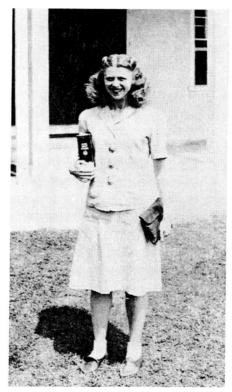

Figure 5 Martha Hill on the Bennington College Campus, circa 1934
Photograph, courtesy of Louis Horst Collection
Dance Division
The New York Public Library for the Performing Arts
Astor, Lennox and Tilden Foundations.

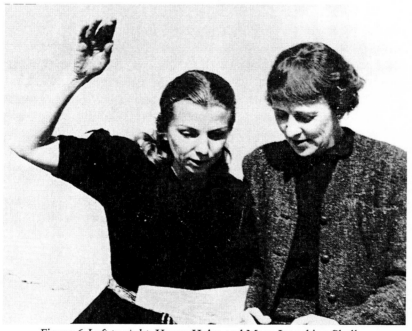

Figure 6 *Left to right:* Hanya Holm and Mary Josephine Shelly,
in the Greek Theater, Mills College,
Bennington-West Summer Session, 1939
Photograph, courtesy of F.W. Olin Library
Mills College, Oakland, CA.

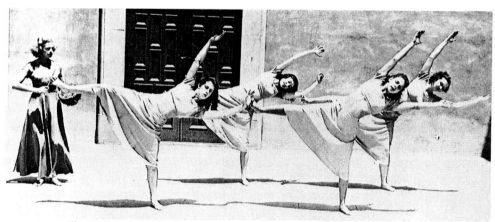

Figure 7 *Left:* Katherine Manning, Teaching Class in the Greek Theater
Mills College, Bennington-West Summer Session 1939
Photograph, courtesy of F.W. Olin Library
Mills College, Oakland, CA.

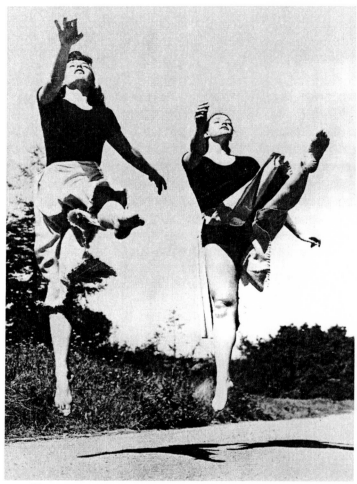

Figure 8 Two Women Dancing-Mills College, circa 1941
Photograph, courtesy of F.W. Olin Library
Mills College, Oakland, CA.

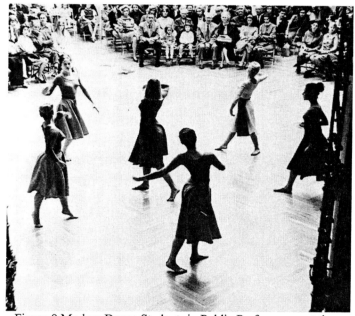

Figure 9 Modern Dance Students in Public Performance at the
Mills College Art Gallery, circa 1963
Choreography by Rebecca Fuller
Photograph by Roy Willams-Oakland Tribune, courtesy of F.W. Olin Library
Mills College, Oakland, CA.

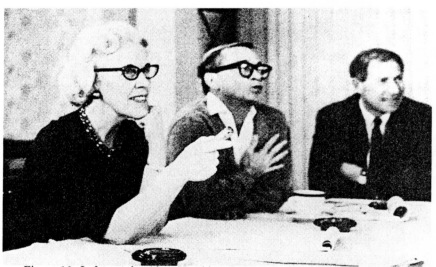

Figure 10 *Left to right:* Alma Hawkins, Eugene Loring and Joseph Gifford
at the Developmental Conference on Dance, UCLA, 1966.
Photograph by Nik Krevitsky, *Impulse* Publications.

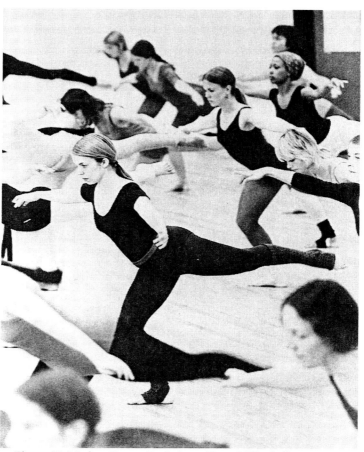

Figure 11 Modern Dance Technique Class, Mills College, 1973
Photograph, courtesy of F.W. Olin Library
Mills College, Oakland, CA.

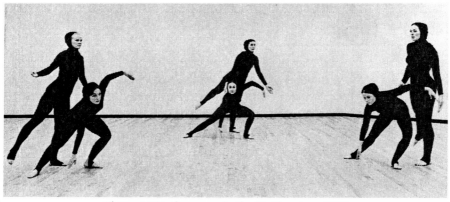

Figure 12 Performance in the Studio, circa 1980
Photograph, courtesy of F.W. Olin Library
Mills College, Oakland, CA.

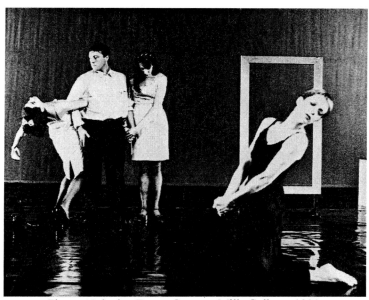

Figure 13 Spring Dance Concert, Mills College, 1991
Photograph by Robert Bryant, courtesy F.W. Olin Library
Mills College, Oakland, CA.

CHAPTER 8

Dance and Higher Education in the 1950's: *Modern Dance in Higher Education*

In the late 1940's, Alma Hawkins was a young woman with a bright future in higher education. She completed the Ed.D. at Teachers College in 1949. Hawkins' dissertation research was the source material for her 1954 text, *Modern Dance in Higher Education.* In this book Hawkins addresses the "current controversy and confusion" surrounding dance in higher education, and provides insights and "Guiding Principles" for reconciling these matters. The first chapter of the book, "Modern Dance: Uncharted Development," clearly states the problems facing the field of dance education and the American university circa 1950. Hawkins opens her text by acknowledging that the conflicts associated with the "rapid growth of modern dance programs in colleges across the country, plus the powerful influence of concert dance on these programs, undoubtedly gives some clue to the cause of the current controversy and confusion." [1] By 1950, dance educators were concerned with the unfocused growth of dance in America's colleges. Educators were confronted with a set of questions that were "raised by a conflict of various points of view":

> Should the teacher be more concerned with working toward good dance or with using dance as a means for the development of the individual?
> Should the teacher direct his efforts primarily toward the skilled students who have artistic ability, or should he have equal concern for all students?
> Should the teacher approach modern dance through technique and body conditioning, reserving composition for advanced students, or should dance provide creative experience at all levels of participation?
> Should the teacher choreograph for all students, or should the students create their own dances even though the resulting dances be at a lower artistic level?

Satisfactory answers to questions such as these cannot be reached through mere acceptance of another person's point of view and imitation of his method. This sort of unreasoned acceptance and imitation as a basis for teaching dance is the primary cause of the confusion that exists today. A real solution to the problem of defining the proper approach to dance in education will be attained only as dance educators acquire a true understanding of the potential contribution of dance experiences to the growth of an individual and establish a philosophy of dance and guiding principles in conformity with the goals of education. [2]

In the next section of *Modern Dance in Higher Education,* Hawkins outlines the history of dance in higher education as this unfolded between 1925 and 1935. Hawkins writes:

The swift development of modern dance compelled teachers to spend much time to keep abreast of changes, and left little opportunity for objective thinking about dance....This new dance world found itself in a perpetual whirl of activity - nothing stood still. Professional artists were busy experimenting and formulating a technical approach to movement that would satisfy their needs as concert dancers. College dance teachers rushed out to learn newly developed techniques during short courses or holiday sessions, then hurried home to teach them to their classes. Seldom did they question or evaluate these techniques as to their appropriateness for college students. It was assumed that anything the artist did was good. Now, as never before, there was a constant interplay between the professional artist and the college dance teacher, both on and off the campuses.

Artists talked about modern dance as a "point of view" and as an art form. So did the educators, although their talk was not always supported by real understanding of art. Their interest in experiencing this new dance and in improving the techniques of instruction took precedence over a serious consideration of philosophy or principles.

In spite of a lack of principles to guide creative work, teachers and their students worked fanatically on composition. Their early dances evolved primarily through imitation of the artists rather than from use of principles. In fact, the artists themselves had not yet clearly defined principles. [3]

Hawkins' discussion provides a clear sense of the dilemma the practicing artist had become for dance in the university: "It was assumed that anything the artist did was good." While this statement may have illustrated the thinking of many dance educators at that time, recall the concern with which the involvement of the professional artist in dance education was viewed by the physical education administrator.

In 1933, at a lecture at the New School for Social Research in New York City, Martha Hill had proclaimed "Anything good in the dance is likewise good in art and education." [4] Hill's comment was included in the introduction to a lecture demonstration she conducted with a group of her NYU students at the New

School. Anonymously reported in the April 1934 issue of Dance Observer, the quotation reads as follows:

> [T]he first was Martha Hill with a small group of college girls. If you had any misgivings about what a college girl could do, this lecture demonstration (if it may be taken as fairly typical) dispelled them completely.
> "Anything good in the dance," Miss Hill said, "is likewise good in art and education, since the dance is no longer removed from life." She stated that the dance can say things in a different way from other arts. It is not entirely narrative; it is not merely body training (the technique of movement is a means only); it is not mere entertainment. It must say something and be more than a system of gymnastics. [5]

Hill may have made these comments in an effort to help push dance towards an artistic meaning in education; however the practical result of her remarks are contained in her first sentence - what the dance artist did in technique and choreography, the educator began to imitate, and if not imitate, import directly into their programs through hiring. By the time Hawkins wrote *Modern Dance in Higher Education*, Hill's sentiment had influenced thinking about dance .in higher education for two decades. Dance educators had placed their alliance with professional artists at the symbolic center of their conflicted experience in higher education. Among physical educators the notion that "anything good in the dance is good in art and education," was viewed with great skepticism. The idealization of the professional dance artist by the college dance educator was an attempt to separate dance from physical education and align more closely with the other arts.

Being 'not physical education' was important to one side of the larger issue of establishing a clear academic identity. But, a clear and separate identity for dance was problematic when dance continued to be contained in physical education curricula and taught in physical education programs. How was an art identity for dance to be established when it was taught between swimming and basketball, by instructors who had never had an "art" experience in their lives? For dance, being 'of art' seemed to foretell the future and negate the past. However, the fact of the matter was that the great majority of dance programs remained a part of a larger program in physical education; part, and yet not part:

loathe to be too like, and not yet unlike enough for everyone to readily see the difference.

For dance in higher education circa 1950 - 1954, Hawkins' text raises the important questions that the field would have to answer if it was to stop displaying academic schizophrenia: Was the study of dance the study of a discipline? Was dance education about dancing as fine and performing art? If dance was a performing art, what were the goals of advanced training in dance in higher education? What would remain of dance if it stayed a part of physical education? What were the goals of liberal learning in dance? Would professional and liberal educational goals be referenced around the making of dance-art? If dance was an academic, arts-based discipline, then how was dance in higher education to be instigated while attending to such matters as a discipline's charge to push back the boundaries of knowledge, forward the cultural legacy, and contribute to society? The field was acknowledging an ever increasing push toward professionalism, yet conflicted about the integrity of dance as a part of liberal learning.

An important step toward academic independence for dance was Hawkins' effort to reconcile the issues impacting dance in the academy. *Modern Dance in Higher Education* picks up where the national discussion on dance in higher education had left off prior to World War II. Hawkins presents a clear rationale for modern dance in higher education in chapters titled "Modern Dance and the Purposes of Higher Education," "Modern Dance and the Body," "Modern Dance and Self Expression," "Modern Dance and Human Relations," and "Modern Dance: New Directions." Hawkins's concluding remarks represent an interesting set of compromise observations about dance in its liberal and professionally oriented contexts, she clearly places the needs of students above the needs of the artist or of the art form:

> The educators work should be guided by a philosophy of education that has been functionally related to the teaching of dance. As dance educators develop a philosophy and begin to use well defined principles as a guide for their teaching, much of the current

166

confusion about dance in education will disappear and the role of dance in education will become more apparent.

In the light of the point of view set forth in this study, the following principles are suggested, with the idea that they should serve as a guide for the selection, planning, and carrying out of dance experiences.

1. The goals of modern dance in the college and university program should be in harmony with the purposes of higher education.
2. Modern dance should make a particular contribution to the development of the individual through experiences that help the student to meet his need for an adequate body, satisfying expression, and effective human relations.
3. Modern dance in education should be considered and taught as an art form, but the emphasis should be on process and growth rather than upon dance as the end product.
4. Modern dance in education should provide experiences through which the students develop an understanding of and skill in movement as a means of expression.
5. Dance experiences should be planned and guided in terms of the abilities and specific needs of students in a particular class or club group.
6. Dance experiences should be planned and guided so that students acquire skill in the use of principles and generalizations basic to effective movement and high quality expression.
7. Dance experiences should be planned and evaluated cooperatively by students and the leader in a learning environment that is permissive and democratic.
8. Dance programs, demonstrations, and concerts should emerge as a natural outgrowth of the regular work of the class or club, and should give each student in the group an opportunity to participate at his level of achievement. [6]

At the start of the text for *Modern Dance in Higher Education,* Alma Hawkins correctly identified the two problems that faced dance in higher education in 1950: "the spontaneous and rapid growth of modern dance programs in colleges across the country, plus the powerful influence of concert dance on these programs..." [7] But, for all the subsequent rationales Hawkins brings forth about dance in the academy, she never directly challenges, or succinctly answers the issues that emerged out of the "cause of the current controversy." The answer to these questions was slow in coming, and even today some of these questions have not been fully addressed by leaders in the field. Some degree of resolution came with the development of professional degree programs in dance (Bachelor of Fine Arts [BFA], and Master of Fine Arts [MFA]), introduced in the 1960's. However, even with the development of professional degrees in dance there remains a lingering indeterminacy in the field. There is a desire to have it both ways - to be for everyone, and yet reserved for the talented few; to be worthy of objectification and the focus of scholarly inquiry, yet remain subjective, enigmatic, and ineffable.

The developing notion of dance as an academic discipline faced a set of issues that confronted it at every turn. There was little agreement among leaders in the field regarding standard approaches to educating through dance. Furthermore there was disagreement over the place of dance in education. The question of whether dance was substantive enough to be on par with the more established academic disciplines was often contentious. Dance educators struggled with their desire to have studies in dance emulate both the conservatory and the academy. The conservatory model was attractive as a reflection of the professional world. The academic model was attractive for its corresponding attention to the intellectual, physical, and creative development of all dance students.

From Hawkins' conceptualization of the needs and direction of dance as a discipline, I turn to other dance related trends in the university and in culture during the 1950's. The 1950's was a deceptively quiet decade for dance in higher education, where much was accumulative in its eventual impact. There were few signs to indicate the coming period of rapid expansion and growth that would characterize the 1960's. However, events and circumstances were happening both in and outside of the university that helped set the stage for the full blooming of dance as an academic discipline.

The 1950's - Dance as Art, Dance as Exercise: A Continuing Struggle for Identity

Dance programs in higher education in the 1950's experienced irregular patterns of growth and development. Most programs remained aligned with departments of women's physical education while others developed separately, in colleges of the fine arts or humanities. [8] Regardless, dance curricula developed haphazardly, without a nationally cohesive vision for content, standards, or disciplinary focus. In some cases students could complete a major in dance with very few credits in the field, or with little or no practice in contemporary dance as an art form. A sequence of one credit courses in the areas of ballet, square dance, folk dance, and social dance was considered a dance emphasis. In other programs, a dance emphasis was 50 percent of a student's major course work. [9]

In spite of these differences, dance educators, and the few who administered separate dance major programs, began to better situate themselves to further their goals and objectives for dance in the university. The National Section on Dance (by 1940 the term National Section on Dance had replaced the more cumbersome National Section on Dancing as the group's moniker), continued to act as the primary national forum for dance educators in academia. [10]

Throughout the 1950's, questions of where dance belonged in the university and its educational mission, continued to frame the discourse on dance in the academy. The discussion among dance and physical educators evolved from physical educators questioning the very idea of dance as art education, to rather grudgingly recognizing the differences between disciplines as each sought amenable means for academic co-existence when academic separation was not a viable option. This led to an edgy kind of separate status for physical education and dance as they continued to occupy the same facilities; an academic version of the "separate but equal" rules of 1950's America. As is always the case, the trouble with such an arrangement is that the dominate party decided just what constituted equal.

In the writings of dance educators, some authors were more diplomatic and patient with the questions and cautions raised than others. On both sides of the "fence" that Mary Jo Shelly had referenced in 1940, the residents were trying to create the academic environment that would best suit their specific needs. Physical educators continued to turn more toward sport and athletics, while dance educators turned their attention more fully toward performance and choreography.

In 1954, in an article for the *Journal of Physical Education, and Recreation*, titled "The Dance Teacher and the Physical Administrator," Elizabeth Hayes clearly and sensitively questions the place of dance in the physical education curriculum. Hayes, NSD President at the time, and director of dance at the University of Utah, writes that physical educators viewed dance as just another form of physical education and recreational activity, and were either unable or unwilling to look at dance through the lens of fine art. She recommended a set of 6 changes for dance:

1) The creation of dance major and minor programs,

2) That the dance major be given equal status in departments of health, physical education, and recreation by adding dance to their titles,

3) Dance educators should be developed through opportunities to minor in dance through departments of physical education, and music, speech, and/or theatre, and that secondary schools should not assume that the PE teacher is best suited to teach dance; real growth in dance could not be expected until dance was taught by people with the education and temperament to do so,

4) Existing physical education minors in dance should be expanded to prepare educators to teach dance as a creative art expression,

5) Elective offerings in lighting for the stage, costuming, and music appreciation must be made available to dance minors, and

6) The department in which dance is housed must secure adequate funds for dance productions that are comparable to productions in the other performing arts.

Hayes cites 13 colleges offering a dance major curriculum in 1950, and 25 in 1954. Her position statement added to the growing concern among dance educators that dance acquire separate recognition as an arts based discipline in higher education. Dance program directors in colleges and universities across the nation were faced with a wide range of practical issues that seemed to confront and challenge expanded studies in dance at every turn including:

      Colleagues, faculty, and administrators: Physical educators had little interest in dance as fine art: Dance educators found themselves playing defense and offense at every turn as their requests for program support fell on deaf ears.

Inadequate dance faculty: Finding educators with the appropriate academic preparation in dance was very difficult. This was true both in terms of numbers and training. Acquiring and keeping FTE (full-time equivalency) faculty without an appropriate terminal degree and clear discipline-based tenure criteria was also difficult.

Small budgets: Budgets for classroom needs and dance productions often depended on projected expenditures and income for athletics and sport.

Limited space: What space was available was often more suited to athletics and sport than it was to the unique needs of dance such as sprung, unvarnished floors, unmarked surfaces, appropriate drapery for stage presentations, mirrored walls.

Limited support personnel: Dance faculty often found themselves performing tasks of accompaniment and production, as hiring personnel solely for instruction or assistance in dance was limited.

Equipment for quality dance performances: Lights, backdrops, drapes for the stage, sound equipment, musical instruments and costuming were expensive, costly to maintain, and limited in their use. Expenditures for these were hard to justify when asked: "Why can't we just turn the lights on, and leave it at that?"

Program facility location: The location of dance programs in women's physical education buildings impacted male enrollments. Until well into the 1960's many campuses did not permit men in women's buildings.

Limited scheduling opportunities: Besides having to schedule dance classes around the larger physical education schedule, the request for what appeared to be odd time requests for studio classes in technique and composition caused scheduling problems. Most physical education

171

classes adhered to the typical university schedule of 50 minute classes three times a week, or one and a half hour sections, twice a week. Dance faculty wanted one and a half hour sections, four to five days a week for technique, and two hour blocks of time for composition classes.

Scheduling and major curricula design: Student schedules and required courses did not allow for elective flexibility to acquaint the dance minor with other aspects of dance as art education. [11]

These practical matters were still minor when compared to the larger and more fundamental issue that plagued the field at a national level: what was dance as a discipline? While the answer to this question may have been clear in the minds of some, there was no broad consensus among dance educators in colleges and universities nationwide. However, consensus, was beginning to take shape and the development of common ground was apparent in some quarters of the field. In the developing field of dance scholarship new ideas were emerging that had a profound effect on the field's sense of identity and academic substance. This is evidenced in the mature level of discourse that appeared in a new journal for dance *Impulse*; initiated by students of the Halprin-Lathrop Dance Studio in San Francisco in the summer of 1948.

Impulse: A West Coast Annual

Ann Halprin and Welland Lathrop had enjoyed success in the professional world of dance in the 1930's and 40's. Ann, "Anna" Halprin was a graduate of the University of Wisconsin-Madison, where she studied with Margaret H'Doubler. After college, Halprin went on to a career in dance performance with the Humphrey-Weidman Company and on Broadway. Welland Lathrop was a former member of Martha Graham's company and also danced on Broadway. In San Francisco Halprin and Lathrop opened a school for dance which attracted students from all over the country. At first *Impulse* was a yearbook for students of the Halprin-Lathrop studio. The 1948 inaugural issue was edited by Murray Louis, a young drama major at San Francisco State University. [12] In 1951, *Impulse* was

172

reborn as "West Coast Annual" under the editorial leadership of Marian Van Tuyl.

Van Tuyl had studied with Martha Graham in the 1930's, and enjoyed a teaching position in dance at the University of Chicago. In 1938, she was selected as one of three Fellows accepted into the Bennington Summer School of the Dance. That fall, Van Tuyl traveled to Oakland, California to teach at Mills College. Van Tuyl received an offer from Mills College President Aurelia Rheinhart to help develop a dance major program at Mills. She accepted Rheinhart's offer and subsequently established a fine arts major program in dance at Mills College in 1941. In 1951 Anna Halprin convinced Van Tuyl to resurrect *Impulse* as an annual journal for dance. She remained its editor until the journal's final publication in 1970.

In her inaugural editorial for *Impulse* Van Tuyl writes:

> With this issue *Impulse* moves out onto a broader horizon. The magazine was initiated in 1948 by the workshop group at the Halprin-Lathrop Dance studio in San Francisco as a student publication. In 1949 the second issue of the magazine appeared under the sponsorship of the same group. Since so much interest has been evidenced in the magazine, we have decided to expand from the category of a student publication to the wider scope of a West Coast Annual.
> In this issue the editorial board has selected the broad topic of "Dance in Relation to the Individual and the Community." We invited well-known and well-qualified persons in the area to contribute articles which are appearing in the present volume. Various points of view are represented, which, we hope, will stimulate some lively, and perhaps controversial, discussion among our readers. In future issues it is planned to consider dance from other aspects such as production, techniques, critical analysis, etc. [13]

Under Van Tuyl's leadership *Impulse* went on to become much more than just a West Coast Annual. It assumed a respected place in dance scholarship as a forum for comment on educational policy, original research, historical analysis, and practical matters in dance education. *Impulse* helped the field focus on the areas of knowledge and understanding upon which an independent discipline of dance could be established.

In addition to her editorial contribution to the first issue of *Impulse*, Van Tuyl authored a separate article titled "Creative Dance Experience and Education."

Here, Van Tuyl presages the basic message of Hayes' 1954 article for JOPER previously mentioned. Speaking to an audience of fellow dancers, Van Tuyl's commentary lacks the diplomacy Hayes used to address physical educators. Van Tuyl's candor is refreshingly honest and straight forward. The capitalized introduction to each paragraph suggests a tone of deserved exasperation:

> AFTER twenty-odd years of honestly taking the positive, or "Pollyanna," approach to the teaching of so-called creative or modern dance at the college level a deep discouragement with the art as it is presented in the American schools overwhelms me. It is not in the spirit of reminiscing about the good old days that we review briefly the background of this modern dance in the colleges and universities, but rather as a means of evaluating our present situation. The excitement generated by Isadora Duncan's whole point of view was carried on into the schools by such inspiring and selfless teachers as Margaret H'Doubler, Martha Hill and a few others. In the twenties and thirties artists and teachers such as Graham, Holm, Horst, Humphrey, Weidman, and Wigman stimulated the entire movement. In the thirties the Bennington School of the Dance, WPA projects, dance clubs such as Orchesis, each contributed to the maintenance of the exhilaration of the college groups. Concert companies toured what was known as the "gymnasium circuit."
>
> HOWEVER, teaching movement at the college level in our culture is basically a remedial proposition. We are trying to make up for the fact that in our society education is almost entirely verbal. We have come to realize that we must educate the total individual in the environment. We recognize that movement is a fundamental experience, that rhythmic movement in a group is enormously satisfying, that the "resultant release" is therapeutic; but we are in a vicious cycle in our schools. Since so little creative dance experience is available in the early years we are constantly struggling with "motor morons" at the college level.
>
> WITH few exceptions dance education has been incorporated in physical education throughout the schools. One leader in physical education has remarked that the only reason for this phenomenon, in the beginning, was that the physical education departments had showers and floor space needed for dance. On the other hand the leaders in physical education were often women with broad vision and sensitivity who realized the importance of vital dance experience for students. For the most part, however, physical education students have shied away from dance as from the plague; and the most adroit salesmanship has been needed to convince them of its worth and attainability for them. Curricula have been formulated on the premise of keeping everything equal; hockey, badminton, swimming, tennis, dance, basketball, etc., etc. Needless to say, dance presented in this context would offer a meager and frustrating experience. The minimum requirement for dance experience as a background for teacher training would seem to be a block of dance activities comparable to the total sports schedule. In the physical education setup one could then hope for minimum adequate training in movement technique, rhythmic form, basic compositional experiences as well as fundamental understanding of and experience in folk and recreational materials. The trend toward transferring dance to the departments of fine arts where it rightfully belongs can serve the small group immediately involved, but under the present setup does little to help in teaching in elementary and secondary schools. [14]

In addition to providing a forum for the intellectual community in dance, perhaps the most important contribution of *Impulse* was the editorial decision to address a specific topic in each issue. The implicitly understood, and perhaps politically wise, policy of self-regulation dance educators held to when writing commentary for *JOPER*, was not an issue in their work for *Impulse*. Within the safe confines of *Impulse*, academics had a national forum for focused and rigorous discussion and debate. They did not have to labor through endless clarification's of the basic tenets and needs of dance education to a skeptical readership. Van Tuyl's 1951 comments on issues regarding the sorry state of dance education was a breath of fresh air for many dance educators. Certainly Van Tuyl's inaugural article for *Impulse* set the tone and stage for less compromised discussion on the matter of separation for dance and physical education.

The editorial decision to focus on a specific topic with each issue stimulated a positive and more focused way of looking at dance. Frames of reference for each issue were new and exciting; "Dance in Relation to the Individual and the Community" (1951), "Production Issue" (1952), "Dance as Communication" (1954), "Theories and Viewpoints" (1958). In *Impulse* one could expect to find the best contemporary thinking on the featured topic. Through her leadership Van Tuyl contributed to the maturation of dance related writing, helping to establish the intellectual bedrock upon which would stand a new generation of dance "scholars," a term rarely used in connection with dance education.

While dance in higher education made fitful gains in its academic standing in the university throughout the 1950's, other developments in American education and culture began to set the stage for a radical evolution for dance in the 1960's. The "baby boom," the "Red Scare" and Sputnik, the Beat generation, increased personal wealth, the suburbanization of America, television, and an expansion in the number of state and junior colleges during the 1950's; all had an influence on dance and influenced the development of dance major curricula in the American university.

Cultural Factors Influencing Dance in America in the 1950's

As a result of political, economic, and social factors following World War II, higher learning in America in the 1950's experienced a period of tremendous growth, self examination, and a significant redistribution of resources. The development of a "Cold War" between capitalist and communist societies led to the perceived need for a large research and development capacity in the university. Huge sums of money were subsequently allocated for industrial, agricultural, energy, weapons development, and applied science programs. Expansion resulted in major increases in capital spending on facilities and technology, an increase in administration personnel and staffing, and changes in the internal allocation of funds for other university programs and personnel. Budgets became lopsided as internal spending increased for some programs. Faculty in disciplines not directly related to the goals of national security pressured college administrators for equity in program enhancement and capital expenditure.

American politics in the years of the Soviet Union (1917 - 1989) were shaped by fear of the "Red Menace." In the 1920's, Isadora Duncan's open affiliation with communism colored her reputation in America a bright red. In the 1930's, with the social and political unrest that emerged out of the Great Depression, some dancers were inspired to work toward socialist, and communist agendas. Dancers, like other artists in the 1930's, represented a broad palette of political opinion and activity. Companies like the "Red Dancers," the "Nature Friends Dance Group" the "New Dance Group," and "Theatre Union Dance Group," brought an energized ideology and political aesthetic into dance. The House Un-American Activities Committee (HUAC), formed in 1938, was well aware of the leftist orientation of some in the concert dance world. Following the Second World War the HUAC was re-activated. In 1950, Republican Senator Joseph McCarthy (Wisconsin), began his public terror of investigation of prominent Americans in politics, science, education, and the arts; playing havoc with the idea of intellectual, artistic, and academic freedom. [15]

In post-war America the "Soviet Scare" had everyone on edge. Communist youth were portrayed as focused, driven, and intellectually and physically superior to Western youth. American educators responded by tightening academic standards in the traditional subject areas of math, science, and language. The progressive education ideals of socialization and learning life's skills, so eloquently referenced by physical educators in decades past, fell prey to a demand that the body be as hard as the mind. The field turned away from the social adjustment and leisure education goals popular in the 1930's and early 40's, toward goals of individual physical fitness and conditioning through sport and play. Physical education's interest in fitness and athletics begged the question of including dance in their programs, further highlighting the difference between dance as art expression and dance as physical activity. Physical educators turned ever more fully toward athletic skill and personal fitness as central to their mission in the schools.

Colleges increased their range of offerings in teacher education as school enrollments grew. Physical education teacher programs enjoyed a respectable growth throughout the 1950's as requests for PE specialists increased. Physical educators strengthened their position in education by promising to make America's students strong and athletically skilled.

Meanwhile, professors and administrators were pressured by legislatures and government agencies to toe the line in matters of patriotism and a rejection of the political left. Fear of government investigation and endless accusations led to pressures from the professoriate for administrators to protect academic freedom and to defend the place of the academy as a center of learning and knowledge for all of society. The faculty's vision of the university as a cultural repository had a spill over effect in that this helped contextualize the developing argument for comprehensive programs in the fine arts.

By 1954, the Korean Conflict had come to an uneasy close and the bitter accusations of McCarthy had been proved false. The American public seemed ready for a rest from the perpetual "Commie" fright. However, the Cold War was not over and communist hegemony remained a very real threat in the minds of many of the nation's leaders. President Dwight Eisenhower took the bold step of requesting Congressional funding for "The President's Emergency Fund for International Affairs": a Presidential discretionary fund to be used to enhance overseas opinion of America's cultural dynamic. Part of these monies were used to send the first federally sponsored dance company abroad; a tour of Latin America by the José Limón Company. [16] Federal subsidy to American cultural organizations for overseas travel and performance in the mid 1950's originated in a political effort to represent a dynamic and culturally exciting America to the rest of the world. If America had to confront the Communist block on all fronts, then the cultural diversity and richness of the West would outshine the stifled, single voiced cultural expression of states within that block. Federal support for dance company touring overseas had its own effect on popular and academic notions of concert dance. Government recognition of dance as an important cultural export helped dance educators argue the case for expanded recognition of dance as a fine arts discipline in higher education.

Perhaps the most important symbol for rethinking the educational, political, and cultural role of the American university in the 1950's was the launching of the Soviet Union's *Sputnik* ("little traveler") satellite and the ensuing "space race." Throughout the decade both the Soviet Union and the United States had worked to refine rocket science and technology. The Soviet Union was first to access the potential of Earth's outer space, sending Sputnik into orbit in 1957. A renewed Soviet challenge to American technological prowess sent a reverberation through all aspects of American education. Such a blatant technological/military success enhanced the prestige of science in education and led to a renewed examination of other areas of education that had an impact on democratic life; areas like physical fitness, the fine arts, and the humanities. Academic historian Lawrence Vesey (1973), writes:

Then came the second major shock wave; the nationwide season of fear of Russian technology as a result of Sputnik. This mood of panic, traceable to the thriving spirit of competitive nationalism in the modern world, gave further leverage to professors of newer ethnic backgrounds, and more demanding intellectual expectations. Everywhere standards of performance were raised, and actual course requirements were made tougher. Meanwhile the national temper, as it affected both private endowments and governmental appropriations at state and federal levels, brought about a temporary academic boom (lasting from about 1958 to 1966) whose only parallel had been the boom during the greatest revolutionary expansion in the 1890's. [17]

Student applications for college dramatically increased as a result of the GI Bill of Rights. Federal support for returning GI's - through educational loans and programs - induced state legislatures to authorize the construction of new public university, college, and community college campuses. Undergraduate enrollments were enhanced both by the returning war veteran and by a growing middle class belief that a college education was necessary for future success in the job market. State supported four-year, and two-year colleges grew the quickest and these were much more willing to experiment with the curriculum than were the older and more established research universities. The new universities offered vocational classes and developed programs that were viewed as a means toward upward mobility for lower middle class whites. [18]

Regional Activity in the Arts and in Dance

An important cultural influence on dance in education in the 1950's may be traced to the development of regional dance in America throughout the decade. A robust economy and an increasingly sophisticated and mobile population led to urban and suburban expansion. Cities outside the province of the major urban areas on the east and west coasts began to form their own cultural institutions. The first of these were regional art museums and symphony orchestras. Opera, theatre, and ballet companies followed suit and began to sprout up, bringing the other performing arts to local audiences. Regional ballet has its origins with the 1929 creation of the Atlanta Civic Ballet, and by 1955, 30 regional companies existed. In 1965 the number of regional, or civic ballet companies, was over 200.[19] Throughout the 1950's ballet found new audiences through the fresh approaches to choreography exemplified by the work of George Balanchine and Jerome Robbins. Ballet artists such as Ruth Page (Chicago), William and Lew Christensen (San Francisco, and later Utah), and Eugene Loring (Los Angeles), brought dance to America's urban/suburban populations. Ballet appealed to the basically conservative tastes of American audiences. While the ballet absorbed many of the contemporary sensibilities that had previously been associated with the modern dance, it kept enough of its tradition to appeal to white, middle, and upper-class values. Ballet was viewed as a dance art that reinforced community ideals of social order, power, beauty, and gender (particularly femininity). Ballet brought a sense of old world glamour for many of its supporters. With the ballet's popular acceptance as a serious art form in communities, dance educators and administrators found it easier to argue that dance in the colleges should be considered a fine art and not an aspect of physical education.

The advent of television in the 1950's also helped educate the American dance audience and stimulated the interests of future dance students. Television allowed millions of viewers to see performances that previously had been viewed only by hundreds, or several thousands at live events. Throughout the 1950's and into the 1960's *Dance Magazine* featured a "Looking at Television" column, reviewing the most recent appearances by dancers on television in Europe and in the United States. Not only did television provide a greater opportunity for many to enjoy what had been reserved for live audiences in the past, it also stimulated Broadway and Hollywood to reach new heights of visual excitement as a means of competing with TV. On the theater and sound stage, dance played a central role in the visual, often "over the top," extravaganzas created to bring a paying audience back to the theaters in such productions and films as *Brigadoon, An American in Paris, Royal Wedding*, and *On the Town*. Popular notions and ideas of art and entertainment, which for decades had been greatly impacted by the cinema, experienced a second wave of evolution as a result of the ability of television to expose the performing arts and artist to millions of viewers.

The decade of the 1950's set the stage for a "great leap forward" for dance in higher education in the 1960's. Between 1960 and 1970 dance emerged as an academic discipline in the American university. A unique aspect of this history is that it happened largely as a result of group activity. The efforts of individual dance educators had made great progress possible in the past. And while lone educators continued to play a significant role in gaining acceptance for dance on their campuses, formal group activity increasingly provided a forum for national change. Throughout the 1960's the numbers of private, local, state, and federal agencies and organizations for the arts grew steadily. Dance educators in America's colleges and universities came together in a series of conferences and group meetings to articulate their thinking, develop their positions, and prepare for academic independence.

CHAPTER 9

A. A Culture in Transition - New Developments in the Arts

The decade of the 1960's was a decade of extremes. Possibilities and lost opportunities in American politics and culture seemed to come and go on a daily basis. Events and circumstances in the arts and education were no different. What appeared to be a rich and materially endowed society was shadowed by economic disparities between classes, racial tensions (as laws for enforced segregation were dismantled), and the constant threat of nuclear annihilation. Legislation meant to assist the poor and empower the politically disenfranchised unleashed decades of resentment, anger, and frustration that were manifested in acts of rebellion against "the establishment." The definition of which establishment would bear the brunt of protest had specific meaning for each group demanding recognition. Students, women, African-Americans, Native-Americans, gays, lesbians, and other newly empowered sectors of the larger population emerged in strength over the decade. They challenged social, political, and educational authority and norms through protests, "sit-ins," riots, and other acts of social confrontation. The potential of humane and visionary leaders was abruptly ended by the assassin's bullet. Art turned its back on tradition and found its voice in confrontation and commercialism. In America, the seeds of the foment of the 1960's grew out of the fertile soil of a Cold War.

With continued industrial and consumer domination of world markets by American businesses, and as a result of the West's political-economic rivalry with the Communist block, America found itself labeled Leader of the Free world. The mantle of responsibility suggested by this title was created externally by the expectations of other nations, and internally by powerful political, economic, and military forces. America's actions on the world stage, and its internal qualities and contradictions, quickly came to represent the best and the worst traits of the West.

As the role America played on the world stage took on more importance, social scientists and other scholars began to analyze and consider the symbols and artifacts of American culture. America was not only represented internationally by its military might, technological innovations, and commercial products, but also by its developed systems for higher education, by art products and art ideas. A new "boom" in building and campus development started in the late '50's and lasted into the middle years of the 1960's. According to Vesey:

> The exhilaration of this peculiar boom period [1958 - 1966] produced certain undeniable excesses. Giddy statistical projections were made for the long-range future expansion of American higher education which apparently went so far as to misread the birthrate to a serious degree. Universities were seen to be replacing business corporations as the principal handmaidens of a benign technocratic government. [1]

The boom period spawned capital expense in the creation of new, specialized state systems. State University systems such as the Univeristy of California and State University of New York expanded to meet projected increases in student enrollments. Some public colleges and universities took on specialty roles as technological campuses, teaching colleges, or professional schools.

The fine and performing arts gained from a new sense of their social and academic worth. In 1961, a young and dynamic President John F. Kennedy assumed the mantel of US. President and with his wife Jacqueline, referred to America's artistic vitality as an important symbol of cultural health. Dance gained in its prestige as an important performing art in its own right. The attention paid to dance by Mrs. Kennedy was significant. She delighted in bringing professional ballet performances into the White House:

President and Mrs. Kennedy's patronage lent the arts a refreshed cache and
importance as a vital product and symbol of democratic civilization. The social
and political importance of American culture was reinforced in government and
business circles following Kennedy's tragic assassination in November of 1963. In
certain respects, Kennedy's death strengthened the desire of politicians and
community leaders to fulfill his vision for an America that was different from, and
greater than, threatening communist societies, largely because of its cultural
vitality. Kennedy's legacy provided a certain political edge to the arts related
aspects of the Great Society programs of Kennedy's successor in office, Lyndon
Johnson.

In the summer of 1964, Congress established a Federal Arts Advisory
Council.[3] The Council's formation led to further legislation submitted in the
House (by Pennsylvania Representative William Morehead), and Senate (by
Claiborne Pell of Rhode Island), in support of the creation of a National Arts and
Humanities Foundation. Their efforts were successful in 1965 with the creation
of the National Endowment for the Arts and the National Endowment for the
Humanities. The creation of a bureau for federal subsidy for the arts had a
positive impact on subsequent academic recognition for the arts in higher
education.

On September 29, 1965, President Johnson signed the Arts and
Humanities Bill. The following is the text of Johnson's speech on that occasion:

In the long history of man, countless empires and nations have come and gone. Those
which create no lasting works of art are reduced today to short footnotes in history's
catalogue.
Art is a nation's most precious heritage. For it is in our works of art that we
reveal to ourselves, and to others, the inner vision which guides us as a nation. And
where there is no vision, the people perish.

We in America have not always been kind to the artists and the scholars who are the creators and the keepers of our vision. Somehow, the scientists always seem to get the penthouse, while the arts and humanities get the basement.

Last year, for the first time in our history, we passed legislation to start changing that situation. We created the National Council of the Arts.

The talented and distinguished members of that Council have worked very hard. They have worked creatively. They have dreamed dreams and they have developed ideas.

This new bill, creating the National Foundation for the Arts and the Humanities, gives us the power to turn some of those dreams and ideas into reality.

We would not have that bill but for the hard and the thorough and the dedicated work of some great legislators in both Houses of the Congress. All lovers of art are especially indebted to Congressman Adam Clayton Powell of New York, to Congressman Frank Thompson of New Jersey, to Senator Lister Hill of Alabama, to Senator Claiborne Pell of Rhode Island, to many Members of both the House and Senate who stand with me on this platform today - too many names to mention.

But these men and women have worked long and hard and effectively to give us this bill. And now we have it. Let me tell you what we are going to do with it. Working together with the state and local governments, and with many private organizations in the arts, we will:

Create a National Theater to bring ancient and modern classics of the theater to audiences all over America.

We will support a National Opera and a National Ballet Company.

We will create an American Film Institute, bringing together leading artists of the film industry, outstanding educators, and young men and women who wish to pursue the 20th century art form as their life work.

We will commission new works of music by American composers.

We will support our symphony orchestras.

We will bring more great artists to our schools and universities by creating grants for their time in residence.

But those are only a small part of the programs that we are ready to begin. They will have an unprecedented effect on the arts and the humanities of our great nation.

But those actions, and others soon to follow, cannot alone achieve our goals. To produce true and lasting results, our states and our municipalities, our schools and our great private foundations, must join forces with us.

It is in the neighborhoods of each community that a nation's art is born. In countless American towns there live thousands of obscure and unknown talents.

What this bill really does is to bring active support to this great national asset, to make fresher the winds of art in this great land of ours.

The arts and humanities belong to the people, for it is, after all, the people who create them. [4]

Johnson's reference to a "National Ballet Company," and call for support from "our great private foundations," alluded to events that had transpired in the professional world of dance in late 1963. In December of that year a development grant of $7,765,000.00 was provided American ballet by the Ford Foundation. The majority of the funds were to be managed through George Balanchine's New York City Ballet (NYC Ballet), with additional monies awarded to regional ballet companies. An event of tremendous import, the Ford Foundation's grants signaled corporate America's interest in expanding the notion of recognition and support for dance. Ballet's windfall had other implications too, as reported by Donald Duncan in a rather 'tongue-in-cheek' manner in the January 1964 edition of *Dance Magazine*:

> On the morning of December 16 [1963], the professional ballet world awoke to discover that Christmas had arrived ten days early. A super - Santa Claus, the Ford Foundation, had left under the tree 9 beautiful bundles in the form of 9 grants totaling $7,650,000! As the gift wrappings were removed there were many squeals of delight, with the obligato of wails on the sidelines from some who were bypassed....
> ...[T]his staggeringly lavish subsidy amounts to the largest sum any foundation ever allotted to any one art form at any one time. It compares in significance to, but even exceeds, the Ford Grants last year of 6.1 million dollars to theater groups. [5]

Duncan's article provides a bit of background information and outlines the grant's distribution. The Ford Foundation had been investing in and supporting ballet since at least 1959 when $25,000 was given to Ballet Society (sponsoring organization of the New York City Ballet), to conduct a survey of metropolitan schools and regional companies for the purposes of identifying new talent. This award was followed by $150,000 for a scholarship program for those fortunate enough to be chosen to study at either the School of American Ballet (the school of the NYC Ballet), or the San Francisco Ballet. Faculty from both schools traveled around the country identifying promising young dancers and awarding scholarships.

After the first two phases of the grant process had been completed, the Ford Foundation's W. McNeil Lowry, Director of Ford's Humanities and Arts Program, came up with a new and expanded plan which led to the award of the 1963 grants. The grants were to be managed in a 10-year plan, and were divided as follows:

$2,000,000 was awarded the NYC Ballet, with an additional $1,175,000 to be given by the New York City Center of Music and Drama.

The yearly $200,000 from Ford was assigned specific purposes: $50,000 for extended rehearsal periods, $50,000 for company members performances with regional ballet companies, $50,000 for costumes, and $50,000 for scenery.

In addition to the monies given to Balanchine's NYC Ballet, San Francisco Ballet received $450,000 over 10 years, the National Ballet of Washington received $400,000, the Pennsylvania Ballet received $295,000, the Utah Ballet received $175,000, the Houston Ballet received $173,750, and the Boston Ballet benefited from $144,000. [6]

These figures were, at the time, "staggering" indeed.

The other staggering aspect of the story was the list of companies left out of the grants structure, most noticeably the NYC Ballet's chief rival, the American Ballet Theatre. The fact that modern dance was not included was clarified by Lowry in an article authored by Lydia Joel for the February 1964 issue of *Dance Magazine*:

> Now add to this configuration the surprise move in which the Ford Foundation has completely bypassed a vital element in American art achievement - the modern dance - an area quite desperately in need of economic assistance. Upon questioning, Mr. Lowry says, "There are minor grants possible in the future." The idea of major assistance to modern dance seemed to have withered in his office for its "lack of definable technique" and the fact that "modern dancers cannot get together." It seems to us that had Mr. Lowry cared as much about working with American modern dance as with ballet, he might also have been able to do a tailor made job for that obviously difficult area. [7]

Joel's article includes a number of responses and reactions to the Ford Foundation's largesse. Among those commenting were George Balanchine and Lincoln Kirstein, NYC Ballet choreographer and founding officer of Ballet Society respectively, modern dance pioneer and Denishawn founder Ted Shawn, Dorothy Alexander of the Atlanta Civic Ballet, impresario Sol Hurok, and critic Walter Terry; with each taking his or her pro or con position.

The Ford Foundation's decision to subsidize ballet in America had repercussions in both the professional and academic worlds of dance. Certainly corporate funding of this magnitude raised the bar for other foundation and corporate gifts. It also changed the budget expectations of companies applying for federal and state support. In addition, corporate-foundation recognition for dance lent a validity to dance that made dance that much more significant and individual in the eyes of educational institutions. One is left to wonder if the Ford Foundation's monies for the non-scholastic education of young ballet professionals didn't have a negative effect on the development of programs in ballet in higher education that might have been in the works at the time.

Integrating the Arts into Higher Education

In the world of the arts in education, a desire for exposure to the arts had steadily gained steam with the middle class throughout the 1950's. In the 15 year period 1945 - 1960, public schools increasingly promoted the arts as part of the curriculum. According to author Gertrude Lippincott, reporting on the state of the arts in American education for the 1965 issue of *Impulse*: "Since 1945, the problems of integrating the creative arts into educational institutions [content, facility, personnel] have mushroomed enormously."[8] In 1960's academia, the arts began to take on a new and much more central role as a symbol of the university's cultural offerings both to the broader society and to the local community. Clark Kerr, then President of the University of California system, is quoted by Lippincott from his 1963 book "The Uses of the University":

> Another field ready to bloom is that of the creative arts, hitherto the ugly duckling of the Cinderella's of the academic world...the universities need to find ways also to accommodate pure creative effort if they are to have places on the stage as well as in the wings and the audience in the great drama of cultural growth now playing the American stage. [9]

"The ugly duckling of the Cinderella's..."; the lowest of the low? Kerr suggests two issues - the shedding of the Cinderella mantel and accommodation of artists in the academy. The creative arts, we may assume by his latter reference, include the performing arts. In 1963, as areas of serious scholarly pursuit, the arts may not only have been the "lowest of the low" in the minds of traditional academics in their content, but their accommodation at the professional level was also problematic. How was the university to offer tenure to professionals whose work

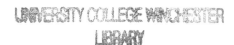

was entirely subjective? Accommodating creative effort in terms of promotion and tenure for faculty was no easy task, particularly when there were no objectively recognized means of quantification and evaluation.

Dance in Higher Education: 1960 - 1970

By the early 1960's the idea of academic separation for dance from physical education was gaining adherents and supporters from both sides of the "fence" so aptly described by Mary Jo Shelly two decades earlier. Where only 13 dance major programs existed in American colleges in 1950, by 1963 there were 65. 80 other schools offered a minor in dance; 27 offered a dance specialization within physical education; and 4 institutions offered a doctorate in physical education with an emphasis in dance. [10]

At the start of the 1960's, members of the National Section on Dance were planning their first Section conference devoted exclusively to dance in academia. The NSD's "Conference on Movement," was held June 11 - 18, 1961 at the Women's College of the University of North Carolina at Greensboro. The Conference on Movement was organized by Virginia Moomaw, director of dance at Women's College, and was an important step in building consensus in the field regarding how the discipline of dance might be conceptualized. The conference report included chapters on "Theories of Movement," "Dance as a Performing Art," "The Role of Dance in Human Society," "Educational Values of Dance," a variety of articles, and reports of discussion seminars on art making, related research, philosophy, and the future of dance in the academy. [11] In a personal correspondence, Miss Moomaw remembered the conference being organized and carried out with little interest or help from the larger AAHPER Association. The desire to clarify the meaning of dance in higher education was coming from the field itself. [12]

In September of 1964 the Conference of the National Council on Arts in Education (NCAIE), was held in at Oberlin College, Oberlin, Ohio. In the 1965 issue of *Impulse* (referenced above), Gertrude Lippincott reported the results of the conference and issues affecting dance in education in "Report of the Arts; In Government, Education, Community 1965." At the NCAIE conference a "Statement on Dance" was developed by 17 professionals representing members of the National Section on Dance, the National Dance Teachers Guild (the moniker used by the American Dance Guild at that time), Dance Notation Bureau, Dance Films, and *Impulse* Publications. Lippincott quotes their statement and writes:

> The Dance Section of the Third Conference of the Arts in Education affirms that dance is an independent art and should be considered as such. While dance can contribute to music, theatre, and physical education, to function most effectively at the several educational levels in today's expanding program of the arts in education, dance needs to be free from administrative subordination to the other professional fields.
>   The statement is highly significant because it marks the first time that dance educators, whether they were attached to dance in physical education, fine arts, or in separate departments, have agreed on the place of dance in education. And the statement is of further significance because it shows clearly that the time is ripe for such a pronouncement. Fifteen years ago there were few voices testifying to the need for dance to affirm its place as an independent art in education. Now there is general agreement that dance has a vital and self determining role in the educative process. [13]

While the "Statement on Dance" is important for the reasons Lippincott cites, it was the first statement of agreement concerning the independent art status of dance in education, it is also significant because it represents the beginnings of inter-organizational agreement and unified group efforts toward common goals. Having organizations with an interest in educational dance in agreement on academic independence for dance was a major step toward a unified field.

The rest of the "Report on the Arts" makes interesting reading as Lippincott looks at the state of dance in America, circa 1964 - 65. After reporting on the work of the dance section of the NCAIE conference, Lippincott continues with information on the NCAIE itself. The NCAIE was founded in 1957 as an off shoot of the American Educational Theater Association. It was incorporated in 1959 as a council of constituent arts groups representing 13 separate fields in arts education. Lippincott contextualizes the Third NCAIE conference with some background on the cultural, educational, and political events that informed the changes arts educators were experiencing in the 1960's. Finally, Lippincott turns to the subjects of dance in education and dance in the community. Concerning dance in education, Lippincott recognizes that while an increase in the number of university dance programs is a sign that a dance "boom" may be under way, increased numbers of programs should not be confused with a corresponding increase in quality. Variations in the range, quality, and scope of independent dance curricula was still a concern for educators interested in finding a means to standardize the study of dance in higher education.

Lippincott discusses the upcoming "Dance as a Discipline Conference" that the National Section on Dance was planning to hold in June of 1965, hoping that the conference would produce a cohesive vision for dance as an independent academic discipline. Commenting on dance in the community, Lippincott mentions a number of positive developments in government. She anticipates the opening of the Kennedy Cultural Center for the Performing Arts in 1967, and commends recent attention paid the arts by the American Council on Education and the Association of Land Grant Colleges. Lippincott concludes her Report with a quotation from President Kennedy, delivered at the ground-breaking ceremony for the Robert Frost Library at Amherst College in 1963:

> I shall look forward to an America which will reward accomplishments in the arts as we reward achievement in business or statecraft. I shall look forward to an America which will steadily raise the standards of artistic accomplishment and which will steadily enlarge our cultural opportunities for all citizens. And I will look forward to an America which commands respect throughout the world not only for its strength but for its civilization as well. And I look forward to a world which will be safe not only for democracy and diversity, but also for personal distinction. [14]

In 1965, Gertrude Lippincott also authored an article for the premiere issue of *Dance Scope*, a publication of the National Dance Teachers Guild. Titled, "A Bright Future for Dance," this article reiterates the substance of Lippincott's writing for *Impulse* but goes several steps further. Lippincott's anecdotal information is interesting here because she is not as upbeat as she was in her previous writing for *Impulse* ; pointing out some of the lingering problems for dance in culture and in education:

Unhappily the cultural explosion has not benefited dance as much as it has the other arts. There is still prejudice, antipathy, apathy, and unenlightenment toward dance in communities and in education. This writer was recently refused an interview in a Southern newspaper on the grounds that modern dance was sinful. Dancers still are smarting over the attacks of Congressmen Peter Frelighuysen and Edna Kelly on Martha Graham's "Phaedra" as it was performed in Germany two years ago [on a federally sponsored European tour, the two Representatives had the occasion to see Graham's "Phaedra" and found it too "erotic." They subsequently brought their complaints to the House floor]. Dance is considered merely entertainment by many observers, and not very high-class entertainment at that....

In many academic institutions dance is not taken seriously as an art form and is still considered a "frill." From 1957 we remember Professor Athelstan Splihaus' often quoted remark, "Get rid of typing, tap-dancing, and tom-foolery in the schools." Even at the first National Arts Council Conference one of the august deans kicked up his heels in high glee each time he saw the dancers pass. After three years of indoctrination, he now salutes us. James Conant's recent book "The Education of the American Teacher" lumps music, art, foreign languages, and physical education together and relegates these subjects to a low status in the academic hierarchy. There is no mention of dance whatsoever in the volume. [15]

Lippincott ends this article, however, on a high note, quoting Dr. William Doty (Executive Director of the New York City Cultural Affairs Office), in his address to the 1964 National Dance Teachers Guild convention. Doty said dance had perhaps the brightest future of any of the arts in the 20th century, and suggested that dance could set the artistic climate for the latter 20th century, as had art and architecture for the Renaissance and music for the 19th century.

Dance in culture and in education experienced a number of dramatic changes in the 1960's. Two major conferences during this period highlight the significant and transformative changes that were in store for dance in the American university.

The Dance as a Discipline Conference - 1965

Following their success in organizing the 1961 Conference on Movement, National Section on Dance leaders began planning a second conference for dance educators under the working title, "Dance as a Discipline." In the years between 1961 and 1965, when this conference was held, the NSD evolved from a Section within the General Division of the American Association for Health, Physical Education and Recreation (AAHPER), to a separate Dance Division of AAHPER.

The struggle for Divisional status within AAHPER was not easy. At the 1963 National Convention, when the petition for divisional status was presented to the AAHPER Assembly, the NSD leadership had to make a forceful appeal to Association members for their vote. [16] NSD members recognized that their colleagues in the larger Association were not interested in the success of dance at this time. NSD members who were interviewed for this history, some of whom helped plan and execute the "Dance as a Discipline" conference, recall that there was very little interest or help coming from the NSD's parent Association - AAHPER. Despite little support coming from AAHPER, the "Dance as a Discipline" conference was held at the University of Colorado-Boulder from June 20 - 26, 1965. Organized by Charlotte Irey and Miriam Gray, the conference was a milestone in the history of dance in American higher education.

Walter Terry described the Dance as a Discipline conference in an article titled "New Spirit In the Colleges," published in the *New York Sunday Herald Tribune Magazine* on July 11, 1965. The following excerpts from Terry's article provides a sense of the importance of this event:

> Dance history is not always made by glittering performers and choreographic innovators on the great stages of the world. Sometimes it is made behind ivied walls in administrative offices, in gymnasiums, in assembly halls on college campuses... This summer, again in ivied halls, dance history has again been made... The site of this significant event in dance education was the campus of the University of Colorado; the sponsoring agency was the Dance Division (until last March only of "Section" status) of the American Association for Health, Physical Education, and Recreation; the topic of the conference was "Dance as a Discipline."
> ...The need for joint re-appraisal (agonizing or otherwise) was recognized by dance leaders of the AAHPER as far back as a meeting held four years ago [the NSD's 1961 Conference on Movement], but the determination to hold such a conference was sparked at a legislative meeting two years ago. At this meeting of the dance members of AAHPER, Dr. Alma Hawkins, the powerful, persuasive, and highly respected chairman of the dance department at the University of California-Los Angeles, posed the blunt question, "Is dance a discipline of college caliber?" Dr. Hawkins, naturally, was certain it was. But how about academic leaders - college presidents, deans, department heads, boards of regents? The time had come for dance to prove its right to a place as a vital and valid discipline in our educational system.
> "We all felt," says Mrs. Irey, [director of dance at the University of Colorado-Boulder] "that we were at the crossroads. We couldn't stay still, we had to move forward. Certain teaching methods were outmoded. How to explore new uses for dance as a discipline? Departments of physical education opened the doors of colleges to us years ago. But should we stay there? Or move into Theatre arts departments (and would we be regulated there to minor duties) or fine arts? Or should we fight for independent

dance departments and if we got them on paper would we get any facilities (space, space, space!) to go with them?"

Mrs. Irey summarized what the delegates to this recent conference, with its many addresses and seminars and specialty working groups, hoped to do. "All of these delegates, having pooled experiences and opinions and knowledge, hope to take back to their colleges and their presidents concrete proof of their reason for being."

All manner of problems had to be faced, and if possible, resolved....[O]ne, perhaps, represents the direction desired. No longer do these educators want dance in college viewed merely as a physical activity within a physical education....That, the teachers, felt, would not do, for dance must be treated as an art as well as an activity and that would necessitate periods beyond the simple warm-ups, periods for study of styles and history and purposes and esthetics; periods for the relating of dance to the sister arts, to the sciences, to the disciplining of the total man himself.

...[V]arious panels tore into such heady subjects as "Identification of Factors Related to the Development of Creativity Through Dance" and "An Experimental Investigation of the Phenomenology of Kinesthetic Perception in its Relation to Certain Measures of Movement Capacity."

...The results of this historic conference - and it will be historic whether or not every goal is achieved - will be published in early 1966 by Focus IV, a comparatively recent publication of the now militant and seemingly rejuvenated Dance Division (the conference witnessed some battles between the old and the new guards in college dance methods) of the AAHPER...[T]he American dance world awaits its publication. **17**

The 1965 Dance as a Discipline Conference marked the beginning of academic independence for dance in the American university. Never before had so many dance educators in higher education been so united in their thinking about the scope and substance of their field. In the forward to the conference document "Focus on Dance IV," proceedings editor Nancy W. Smith writes:

The stated purpose of this conference was "To consider the academic implications of dance as an artistic discipline, a performing art, and a nonverbal form of learning." ...the conference was attended by 235 participants of varied geographic and professional representation. Specific aims of the endeavor were to (1) To clarify the status of dance as an area of learning in the academic environment; (2) To support the premise the arts, and therefore dance, are significant to the development to the individual in society; and (3) To prepare the case for dance as a full partner in the academic enterprise. **18**

In preparing "the case for dance as a full partner in the academic enterprise," conference participants broke off into a number of working groups to prepare policy statements that would represent a significant shift in the field's academic orientation. They were no longer interested in discussing the need to accommodate their work in the context of programs for physical education. The time for change was upon them and out of their efforts came clearly worded statements of academic independence. A report from the working group on "The

195

Place of the Dance Curriculum in the Academic Structure," illustrates the tone of these conference proceedings. Chaired by Alma Hawkins, this group made a series of 9 recommendations for the "further development of dance":

1. Dance should be recognized as a distinct discipline.
2. The body of knowledge related to the discipline of dance should be used as the basis for determining areas of study and the curriculum plan.
3. The curricular offerings in dance should be broad enough in scope so that they will meet the interests and needs of the students in various fields of study.
4. Administrative procedures should be established in such a way that they allow and encourage dance to flourish as an art.
5. A dance faculty, adequate in number and in competence, should be provided to teach the body of knowledge.
6. The institution should provide adequate support in the way of budget and facilities needed for the development of dance.
7. Faculty who assume responsibility for the dance discipline should seek to establish appropriate working relationships with other disciplines, especially in the fields of the arts and behavioral sciences.
8. Fragmentation of the discipline should be avoided.
9. Constant reexamination and reevaluation of the dance program should be accepted in practice, in order that continued growth may be assured. [19]

The above quotes from Walter Terry, Nancy W. Smith, and Alma Hawkins, et.al., essentially stand as a declaration of rights and responsibilities for dance as a separate, arts-based curriculum in the university. With the majority of members in the field newly united in their desire to defend this position, the time was ripe for significant change. The Dance as a Discipline Conference set the stage for the professoriate in dance to effectively argue the merits of their strengthened commitment to, and academic identification with, the arts. They defended their rights ("lehrfreiheit"), as the experts and professionals in the field, to articulate the parameters of studies in dance. The conference also helped begin the task of standardizing the curricular design for dance in higher education.

The Dance as a Discipline Conference was an extremely empowering event for its participants. Not only did academics who attended the meetings in Boulder return to their campuses with a new commitment toward acquiring the rights and resources for an independent dance program, educators in the public schools and even in the private sector were empowered to act also. In Wisconsin for example, the current Wisconsin Dance Council (WDC), an advocacy organization for dance-arts education, traces its origins back to the Boulder conference. Virginia Weiler, the WDC's founder, returned to Wisconsin with a vision for a state wide dance organization that would bring together separate organizations already in existence; local "dance councils" in Milwaukee and Madison. Upon her return Weiler organized a "Conference on International Understanding Through Dance," held at the University of Wisconsin-Stevens Point, in June of 1966. There, the idea of a state-wide dance organization was put forward by Weiler and out of this meeting was created the Wisconsin Dance Council. The WDC was developed as an advocacy group for dance at the state level. It continues to play an active role in state arts policy initiatives that affect dance. [20]

College Dance: Aesthetic vs. Professional

By the middle years of the 1960's dance in higher education was beginning to benefit from the organized actions of its leaders, and from information about dance that was getting out to the general public, helping to shape the thinking of potential students (and their parents). In 1964 *Dance Magazine* began a series of articles on dance in higher education titled "College or Career for Dancers?" and authored by Ernestine Stodelle. Each article focused on a university or college dance program; e.g. Bennington College (September 1964), UCLA (May, 1965) and the University of Illinois (April 1966). Later, Stodelle's column was augmented by articles written by a variety of other authors. Titles like, "Project for the 'Farthest-Out' College" (February 1969), and "A Dance Department with the Aloha Spirit" (December 1969), illustrated the unique characteristics of independent dance programs in higher education. One set of three articles in this series, however, is of particular interest to the discussion regarding the nature of dance as a discipline in higher education.

Olga Maynard authored three articles on dance educator Eugene Loring for *Dance Magazine*. The first two articles seem harmless enough, "Eugene Loring Talks to Olga Maynard, parts 1 and 2" published respectively in the July and August 1966 issues. [21] Here, Maynard talks to an iconoclastic Loring, a performer and choreographer of the ballet who made a name for himself (along with Lew Christensen), by developing the "American style" of ballet, through such works as *Yankee Clipper* and *Billy the Kid*. In Part 1, Maynard talks with Loring about his past, about his work in Hollywood films, and about his Los Angeles based "American School of Dance." In Part 2, Loring and his assistant James Penrod, discuss their vision for a new kind of dance curriculum centered around their idea of "freestyle": modern dance technique classes that actively fused concepts of ballet, modern and jazz dance in the training of the "whole" dancer. At the end of her second article Maynard leads up to discussing Loring's recent appointment as director of the dance department at California's newest campus; the University of California at Irvine. In the third article Maynard gets to the heart of the matter of what it is Loring brings to his directorship, and to dance in higher education. Titled "College Controversy: University of California at Irvine," the third installment was published in the September 1966 issue of *Dance Magazine*. [22]

Before exploring Maynard's article, important to note is the fact that while *Dance Magazine* was running a series on dance programs in higher education, its editorial tone on the benefits of studying dance in college was mixed, at best. Agnes de Mille put the professional's disdain for dance in the academy into words in testimony to the Congressional Select Sub-Committee on Education (reported in the May 1970 issue of *Dance Magazine*), when she said she thought dance in higher education was "largely fraudulent." [23] Dance programs were not training dancers as much as they were training "dilettantes." There is an aggressive anti-intellectualism in the tone of many of the dancers quoted in *Dance Magazine* throughout the decade; 'dance should be done, not thought about,' 'I hate academic dance,' 'dancers in college aren't prepared to dance, they're only prepared to talk about dance.' With that said, Maynard's report on the kind of dance program envisioned for the University of California-Irvine, takes on a more subtle shade of meaning.

The University of California campus at Irvine (UCI), is located in a suburban community south of Los Angeles: "geographically half way between the University of California-San Diego (USCSD), and the University of California-Los Angeles (UCLA)." [24] In developing the dance-arts curriculum for the new campus, Loring transplanted the curricular model that he had developed for his American School of Dance to the university. The byline for Maynard's article states; "The University of California at Irvine causes a major stir by its 'totally professional' approach to dance in college." Maynard begins with an introduction to Loring and then continues:

[C]urrently as head of the dance department at UCI, he is involved in an unusually fierce controversy - one which forces all those concerned to formulate their concepts of what sort of dance training a college should provide.
    This is a problem which, today, very much concerns both educators and dancers. A famed modern dancer, whose opinion commands respect   recently complained, "Dance has a double standard in America. Colleges hire professional dancers to teach and perform, but what is known as 'college dance' is a dilettante cult, not dance training." The dancer insisted that he spoke "not in contempt, but in genuine concern for college dance majors who leave campus with romantic ideas about dance. College dance is a form of arts appreciation. This is inadequate for professional dancers. In justice to their students, college dance departments must qualify their attitudes and approaches."
    "We do qualify our approach as a creative, not a critical one," says the Dean of Women of a physical education department, under which dance is taught at a major university. "Our attitudes to dance are aesthetic, not professional."
    "But aesthetics are ethics in professional dance," argues the aforementioned modern dancer. "Dance is a profession for the dancer, and a hobby for the audience, but college dance majors come off campus starry eyed, seeking careers with dance troupes, totally unprepared for the realities of the field. College is usually a waste of time and energy for potential dancers." [25]

Here, in the verbal 'back and forth' between two anonymous voices, are the points of concern and discussion that framed the discourse on dance in higher education since the Bennington Experience of the 1930's: the liberal, "aesthetic" approach vs. professional preparation. These comments also reflect the growing tension and dynamic of encroaching professionalism in all of the academy, a professionalism that gained considerable steam in the 1960's: an encroachment that had been building steadily in the American university and in the public's appreciation for the purpose and nature of higher education since the days of the Yale Report of 1828.

What follows in Maynard's article expresses a kind of "certain-uncertainty"; "certain" in the sense that what was wanted was known; dance-arts education; agreement by the field as to how to prepare for it, on the other hand, was still very much an "uncertainty," in interesting and predictive ways. Clayton Garrison, newly appointed Dean of Fine Arts at UCI, and driving force behind this "college controversy" is quoted by Maynard as saying:

> The university is no longer a thing apart, existing on the fringe of society. The decade of the '60's has brought a new perspective wherein the university is seen as part of contemporary society. Ivy may still grow on the walls, but the walls no longer shut out the world. The men and women who come to us want the university to prepare them for life, not to be an end in itself. When the university fails the student, it defrauds them. Worse, the university deludes itself. [26]

Garrison's statement rings of a Deweyan progressivism in higher education "squared"; multiplied by itself twofold. Garrison's concern for the student's preparation for life through professional experience seems to ignore Dewey's caution that experience in and of itself is not necessarily in the best interests of education. And in Garrison's statement, experiencing the professional's "world" seems to supersede the university's traditional charge which is to preserve and pass on the culture's heritage, prepare the learner for participation in a democratic society, and expand the boundaries of knowledge. Certainly Garrison's views were not accepted by most in the academy. The majority of institutions would not have considered themselves existing "on the fringe," but rather existing above the ebb and flow of popular trends and societal upheavals. Garrison's points, admittedly unqualified here, have an edge of rejection for academic tradition that clearly sets the stage for experiment and change:

> [T]he controversy that rages around Garrison centers on his revolutionary plan for separating the arts from the humanities at UCI and taking a totally professional approach to education.
> Garrison told me, "Every teacher in my department is a professional who has earned a living in the art form he is teaching. After all, the American artist practices a profession, just as the American scientist, industrialist, or businessman. Law, medicine, the ministry, and the arts are all parts of our modern society, and therefore should be parts of our educational concepts." [27]

Loring was brought into the mix to fulfill Garrison's vision for a 'conservatory within the university.' Lacking a formal college education, but having had a lengthy professional career, Loring represented the kind of artist-educator Garrison and professional dancers wanted to see managing college dance programs. Loring's curricular contribution to Garrison's vision for dance, modeled after his American School, exposed students to training in multiple forms and techniques. Ballet, jazz, and dance for musical theatre were studied in concert with modern-creative dance. In the majority of other college dance programs modern-creative dance dominated the curriculum. Few dance programs allowed the student to take ballet or jazz dance classes and count them toward their major program credits. A few programs, like Butler University in Indiana, Texas Christian University, in Fort Worth, Texas, and the University of Utah in Salt Lake City, offered a major curriculum in ballet. But the vast majority of college programs in dance in 1966 were still curricularly and conceptually tied to H'Doubler's educational philosophy, with a taste of Bennington's compositional and technical standards thrown in for arts sake:

> The majority of college programs teach modern dance. A few add ballet, but the tendency is to qualify it as being of lesser significance than modern dance. For example, UCLA's dance department, under Dr. Alma Hawkins, recently added ballet, but ballet courses cannot be applied as credits for degrees. When another west coast university, after many student requests, included ballet, it was taught by a regular physical education faculty member, without barre. Some college teachers still consider ballet effete, term jazz vulgar, and maintain that modern dance is the only "good and proper" college dance.
>   "But I have had eight years of ballet," a UCI dance major told me, "and while I want to study several dance forms, so that I will be able to work professionally in them, I feel myself altogether better suited to ballet and jazz than to modern dance. It is ridiculous to have prejudices in art forms today! Yet college dance teachers incline toward artistic bigotry." **28**

Next, Maynard includes parents in the conversation:

> [T]his young woman's parents are very articulate on the subject of a "professional" university education.,.."When I got my degree, it was more than a piece of paper - I went to work, professionally, as soon as I left the university....[C]ollege dance should be an adequate preparation for a professional career."
>   Another UCI parent...told me..."Frankly, I would not pay university expenses for our son to take a theater arts degree if the school were taking a purely aesthetic, and

not a realistic, approach to it...As a businessman I deplore amateurish attitudes, and I insist upon a professional quality of excellence. Naturally, I also want this professional quality in education for my children. I am glad UCI has returned to fundamental educational values." [29]

In just a few short years, considering the history of the university in Western culture, "fundamental educational values" now represented the practical knowledge and skills, and vocational preparation one needed to survive *after* college. The implication that vocational professionalism was a "fundamental educational value" was anathema to many in dance in higher education. Recall the debate in the field in the 1930's and '40's. The physical educator's were no longer the one's complaining about professional dance artists corrupting the curriculum, the newest round of complaints was coming from the dance educators themselves. The purposes of the university were being undermined by professionalism where product was all and process was set aside. In the view of parents, the university was "returning" to a way of thinking about vocationalism. Historically, this was a relatively new perspective for disciplines outside the professions of law, medicine, and theology.

Garrison's appointment of Loring caused quite a stir in the University of California system:

I was informed that this appointment is overtly opposed by members of dance departments in other colleges because Loring is a professional and will take a professional approach to university dance training....One college dance teacher objected to me, "Loring is violating college dance concepts by making them professional instead of aesthetic." [30]

Student showed great interest in professionally oriented major programs. This was true because studies were focused on the acquisition of skills that would prepare them for professional careers and because the new curriculum freed them from the rigors of liberal learning:

The students there now seem particularly in favor of UCI's principle of awarding degrees on the basis of arts related courses, rather than as the result of having accumulated a specified number of required units. A drama student said "Isn't it far more sensible to work as we do here, than to be compelled to take 'college units' that have little or no relation to one's major? I am required to take the dance courses and music course which will serve me as an actor, but not science courses which are useless to me, yet which would consume time and energy."

"Garrison's is not simply a one man revolution in the fine arts," a professor from another college told me, "UCI is part of a new trend concerning theater arts in education, a very necessary trend if we are to establish an American theater comparable to the European and Russian theater traditions." **31**

These last two quotes are particularly revealing. The former is symbolic of an anti-intellectualism that pervaded the rationales generated in the struggle to identify and validate the fine and performing arts as curricula worthy of advanced study in the university. The rejection of such an important tenet of higher education; that the value of the college experience is realized in the individuals broad understanding of, and appreciation for, the breadth of human thought and application, is an aspect of the previously mentioned "certain-uncertainty." To me, the first paragraph quoted above seems representative of a kind of "art-ism" that was a byproduct of separating the fine arts curricularly from the arts and humanities. The most accessible model for reference was the conservatory; a term which, in its literal definition, references a specialized and rarefied enclosure for the breeding of delicate plants. The incorporation of the conservatory within the university inspired a new perspective for curricular design for dance. The latter comment is also revealing in its sentiment; that an "art-ism" is necessary in order for the American theater (performing arts) to emerge from its cultural backwater (seemingly of its own making), via the conduit provided by higher education: to compete with the more refined "European and Russian" traditions. The latter quotation represents a cultural inferiority complex that has kept the American public and artists on edge, and second guessing themselves, since the founding of the Republic.

Maynard's article exposes the educational dialectic for dance in the opposing contradictions of dance as an academic discipline. This new thesis for dance, coming as it was from within the field and building in dynamic since Bennington and the scholarly battles in the discourse of the 1930's and '40's, was firmly "out of the academic closet." As revealed in the institutionalization of professionalism in a public university, and not in some prototypical college or conservatory, this represented as Maynard so aptly puts it, a "College Controversy."

In November of 1966, Loring was a key participant in the Developmental Conference on Dance (1966 - 1967), the next important meeting for dance educators who were looking to frame and articulate dance in the academy. This important meeting clarified a number of issues that challenged the field. However, Maynard's article of September 1966, provided an interesting introduction to the Developmental Conference and may have stimulated some interesting discussion among Conference participants. At the Developmental Conference Alma Hawkins gathered a group of professionally trained and academically prepared leaders in the field to sort out the business of the future of dance as a discipline.

The Developmental Conference on Dance 1966 - 1967

Following the success of the Dance as a Discipline conference, Alma Hawkins returned to her position as Chair of the dance department at UCLA. Knowing that the momentum of substantial change was in the air, in the summer of 1965 Hawkins submitted a grant proposal to the United States Office of Education-Arts and Humanities Program for $10,000 to support a two-part conference planned for the fall of 1966 and spring of 1967. The Office of Education-Arts and Humanities Program had already subsidized developmental conferences for the disciplines of music, theatre, and art. Jack Morrison, Professor of Theatre Arts at UCLA had recently been appointed Director of the Arts and Humanities Programs, and let it be known that funds were available for the arts disciplines to further their academic goals. In early 1966 Hawkins' request for federal support was granted. Upon being awarded funding, the two-part "Developmental Conference on Dance" was planned and held at UCLA, November 24 - December 3, 1966, and May 28 - June 3, 1967. Conference meetings were organized to further the work begun at the Dance as a Discipline Conference, but with a smaller, more manageable, group of invited participants representing professional and educational interests in dance. The Developmental Conference was planned to allow, "a representative group of experienced and knowledgeable artists, scholars, and educators to explore together the role of dance in education, and to evolve a point of view that would give direction to the immediate as well as the long range curricular and research developments in dance." [32]

Phase One of the Developmental Conference was organized to consider the nature of dance instruction in higher education and to develop guidelines for dance curricula. Conference sessions included discussions on philosophy, creativity, the nature of movement, and artistic/intellectual growth. Phase Two was concerned with developing a 25-year projection plan for undergraduate and graduate programs, and with the role of the professional dance artist and performer in education.

In the spirit of the Dance as a Discipline Conference, the Developmental Conference broke new ground in the conceptualization of dance in higher education. At the Developmental Conference professional artists and educators met to discuss common ground in support of dance as an independent, arts based discipline. In an interview conducted with conference participant Helen Alkire in the spring of 1989, Alkire recalled:

> In 1966 Alma Hawkins initiated the first developmental conferences on dance. This event was one of the most important ever held for the professional and academic dance worlds. It was the first time leaders from both arenas sat across from one another and spoke freely and frankly. This was a time when dance (through government grants and sponsorship) was "exploding." At the same time dance educators were separating themselves from programs in physical education and joining programs in fine arts, music, theatre, or moving into their own departments. The conference evoked a new freedom of thought and a confidence that had not existed before. The conference provided the impetus for many of the attendees to return to their institutions and establish dance as an independent artistic and educational medium. [33]

Conference members put forward a manifesto articulating the independent and arts related nature of dance in education. Published by *Impulse* in a 1968 special issue; "Dance: A Projection for the Future, " the manifesto states:

The purpose of education is the full realization of the total man and his understanding and communication with others.

Art experience is an ingredient of that total realization.

This ingredient in dance is a unique, non-verbal revelation of an aspect of living.

Incisive and specific information from the behavioral, medical, psychological, and social sciences is providing us with the strongest evidence that dance as a basic art is vital to the development of the whole individual. In our period of rapid change and fragmented experiences, the development of the whole person becomes increasingly difficult. The education of the senses and the objectification of feeling through the arts provides one way by which man is able to know himself, and to shape and bring order to his world.

Most educational systems at the present time do not afford an opportunity for growth in these areas. For that reason, we, the participants in the Developmental Conference on Dance, believe that dance should become an increasingly integral part of society and, therefore, of education.

There should be:

The opportunity for every child, male and female, to have a dance experience.

A skilled dance teacher in every school at every level.

Space and time and the financial support necessary to dance education.

Available resources such as films, books, recordings, and notation.

Exposure to the best of all types of live dance performances.

An honors program for the gifted individual.

The climate and conditions that will interest men in dance as an avocation and profession.

Representatives of dance in education on all councils, boards, and faculties dealing with the education of our people. [34]

The manifesto clearly illustrates the particular confidence and bravado conference participants must have felt as a result of their time together. Yet thirty years later, much of what was asked for in the manifesto is still needed. Skilled teachers, opportunities, resources, and the requisite climate and conditions are not yet in broad evidence in today's educational systems. This is particularly true for elementary and secondary education. However, change had been made and these demands mark a certain academic and disciplinary maturation among dance artists and educators in 1966 - 1967: a time when many things seemed possible and real change for dance, and the arts in general, was just around the corner.

The Developmental Conference added greatly to the field's impetus toward separation from physical education. Between the Dance as a Discipline (1965), and the Developmental Conferences (1966 - 1967), much progress had been made in making the broad argument for an independent, arts-related discipline and identifying the specific characteristics and elemental properties of the discipline's nature as expressed through the dance curriculum. There was, however, still a lingering uncertainty as to how the field should go about resolving the issue of the "aesthetic" vs. the "professional" focus of the curriculum. The tension indicated in Olga Maynard's *Dance Magazine* article on the "College Controversy" was addressed, at least in part by conference attendees in comments on minimum standards for dance:

> The conference participants felt that it was important that professional and educational leaders in dance give consideration to standards of quality that should be used as a guide in the establishment of new dance curricula. They recognized that all major programs will not be the same. In fact, curricula will vary markedly because of the uniqueness of each situation. For example, one would not expect the dance major in a small liberal arts college to be the same as the program in a large university....[D]iversity among our institutions will give strength to the total effort in dance. But undergirding all of the differences should exist the standard of quality. [35]

There is a thread that ties these conferences, and the discussions and ideas that evolved out of them, to the earlier work of H'Doubler and Hill. H'Doubler shaped the component parts of the contemporary dance curriculum, while Hill assigned instruction in specific areas of the dance curriculum to specialists. Now, several decades later, the acknowledged new leaders in the field, organized as never before, were breathing administrative and conceptual life into the dormant notions developed by the earlier pioneers.

Consider the following statistics for 21 separate institutions surveyed in 1976 when asked to provide a date for "departmental status achieved":

Table 1: Institutional Development of Independent Dance Major Programs by Year

| Column A | | Column B | |
School	Year	School	Year
Adelphi	1938	U. of Southern Florida	1972
Mills College	1943	SUNY Purchase	1972
Julliard	1951	University of Michigan	1974
George Washington U.	1964	NYU - Creative Arts	1974
New York University-Arts	1965	Arizona State University	n/a
University of Utah	1966	CA State U. - Hayward	n/a
University of Maryland	1967	Connecticut College	n/a
Ohio State University	1968	University of Hawaii	n/a
University of Illinois	1969	Hunter College	n/a
Southern Methodist U.	1970	University of Wisconsin	No separation achieved [36]
Ohio University	1971		

37

The number of dance programs achieving independent status in the period 1965 - 1975 is illustrative of the rapid progress dance made in its development following the Dance as a Discipline and Developmental Conferences of 1965 - 1967.

The special issue of *Impulse* dedicated to the proceedings of the conference is a time capsule of this moment for dance in higher education. It is an invaluable document for appreciating the tenor, tone, and flow of the group's dynamic. Of special interest is a chapter titled: "Dance in Education - Four Statements." Here, four noted dance professionals, Jean Erdman, Alwin Nikolais, Patricia Wilde, and José Limón, discuss their views on the nature and substance of dance in education.

Jean Erdman, a former student at Sarah Lawrence College became a featured member of Martha Graham's company, and later married the noted philosopher and scholar of mythology, Joseph Campbell. At the time of the conference Erdman was chair of the dance program at New York University's newly formed School of the Arts.

Erdman's comments to conference participants focus on the developing relationship between creative dancers and the colleges. She praises the colleges for having instilled a professional level of excitement into the curriculum declaring that:

> It *is* possible for college teaching to prepare young dancers properly because the body of technique is well enough articulated to make the day of the studio-trained performers as the *sole* source of new dancers a thing of the past. The advantage of this broader base and wider range of points of view carries with it, however, one very real danger. If the training program becomes "academic" - organized so that: "This term we shall learn to fall, this term we shall learn to skip," and that sort of thing - it becomes merely an objective body of material to be learned, and there is no excitement
> ...[I]n the college dance department precautions must be taken to preserve the excitement and the true meaning of what an art is, the significance of handing the art down from one individual to the next through the generations. The dance program must be carefully planned so that individual, excited dancer-teachers are there to inspire students. **38**

Erdman believes that the artist-teacher need not necessarily be a professional performer or choreographer, but that she *must* [author's emphasis] have had a transformative experience in the doing or making of dance, in order to teach dance as an "organic self-generating creative activity." [39]

Following her discussion about the nature and intent of the artist-teacher, Erdman then asks: "Knowing that we must have the artist in the teacher, what about the teacher in the artist?" [40] The teaching artist is warned that working in the college environment is a very different thing than having the pleasure of working with young professionals in one's own studio. Erdman compares the "spirit of pedagogy" with a "spirit of sympathy":

> If the professional dancer - choreographer is going to be involved now in teaching in colleges, a set-up with a broader base than his own individual studio, he will need to develop this spirit of sympathy, for not every student will be slated automatically for his own company as those in his studio might have been. And he has to function in a wider field with varying points of view coexisting. In such an environment it will constantly be apparent that the discoveries of one generation become the sentimentalities of the next. It may be hard for the artist to realize that the things he discovered, those things that he shaped and gave form to, are now everybody's property. But the artist who follows, the younger one, is going to have to find a new way. [41]

Here Erdman takes the second tack in her discussion: while the artist-teacher must be one who has had a transformative experience, she must also be resilient enough to release personal discovery to the machinations of others and stimulate an environment where the student is "allowed to create something new." [42] Creating something new is internally focused as the student is encouraged to take physical and artistic risks, and externally focused as the product of risk taking is allowed to come to some end product. Finally the student is thoughtfully critiqued and helped to find the best means toward development and further maturation.

In retrospect Erdman's statement is most thoughtful and evocative because it is simultaneously both professionally and liberally focused. Erdman clarifies the "College Controversy" previously mentioned by Olga Maynard in an intelligent and insightful manner. Her point of view is expansive and her cautions regarding the dual nature of the kind of pedagogue she envisions will be best suited for a program of study in dance still ring true.

The second Statement by Alwin Nikolais is much more anecdotal and self-reflective. In his youth, Nikolais was an aspiring music student. He turned to dance following his attendance at a concert by Mary Wigman in 1933. According to Nikolais this was his first encounter with an elemental, artistic, "source." Following his exposure to Wigman, Nikolais began serious training in dance, attending the Bennington summer programs and finding he had a "stomach" for the whole range of thinking and doing indicative of the Bennington Experience. In the years after Bennington, and following service in the military, Nikolais struck upon a lasting relationship with Hanya Holm and ultimately found his own fame through the creation of dance works that stretched the visual, aural, and kinetic imagination of his audiences.

Nikolais' approach to dance education was very much influenced by the German School of Dance through Holm. Improvisation, technical problem solving, and sensitivity to space and rhythm were some of the attributes dealt with by the German modern dancers in classes and in training. In many ways the following quotation, an encapsulated statement of Nikolais' philosophy, is reminiscent of H'Doubler:

> In teaching...I have been trying to get down to some germinal things. I'd like to provide a basis on which any student could build according to his unique experiences. I don't know if it is possible. We talk about ballet, about Graham technique, about Holm technique, but is there a possible technical basis which rests *underneath,* and which we can offer to a student, so that he can then be equipped as an instrument to carry out his vision?" [43]

Nikolais' statements are infused with the intellectual wanderings of one of the true renaissance men of 20th century dance. Nikolais' interest in education, to "get down to some germinal things," was also his interest in his art making. In reading this statement one gets the sense that Nikolais is intellectually and artistically restless. Yet Nikolais was no jack of all trades, he became a master: of sound design, visual image, kinetic phrase and motion; creating a kind of total theatrical 'art' event unlike the work of his peers and contemporaries.

Patricia Wilde writes the third Statement in this chapter. A former soloist with the New York City Ballet, and past-director of the Harkness House School of Ballet and Dance (also in New York City), Wilde brings a professional's focus to the discussion. She does not wax philosophic, nor does she envision broad educational contexts for dance; and she does not question and talk to herself at every turn in the charming manner of Nikolais, Wilde issues her opinion directly:

> [T]hey should start their training to be teachers in the universities. Except in rare cases, students in dance in universities will become teachers or people who write about dance - sometimes choreographers - but more often than not they will be teachers, so that the more experience they have under guidance, before they go out on their own, the better. They are going to make mistakes anyway, but its better if somebody is around to say "careful, you're not on the right track," or "take it a little slowly in this area."
>
> These are my beliefs: first of all the technique that they should have to prepare them, and then the opportunity to work with great artists. Together, these experiences will allow the young dancers to go on to become complete artists themselves. **44**

Wilde's ballet pedagogy was typical of the period. The explicit understanding that performers are not trained in the university pervades her discussion. But, if dance is to be done in the academy, her advice is: find your skill and mastery over an aesthetic form, perform the work of the masters, and the artist within will bloom.

The last Statement was delivered by the most celebrated of the Developmental Conference professionals. At the time of these meetings, José Limón's name loomed large in the professional dance world. Like Nikolais, Limón stumbled onto dance. He spent his youth in Mexico and in the cities of the southwestern United States. Limón briefly attended the University of California-Southern Branch, the original title for the University of California-Los Angeles, as an art major. Unhappy with the general education studies he was expected to master, Limón left Los Angeles and hitch-hiked to New York City. There he "was taken" to a dance concert and was transformed by the work of Harald Kreutzberg, having his first exposure to a kind of art dance he could identify with:

> Now, I was in New York City, and I was going to be Michelangelo and Picasso rolled into one. My destiny was clear as daylight. Then one afternoon I was taken to a matinee concert by Harald Kreutzberg and his partner, Yvonne Georgi. There were no transparent Greek tunics, no soft swooning movement and capricious prancing of young bacchantes.

There was a terrible power and beauty and eloquence. There was the compelling drama of the modern dance. I saw, with a searing clarity, something a man could do, because dancing like a proud stallion, or an Angel of Death, or a lover out of a Persian miniature was worthy of a man. There was my destiny. [45]

Limón started his dance career late for a professional dancer, in his early 20's. He sought instruction in the studio of Doris Humphrey and Charles Weidman, and demonstrated real talent. In the 1930's and 40's he was a featured performer with the Humphrey-Weidman Company. Following the break up of Humphrey-Weidman in 1947, Limón began his own group with Humphrey serving as Artistic Director. In 1954 Limón's was the first company to be sponsored in overseas touring by President Eisenhower's Emergency Fund for International Affairs. [46] By 1968, he was an internationally recognized dance artist and was on the faculty of the Juilliard School.

Limón's statement reflects Erdman's, as both are professionally and liberally focused. He comments on Hawkins' request that he address the conference on the matter of dance education, and, in so doing makes the case that the practicing dance artist is an ally of the dance educator. He suggests "a deliberately coordinated concatenation of purpose should be established between the universities (and ultimately, the professional world) and the primary schools" for the purposes of identifying the gifted dancers at an early age. [47]

The statements by Erdman, Nikolais, Wilde, and Limón celebrate a coming of age in dance education, in which dance professionals were asked to comment on and advise dance as an academic discipline. The conservatory within the university was an exciting new opportunity. It seemed to verify the substance of the expanding non-academic and non-utilitarian professionalism. There is a delight in the tone of the discourse, and a lancing of the old myth that dance education was for "dilettante's" or that dance in the college was "physical education's own art."

After the aforementioned professionals conclude their Statements, the text of the proceedings turn toward the practical matters of implementing and managing the dance curriculum and dance department. Here, the academics join

212

the discussion to frame visions for dance within the reality of the systems that will manage dance in higher education. Topics include the content of course work, design for curriculum for undergraduate and graduate programs, the professional dance company in the university, faculty, standards for dance programs, research, and summary comments. Analyzing these categories helped further contextualize the moment in dance education and laid a foundation for the subsequent development of new dance major programs.

In addition to serving as a cauldron for the practical, theoretical, and artistic conceptualization that was necessary for the development of dance as an academic discipline, the Developmental Conference also acted as the catalyst for developing a new dance organization. Following the conference meetings, Hawkins and 11 administrators of dance programs in higher education, met in May of 1968 at the Congressional Hotel in Washington, D.C. to discuss concerns specific to the responsibilities of being a dance administrator. Participants included:

Helen Alkire (Ohio State University),
William Bales (State University of New York, College at Purchase),
Jean Erdman (New York University),
Margaret Erlanger (University of Illinois, Urbana-Champaign),
Elizabeth Hayes (University of Utah),
Charlotte Irey (University of Colorado-Boulder),
Louise Kloepper (University of Wisconsin-Madison),
Eugene Loring (University of California-Irvine),
Dorothy Madden (University of Maryland-College Park),
Nancy Smith (Florida State University),
Shirley Wimmer (Ohio University at Athens). [48]

The Council of Dance Administrators (CODA) emerged from this group. At first CODA was an informal group of like-minded academic administrators who realized a need and benefit in meeting to discuss issues related to dance in higher education. Over time the Council evolved into a significant force for change in dance education, particularly in the area of developing standards for dance curricula in the university. CODA will be discussed more fully in the next chapter as their activities became more important in the 1970's. I conclude discussion of the importance of the Developmental Conference for Dance by quoting John Martin who wrote a statement on May 8, 1968, a few weeks before the conference's second session:

> The Developmental Conference on Dance was one of those essentially organic things that had to happen; it was not just something that somebody thought it might be nice to do. The art of the dance as a whole -- both inside and outside the educational field -- has gone through a half century of phenomenal inner growth and outward expansion and is fairly bursting at the seams; it must accordingly be provided with new and more elastic garments, as it were, not only to cover its present needs but also to allow for its continued growth.
>
> It is actually not very long ago as years are counted that dance in education was little more than a "finishing school" frill concerned with young ladies' grace and deportment. How remote that seems now! The young ladies have been joined by the young men, all equally vital, and together they are devoting bodies, minds, creative compulsions to a total cultural commitment of somewhat overwhelming scope. From recreation the dance has burgeoned, indeed, into re-creation -- into broad social involvement, into psychological as well physical therapy, into the dedicated evolvement of works of art and professional careers as artists.
>
> No wonder that the conference members included philosophers and performers, therapists and musicians, ballet dancers, modern dancers, designers and choreographers along with the specialists in higher education per se. It is well that they were all there, for they are all part of the pressing future. Certainly their animated discussions should provide provocative soul - searching's for practical paths to follow. The prospect ahead and its challenges are excitingly exigent.
>
> John Martin
> Dance Critic Emeritus
> New York Times [49]

The American Dance Symposium: 1968

The last important national conference considered here is one that has often been overlooked in the literature: the American Dance Symposium, held in Wichita, Kansas, August 20 - 23, 1968. The Symposium was planned and organized by members of the Kansas Dance Councils Inc. and faculty of the Wichita State University:

> The American Dance Symposium, sponsored by the Kansas Dance Councils Inc., with the assistance of the Wichita State University, will bring the pioneers of American dance and leaders of following generations to Wichita to discuss, demonstrate, and teach from August 20 - 23, 1968....Walter Terry, dance editor for The Saturday Review, who will moderate all sessions of the symposium, has called it 'the major dance event of the year'.
> [50]

The Symposium's driving force was Mrs. Alice Bauman, a Wichita native and dance educator who, with her twin sister Elizabeth Sherbon, had done much to generate interest in dance in higher education in Kansas. In the late 1920's, Alice and Elizabeth attended the University of Kansas as undergraduates. They went on to the University of Iowa for graduate degrees in physical education and both attended summer sessions at the University of Wisconsin with Margaret H'Doubler. The Sherbon sisters attended and taught at Bennington College during the Bennington summer sessions. Alice Sherbon served as "Sub-Chairman, Section 1," of "The Committee on Percussion Accompaniment for Dance" and reported on "The use of percussion instruments commonly used, with suggested methods for ways to play them," for the 1934 Bennington School of the Dance. [51] Both listed teaching and performance experiences in the mid to late 1930's with Martha Graham and company in their individual vitae. In the 1950's, Alice and Elizabeth returned to Kansas and eventually assumed teaching positions respectively at the municipal University of Wichita and the University of Kansas at Lawrence.

In an article for the *Wichita Sunday Eagle*, dated June 23, 1968, reporter Dolores Hills quotes Bauman on planning the Symposium, "...I had read in one of our trade journals that the National Endowment for the Arts had given the University of California $10,000 for local people to talk about the pioneers and history of dance. I said, 'For $10,000 we could get the artists themselves.' "[52] No one can be certain if Bauman was referring to the Developmental Conference on Dance in the above quote or not. However, Bauman and collaborators did raise money to "get the artists themselves" and invited prominent dance performers, educators, and scholars to an ambitious three-day event that included master classes, concerts, discussions, and demonstrations. Participants of the Symposium included Charles Weidman, José Limón, Martha Hill, Walter Terry, Bella Lewitsky, Paul Taylor, Daniel Nagrin, Jean Erdman, Juana de Laban, Bruce King, and Myron Nadel. Ruth St. Denis had accepted an invitation to be present at the Symposium but passed away at the age of 91, two weeks before the opening sessions. [53]

The American Dance Symposium was significant for dance in higher education in that it brought professional and academic dance leaders together in Wichita, Kansas - the nation's center. This was the first time such a strong presence for dance had come to the nation's heartland. Conference participants remember a feeling of great excitement and possibility following the Symposium. [54] Public Symposium performances marked the first national exposure for west-coast choreographer Bella Lewitsky. The Symposium's organization prompted participant Jean Erdman to return to New York and begin organizing the New York State College Dance Festival, which served as a model for the later development of the American College Dance Festival (discussed in the next chapter). In 1969 the American Dance Symposium was held again in Wichita with a new cast of dance professionals and educators. Unfortunately the Symposium came to an end in 1970 due to a lack of funds and interest. Alice Bauman worked without success for several years thereafter to promote a Mid-America Center for the Dance in Wichita, Kansas.

The 1960's was a decade of significant and dramatic development for dance in higher education. At the beginning of the decade dance educators still questioned whether or not dance was, or could be, an academic discipline. By the end of the 1960's this question was no longer central to their debate. Now new concerns arose from dramatic increases in student enrollments and the development of standards in the curriculum. In the 1970's dance in higher education experienced the full effects of the Dance Boom as the numbers of dance majors in undergraduate and graduate programs increased significantly.

216

CHAPTER 10

The 1970's: The 'Dance Boom' in Higher Education.

The 1960's are regarded as a decade of great change in American culture, but they did not begin and end within the strict time frame of ten years. In the case of national politics, for example, the 60's might be viewed as the years between President Kennedy's assassination in November of 1963, and Richard Nixon's resignation as President in August of 1974. In American higher education, the decade of challenge and change that came to be represented by the moniker "the 60's," roughly corresponds with this political time frame. As a center for social change and political confrontation, the college campus played host to a number of social and intellectual awakenings that began in the early 1960's and lasted into the early years of the 1970's. The Civil Rights movement began in earnest in 1962, and student protests of the Vietnam conflict spanned the period 1964 - 1973. Both issues fed off of, and into, the gathering strength of demands by students and other minorities (people of color and diverse ethnic origin, women, gays and lesbians) for access to the power centers and decision making processes of American higher education. The broad student population pressed for revisions to academic requirements and an expansion in areas of study. Students also wanted a greater say in the organization and governance of the university, desiring input on the range of academic programs, issues of appointment and tenure, and student representation in all aspects of university life. Specific action groups pressured academic administrators and the professoriate for greater opportunity for minorities in hiring and inclusion in the mainstream of scholarly discourse. The tidal forces unleashed in academe in the 1960's are still shaping the landscape of higher education.

For dance, the years between 1965 and 1980 represent a 15 year period that many dance educators affectionately remember as the years of the "dance boom," a period of significant and sustained growth in the numbers of students pursuing a dance major, and in the number of departments offering this degree. Gertrude Lippincott first used this term in "Report of the Arts; In Government, Education, Community 1965," discussed in the previous chapter: "When one glances through the DANCE DIRECTORY issues by the National Section on Dance, one sees lists of many institutions with numerous programs and courses in dance. It would look as though dance in education was 'booming'." [1] As a descriptor for the phenomenal growth of dance in America's colleges and universities during this period her term entered the lexicon rather quickly.

Why was there a dance boom in American higher education? This question has been posed to many colleagues. Paraphrased, their answers focus on three basic premises:

'It was the economy. The economy, especially between 1963 and the oil embargo of 1973, was so good that many students enrolled in majors that weren't typically vocational.'

'The dance boom was largely the result of the "baby boom," there were just more students to go around.'

'The dance boom was stimulated by federal and state funding for the arts. The creation of the National Endowment for the Arts, the Great Society programs of the Johnson Administration, and the creation of State Arts Councils made it possible for dancers to make a living (and therefore made the study of dance vocationally viable).'

All three of these themes factor into developing a rational for the dance boom. Certainly the economy in the United States during the years of the Vietnam conflict, and leading up to the 1973 energy crisis was strong. Real wages and standards of living rose yearly. Blue and white collar jobs paid a wage that

218

permitted workers to support children in college. Fees for higher education, particularly in public institutions were very low. In some states a resident with a high school diploma could enroll in a public university without fee. A college age baby boom generation filled campuses with students, and universities were increasingly willing to experiment with new curricula. Federal and state support for the arts was new, generous, and regular. But there may be more to the phenomenon of the dance boom. To better understand the explosion in the numbers of dance major students during the 15 year period 1965 - 1980, one must also consider other social, educational, and cultural factors.

Robert Roemer discusses shifts in the preferred fields of study for bachelor's degrees in the 1970's and includes data for dance in "Vocationalism in Higher Education: Explanation from Social Theory," for *The Review of Higher Education*. Roemer defines vocationalism in higher education as interest in the pursuit of studies that lead directly to occupational competence. An educational program is vocationally relevant in two ways - mastery of subject matter as prerequisite for entrance into an occupation, and mastery of subject matter leading to occupational competence. The first case may be illustrated by the necessity of a terminal degree for a position in university teaching (the degree is necessary), and the second case by entrance into the occupation of law, where procedural knowledge is necessary and specific tests must be passed.

Roemer argues that vocationalism in the 1970's was closely related to an increased interest in specific preparation for occupational competence. [2] In his study Roemer charts the conferral of degrees for Fine and Applied Arts in the following categories: general, art, art history, music (performance), music (liberal arts), music history, dramatic arts, dance, applied design, cinematography, photography and, 'other.' Referencing data compiled by the National Center for Educational Statistics, Roemer reports that the number of BFA degrees in dance 1970 - 1971, for men and women, was 297. By 1977 - 1978 this figure had increased to 886, a gain over 1970 - 71 enrollments of 198.3%. Of the arts disciplines listed, comparing graduation figures for 1970 - 1971 and 1977 - 1978

219

respectively, cinematography experienced the greatest overall increase in conferral of degrees with an increase of 830.0%, followed by dance (198.3%). Photography is listed next with an increase of 101%, followed by the category of Music History with 76.0%. Breaking down the numbers for dance further, Roemer's figures show a 317.4% increase in degrees awarded to male students in dance during this period [70 - 71 = 23; 77 - 78 = 96], and a 288.3% (see note 3 for explanation of mathematical error) increase for female students [70 - 71 = 274; 77 - 78 = 790]. [3]

Apparently dance had come to be a discipline where the student could expect to acquire an appropriate level of occupational competence in their undergraduate training. From the "Current College Controversy" of 1966, where preparation for occupational competence was hotly debated, to the field moving further away from a purely aesthetic vision for dance in higher education in the early 1970's, a change in educational dance was realized as more and more students felt secure in pursuing a college dance major expecting to have a career in dance following graduation. I am struck by which disciplines are the leaders in increased enrollments in Roemer's statistics: cinematography and dance. As Roemer does not attempt to explain increases in enrollments by academic discipline, the reader is left to posit possible explanations for such increases in cinematography and dance. Besides the competency and preparation necessary for success in either of these fields, or the employment opportunities that may or may not have been waiting for graduates, there may have been other reasons that cinematography and dance lead the arts in academic enrollment during this period.

Both cinematography and dance were new major fields of study in academe. Their respective newness suggested experimentation, individuality, and a holistic approach to art making. A hallmark of student attitudes in the '60's, which spilled over into the early years of the 1970's, was an intellectual and spiritual search for self. This may or may not have been grounded in a considered, strategic plan for a vocational future, but nonetheless, the search for self-influenced decision making in education was a characteristic of student life during this period. This idealism was coupled with a determined effort to connect life's work to one's sense of individuality as that merged with one's sense of shared humanity.

Because I was one of those undergraduate dance majors during the years of the dance boom (1972 - 1978), I have my own views on why so many of us were going to college to dance. I remember students being excited about cinematography and dance, and about other new majors in college, like ecology, political geography, cultural anthropology, dance therapy, and even human consciousness. These new major areas of study were developed by a faculty interested in expanding the intellectual paradigm for higher education. New fields allowed new avenues in discourse and scholarship. Students enrolling in new disciplines felt at the forefront of what was thought to be a new direction in higher education; a sense of vocational preparation and theoretical knowledge coming together to be used to make a difference; we were connecting profession to pleasurable life learning and active involvement with humans and human issues. Study in these areas addressed a popular animosity young people had toward the dogmas of education and profession. The traditional college experience was associated with an image of the complacent student becoming the "numbed office worker," the "mindless bureaucrat," or the "cog"; captured in such films as *The Graduate* (1967). Interest in new areas of study in higher education stemmed, at least in part, from fear that a sentient, exploring, and life-curious youth, would become like their parents: which, in our own archetypal thinking meant dull, conformist, and mindlessly obedient to authority. This is not to suggest that all-American youth in the 16 - 25 age range circa 1971 were of this mind set, but certainly many were. The sense that college preparation was to prepare us for the work we would need to do to change the world or simply make a difference was common. [4]

An important component of the disciplines of cinematography and dance was movement and individual expression through movement. Movement was identified with personal development, societal boundaries overcome, a rejection of the Descartian split of body and mind, and a seemingly unlimited opportunity for meaningful, artistic investigation. In the case of film making the allure of a possible future life in Hollywood and the potential of huge financial rewards did not deter the less idealistic among us. Popular and artistic notions of the expressive, non-conformist self dominated both mediums during this period. In cinema and in dance art makers were exploring ideas of personal and social identification, disregarding accepted boundaries of art, behavior, and class, and deconstructing norms of sexuality, gender, and the body. Images and concepts of the celebrated and disciplined body were infused throughout popular culture. Dance addressed both these concerns, and the dedicated dancer took on a popular image in the 1970's that was unheard of just a few short years before. Popular television shows, as diverse as *Kung Fu* and *Fame*, promised everything from higher consciousness and a natural high, to celebrated stardom through disciplined and aesthetic use the body. Books and magazines opined on the importance of body-language and body-building. The old rules of how we were to 'live' in the body fell by the wayside as the physical-self took on a renewed cultural importance. Such factors may have played a role in enticing students to dance in higher education.

Turning back to more pragmatic issues of occupational-vocationalism in higher education, a number of factors contributed to programmatic growth and increases in enrollments in dance in the 1960's and '70's. Throughout this period the new dance program focused on professional art standards in performance, choreography, and teaching. The word was out that the best dance programs were becoming professional, and that a professional level of training in dance was becoming more and more common and available. More students could expect to be prepared and accepted professionally following graduation. Faculty with academic credentials were needed as departments developed and the number of faculty positions increased. Occupational competence for teaching dance in higher education demanded many abilities and skills. Training in the subject matter of dance could be well attended to in the focused environment of higher education.

Occupational competency outside of education was supported by the college degree, especially in teaching, grant writing and in competition for state and federal funding. The opportunity for students to refine their skills in performance, choreography, and teaching in a quality college dance program helped develop their survival skills outside of the university.

University preparation was much more beneficial for the emerging modern dance performer-teacher-choreographer than it was for the ballet artist. Vocational training in ballet was still viewed as properly taking place in the professional training academy. Because the successful ballet artist was expected to exhibit a greater degree of technical proficiency, as opposed to developing creative or educational skills, training in ballet began well before the student could consider higher education as an environment for occupational preparation. Ballet in higher education in this period focused on training the pedagogue and not the performer. Acquisition of a professional level of ballet technique demanded early training, and the skill of ballet choreography was best apprenticed with a master in a professional company.

The trend toward using one's college education in preparation for life's work gathered steam throughout the 19th century, and became a dominate rationale for the student's pursuit of higher learning by the middle decades of the 20th century. Following World War II, middle class Americans believed that completion of a specific college program was necessary if one wanted to join a corresponding sector of the professional work force. Roemer (1981), writes:

> Thus the growth of vocationalism that occurred in higher education in the 1970's was not just that which derives from the general relevance of a bachelor's degree to securing an occupation of high status, but rather featured an increased interest in the specific preparation for occupational performance found in some fields of study. [5]

In the case of dance, the discipline began to make its break from physical education after discovering its own sense of academic substance in the mid to late 1960's. The new dance department offered the student liberal *and* professional training that had not been clearly defined in the years dance occupied its academic

223

niche as adjunct study in physical education. The independent dance major provided the programmatic framework of academic and professional preparation for the dance artist. Quality dance departments offered dance technique, history, education, kinesiology, repertory, philosophy, and criticism. These courses provided a framework for occupational training and exposure that enabled the student to acquire the requisite knowledge to perform, to create, to teach, and to administrate following graduation. The development and expansion of federal and state sponsored support for the arts, a strong economy, the rapid growth in the number of dance major programs in higher education, and a body conscious, humanistic, educational-art-cultural milieu merged together to create an enviroment for growth. The idea that the college trained dancer could actually use their degree to make a living was not too far off the mark. The dance major's job potential after graduation was part individual initiative and part pioneering adventure.

American College Dance Festival

Expansion in the educational field of dance led to the development of state and regional college dance festivals. As a means for program recruitment and student-faculty development, dance festivals were a symbol of a dynamic new force in college arts. The National Dance Guild [ADG] organized the first regional festival in 1968. The following "PressTime News" notice appeared in the April 1968 issue of *Dance Magazine*:

> College Dance Festival Planned:
> Mid Atlantic Regional Organization for University and College Dance - Festivals, Sponsored by the National Dance Guild and organized by Miss Martha Darby: "As far as we know, we are the first region to organize and hold a college festival of this kind. We hope that, in doing so, we shall contribute to the raising of dance as a performing art in colleges and universities. [6]

Following her experience attending the American Dance Symposium in Wichita, Kansas, Jean Erdman began organizing a national organization for college dance. Erdman and fellow educator Betty Lind presented their ideas to a group of interested individuals at the University of Pittsburgh in 1971. The first pilot

224

festival was held on that campus in 1973. Adjudicators Hanya Holm, Marian Van Tuyl, and Rod Rogers traveled to 65 eastern colleges (representing college dance in New York, Ohio, Pennsylvania and West Virginia) and viewed choreography from which dances were selected for two inaugural concerts.[7]

The ACDF's first regional festival provides a context for further understanding the thinking of the young women and men who chose dance as a college major in the 1970's. The festival was critically reviewed for *Dance Magazine* by Robb Baker in an article titled: "Frisbees and Unicycles Versus the Politics of Paternalism." Baker took the festival's organization and faculty to task for their conservative tastes and paternalistic views. In context with the previous discussion on the goals of students enrolling in college programs during the dance boom, Baker's article permits us to listen in on the thoughts of a dance major circa 1973:

> The first regional American College Dance Festival was held March 9 - 13 in Pittsburgh. It was a good idea - to create the same sense of identity and cooperation between college dance departments across the country that the National Association for Regional Ballet had achieved for civic dance companies....[B]ut the conference had one big, bad flaw right down the middle that threatened to overshadow its more positive aspects - and that does not bode well for the organization....[H]ere was a college dance festival at which the opinions and attitudes of college students were all but forgotten - in the planning, in the evaluation, in almost all the decision making. The organization was instead paternalistic, completely faculty - and administration - oriented (there were also a few outsiders - with no connection to college dance whatsoever - in on the policy sessions)....
> ...The final straw came on the closing day of the conference, at an organizational meeting to set up a permanent college dance association. After a snappy adaptation of the bylaws, which the temporary committee recommended (to the fifty or so college representatives left) a list of thirty one names to serve the permanent executive committee. Not a single student was on the list. The temporary committee members even seemed shocked that the question should be raised. There had been no students on the national planning committee; why should there be now? [8]

The tone of Baker's article is caught between a finger wag at bossy parental figures and a constructive warning. He questions the professional-educational tradition in dance, and perhaps, irritated a few of his targets in the process. At the dawn of wide spread acceptance of dance as an academic discipline Baker harshly took some of its leaders to task for their beliefs. In retrospect, the nature, tone, and substance of Baker's critique is not surprising given campus activities and student-faculty relations in the previous 7 - 8 years. However, 1973 was just on the waning side of the nadir of the years of student confrontation and rebellion. The Watergate scandal was gaining momentum, and the Vietnam War, while winding down, was certainly not over. The kind of student drawn to dance in higher education at this time could generally be classified as liberal. Certainly, those who gravitated toward creative, modern dance had a developed sense of individualism. Baker's article allows us to segue for a moment into the nature of an important cultural shift that, at the same time dance was gaining its academic independence, was impacting and changing the ways in which student's perceived their role in their education.

By the early 1970's, movement among modern dancers and choreographers, exemplified by the work of the performers who held avant-garde concerts at New York City's Judson Church, was gaining in stature and broad appeal in professional dance. The Judson Church, located on the south edge of Washington Square Park in the City's Greenwich Village, gained recognition in the early 1960's for hosting experimental performance works by poets, dancers, musicians, and actors. Post 'Judson,' experiment and a happy deconstruction of tradition in dance theory, performance, and choreography was in the air. In the early 1970's this new dance, was termed "post-modern dance." It was meant to be, "... a lifelike experience where chance, non-sequitur, choice, [and] imagination all come into play." [9]

Until the 1960's and the advent of post-modernism, dance, in both its professional and academic settings, had been about a culture of compliance. In the professional world the dancer is the physical vehicle for the choreographer's kinetic-artistic vision. One doesn't join a company and expect to question or make demands of the choreographer; just as one was not expected to enroll as a dance major and seriously question the policies and practices of the faculty. The transference of professional attitudes of compliance into the university studio was implicitly understood and expected. Subjective opinions about an appropriate body type, levels of technical virtuosity, demeanor, and potential in artistic talent

226

permeated the culture of the professional dance world. By the time Baker attended this first Regional-American College Dance Festival, these cultural norms were well entrenched in the academic world as well. Directive, control, and sometimes ridicule (Louis Horst, for instance, was famous for his ability to embarrass choreography students), were considered means to subjugate, discipline, and shape the dancer. On the other hand, student activism in the 1960's led to an expectation that they would be players in the decision making processes of education. This was as true for college majors in political science as it was for those in dance. Baker's article suggests the conflict in values that was a prominent feature of college life in this period.

Commenting on faculty responses to student choreography Baker reports some positive experiences and some close-mindedness, overt bias, and dismissive commentary: "One gentlemen stated flatly, 'Most of this stuff isn't ready to be shown anywhere. At least it should be put on a gym floor, not a stage'." [10] Baker has praise for faculty that encourage individual interpretation, freedom of expressivity, and student-faculty dialogue, and shows no fear in confronting those who, perhaps, were not so inclined. Apparently, in Pittsburgh, the traditional teacher had run into the new student:

> For years the dance world has been figuratively castrating individual dancers, telling them they have to conform to "ideal" physical types, robbing them of any spark of individualism (hair style, etc.) they may attempt to assert. Young people today have realized the psychological dangers of this and no longer buy such out-dated standards - in art or personal politics. The exciting thing about college dance today is its possibility, its freedom, its openness to new forms and ideas. Students are sick of being told who "should" and "shouldn't" dance, in the same way they're sick of being presented with all the other rules and regulations and taxation's without representation that have led to student dissent over the last twenty years. If an American Regional College Dance Festival is to offer real value to contemporary college dance students, it must go after the freedom, the vitality, the freshness of college life of today...not the paternalistic platitudes of the past. [11]

Mr. Baker's monograph captures the feelings many of the children of the counter-culture had faced when they felt the startling rigidity of their teachers. Relativism, a hallmark of the "I'm OK, You're OK" generation, clashed with the absolutism of the professional dance world as it was transplanted into the academic environment. The dance program's weight contracts, interest in physical types (and the all important issue of hair), and other "out-dated standards" did not sit well with a liberal, relativist, democratically influenced, government suspicious, pre-Watergate dance student. To be sure, not all students were of Baker's ilk, and many were content to buy into traditions, especially if they happened to easily fit the mold. But another part of the student population was ready to generate its own academic *NO Manifesto* for dance. [12]

After a rough start the American College Dance Festival Association (ACDFA) grew steadily. Today the ACDFA is a strong and dynamic organization dedicated to the regional presentation and adjudication of outstanding choreography by students and teachers of dance in higher education. Regional festivals culminate annually in a Regional Gala Concert, and bi-annually at a National ACDFA Festival held in Washington, D.C.. [13]

The Council of Dance Administrators

From the cultural clash between those who would throw Frisbees, and those who would have their student's hair under control, I turn back to organized activity for dance in higher education. Coinciding with the dance boom in the colleges was the development of an organization specifically focused on the issues and matters facing dance as an academic discipline; the Council of Dance Administrators (CODA). Throughout the years of the dance boom, CODA was the only organization with a nationally representative membership to focus exclusively on dance in the university. Because CODA's history and development is so tightly coupled with the evolution of dance in the academy, the Council's function in the 1970's and 1980's reflects many of the key issues for dance in American higher education. For these reasons, the Council's history and progress are important to our story. A detailed look at CODA's process and work provides contexts for understanding the history of dance in higher education in the late decades of the 20th century.

The Council's history begins following the Developmental Conference of 1966 - 1967. Between 1968 and 1970 a small group of attendees who managed dance departments organized and began to sketch out a mission for their organization. In its first manifestation, CODA was meant to be an informal group of like-minded dance educators who, having suddenly found themselves administrating, were in search of their own support group. The informal and closed nature of CODA's membership and function was an important and carefully guarded aspect of their group culture. Members appreciated the small size of CODA. This allowed for detailed discussion and a sense that progress was being made with the issues dance administrators faced. Agenda and summary documents generated by the Council trace its development over time and act as a longitudinal reference for what members attended to in CODA. Agendas list the topics of interest and summary documents outline the substance of CODA meetings beginning in 1970.

In 1972, the original group of 10 dance administrators discussed a greater degree of formal organization and began to call themselves the "Dance Administrators Council." In a memo from CODA President Alma Hawkins to group members dated July 12, 1973 "re: Dance Administrators Council Meeting," Hawkins asks; "How do you like our new name? I think it is a good one." [14] The Summary Notes for the Council's November 1973 meetings is titled "Council of Dance Administrators." Somewhere in the interim, the group changed its moniker (for the sake of consistency the acronym CODA is used for all references to this group).

The CODA agenda for the 1972 meeting lists "limiting incoming majors" as the first item of discussion. Summary notes for the 1972 meetings state, "All departments are concerned about the increased number of students seeking admission to the dance major. Critical aspects relate to limited space, faculty load, and competence of the student." [15] The competency issue was compounded by the fact that most students interested in a dance major knew very little about the discipline, and had never been exposed to the demanding nature of dance in their previous educational experiences. CODA summary notes for 1972 conclude with a listing of current practices in admissions for 6 member institutions, the: Florida State University, Ohio State University, University of Maryland, University of Utah, University of California, Los-Angeles, and State University of New York-College at Purchase. Each program defines their respective admission policies, with some auditioning students, and others having to accept majors through university admissions. The topic of concern over the large numbers of majors and the basis for their admission appears at or near the top of the agenda for CODA meetings again in 1973 and 1974.

By 1975, the Council agenda begins to reveal the developing complexity of the new dance administrators job. As an example of the range of the business Council members attended to, consider the following outline of their 1976 agenda:

University of California - Los Angeles
Department of Dance
CODA Meeting
Marina International Hotel - November 1976
Agenda

Curriculum/Teaching
1. Undergraduate Program - How much flexibility?
2. Graduate - What about the individually tailored program?
3. Standards of written work for majors with performance/choreography emphasis.
4. Grading - How does the department handle it?
5. Course evaluation questionnaire.
6. ·Evaluation of the dance major program.
7. How to establish development and continuity in technique and choreography classes? How to evaluate?
8. Dance theory and philosophy - How do you teach it?
9. How are the developments in society that influence the dance art form related to our classes?
10. New directions in dance therapy.
11. Teacher preparation in public schools.
12. Problems of expanding the dance program in the university.

Administration/Faculty
13. Faculty evaluation and promotion criteria.
14. Tenure - What to do when the department feels held back by a tenured person?
15. Affirmation (*sic*) action guidelines:
   a) employment of faculty and musicians.
   b) promotion/tenure situations,
16. Liability insurance for faculty - other legal aspects of liability?
17. Teaching load - how to weigh different responsibilities i.e. technique, composition, lecture, supervision etc.?
18. Audition/assessment procedure - How detailed? Follow up?

230

19.	How to attract strong TA's for teaching?
20.	How to provide adequate performance opportunities for undergraduates?
21.	Guest artist residency - How to integrate with the regular program? What responsibilities?
22.	Exchange programs
	a) for faculty choreographers in a 4 week period?
	b) for student/faculty in CODA institutions?
23.	Accreditation standards for dance departments? Minimal facilities, FTE, etc.?
24.	Degrees - advantage and disadvantage of BA/BFA.
25.	Ph.D. programs - where - how?
26.	Budget - How can one generate more funds?
27.	Scholarships/grants in the university.
28.	Grants - How to use them in the dance department?

General

29.	National Dance Organization - Is the National Dance Association the answer?
30.	Prospect for an International Dance Convention & Travel/study.
31.	Major dance festival in Hawaii.
32.	Memberships in CODA
33.	Place for meeting in 1977 - coordinator - who?

16

Most items listed above are in the form of questions, indicating the degree to which the Council's members were still clarifying programmatic issues and their individual role's as dance administrators.

Since the establishment of the first dance programs in higher education, standards for curricular quality and breadth had been key issues for dance educators. Recall Walter Terry's admonition to the field to come together on this issue in his 1940 article on "Collegiate Dance": "The diversity of approach is reflected in the collegiate dance to such a degree that a plea for recognized standards of dance education would probably be tossed aside as the ravings of a dance faddist." [17] Other commentary on the need for curricular and programmatic standards followed in the 1950's and 1960's. [18] Necessity finally stimulated real change in this direction in the 1970's.

Item # 23 in CODA's 1976 agenda concerns "Accreditation standards for dance departments...?" This topic resurfaces as discussion item #15 in 1976 CODA summary notes. The pursuit and articulation of dance major standards emerged as the central matter of concern for CODA well into the next decade.

Summary notes for 1976 suggest the tone Council discussions took regarding discipline based standards:

> 15.   Accreditation: -- We recognized that we need standards and guidelines which could help new departments and also be used for evaluative purposes in other departments. It was pointed out that accreditation could have negative as well as positive benefits.
>
> After considerable discussion, we decided that we are not ready for the official type of accreditation. Instead it seems desirable that at this time we establish an intermediate step whereby we set up standards and develop a consulting service within CODA membership. Consultants would be paid an honorarium and travel expenses. The purpose would be evaluation of faculty and program in relation to the standards.
>
> It was stressed that some formal approach to evaluation is critical because if we do not have a plan in the near future some institutions may set up their own scheme. It was thought that a plan sponsored by CODA would probably meet this need. [19]

The comment that "some institutions may set up their own scheme," refers to other organizations that were also considering the topic of standards. Standards had become a concern for studio based, professional-educational programs in dance. Within the field of other educational dance organizations, the National Dance Association of AAHPER (the Dance Division of AAHPER evolved into the National Dance Association of AAHPER in 1974), was taking a position on the need for standards in the undergraduate major in dance, as was the American Dance Guild.

By the early 1970's, schools and programs in dance training had developed as a significant source of income for internationally recognized dance artists and their companies. The Martha Graham School of Contemporary Dance, the Merce Cunningham Studio, and the School of the Dance Theater of Harlem for example, were informed that federally recognized accreditation was necessary for prospective students to be eligible for government supported loans and financial aid. Representatives of the professional schools approached the offices of existing arts-related accreditation agencies for information and help in organizing an accreditation agency for dance. The National Association of Schools of Music (NASM), created in 1924, and the National Association of Schools of Art and

Design (NASAD), founded in 1944, were already well established, and plans to establish a National Association of Schools of Theatre were in progress.

In 1977, members of the Council met twice, in June and again in November, to discuss the issue of discipline based standards. CODA summary notes from the June 23 - 25, 1977 meetings provide an interesting perspective on their desire to play a central role in contributing to the evolution of standards in dance education:

> Guidelines -- agreed that we have a pressing need for updated guidelines and some kind of procedure for accreditation. Established standards would (a) help protect the quality of dance programs and avoid proliferation of inadequate majors, (b) serve as guidelines for established departments who face changes in institutional patterns, and (c) provide criteria for Institutions and official evaluating committees such as internal reviews, state level evaluation, and National accreditation bodies.
>
> Music, Art, and Theater have developed standards and have accreditation plans....The NDA has done some work on standards. The results are published in an AAHPER pamphlet; "Undergraduate Professional Preparation." This publication reaches teachers in physical education more than dance departments. Also, Dance Guild [American Dance Guild] has been talking about standards. Both groups have expressed interest in some kind of approval procedure.
>
> Agreed-- that CODA is the appropriate organization to develop standards and explore approval procedures....Since members of this group are responsible for the original guidelines published in *Impulse* 1968, it seems logical that we continue the process of development and refinement of standards that reflect our best understandings about dance programs for today.
>
> We felt that if dance programs are to be evaluated, CODA is the most appropriate organization, because of our background and relationship to higher education.
>
> 16. Procedure for Working -- Decided on three stages.
>
> First Stage -- Agreed that the first step should be the development of standards and guidelines. The results should be published in an attractive, concise brochure, and sent to colleges throughout the US.
> Funding for publication and circulation needs to be explored. Possible sources might be our universities, Office of Education, or other funding agencies.
> Second Step - After completion of standards, members of our group could be made available to Institutions for visitation and consulting roles. Such a practice could help with interpretation and provide assistance to institutions in the process of developing new programs.
> Third Step - Establish a plan for granting approval and accreditation.
> We were clear about the first step but not so clear about accreditation procedures. However, we felt we should inform the Office of Education Accreditation committee about our current work and projected plan. [20]

This information provides a context and reference for the Council's work during the period 1977-1982. Because CODA was the only organization whose sole mission was to address the vicissitudes of dance in the university, and its membership - albeit small and closed to those not invited - reflected a national sample of leaders in university dance, Council member's felt they were the "appropriate organization" to take on the task of developing standards for dance. While CODA continued to attend to the practical issues of budget, administration, facilities, faculty-staff issues, and program implementation, the need for establishing curricular and programmatic standards for dance major programs was increasingly their central focus.

In November of 1977 the Council met for the second time that year, again in California, "The primary task of this conference was to develop a statement on standards for the dance major program." [21] The draft document titled "Standards for Dance Major Curricula" was completed at this time. Its contents include outlines for undergraduate curriculum, degree requirements, admission practices, faculty, scheduling and support staff, facilities and equipment, budget, advising, library, and publications. Similar considerations were attended to for the "Graduate-Master's Degree Program." [22]

The Council's 1978 meetings, held on November 24 - 25, were devoted to revision and completion of the "Standards for Dance Major Curricula" and discussion on a variety of related issues, including the recent creation of a Joint Commission on Dance and Theatre Accreditation. The existing accreditation agencies for the arts were contacted during the year to offer the Council's assistance in creating accreditation standards, and suggest their cooperation in developing a corresponding accreditation agency for dance. The National Association of Schools of Music and the National Association of Schools of Art and Design, in cooperation with the International Council of Fine Arts Deans (ICFAD), the Office of Arts Accreditation in Higher Education, and the Council on Post Secondary Accreditation (COPA) suggested plans for structuring national accreditation agencies for dance and theater. To facilitate federal acceptance of accreditation agencies for dance and theater, a Joint Commission for Dance and Theater Accreditation (JCDTA) was formed by these groups in 1978, funded in part by a Ford Foundation grant of $14,000.00. [23] 1978 CODA summary notes comment on the creation of the JCDTA outlining the way in which the JCDTA was formed and for whom it would act:

> Alma [Hawkins] reported on correspondence and reviewed the document which set forth the purpose and the plan of the Commission. The Commission is sponsored by the National Association of Schools of Music and the National Association of Schools of Art [and Design]. This accreditation plan is designed for professional (non-degree granting) institutions and does not cover mutidisciplinary degree granting institutions.
> Agreed that CODA should keep in touch with the Commission and be available for discussions and meetings.

Council members also considered the impact of more formalized relations with other organizations in the field on the Council's structure and process:

> [W]e reaffirmed our strong feelings about protecting the structure of CODA and our way of functioning as a process oriented group. However, we did agree that it seems appropriate at this time for us to establish some minimal organizational pattern which might facilitate our working with national professional groups....
>
> We agreed to take the following steps:
> a.   To identify CODA as an unincorportated association.
> b.   To develop a statement about CODA which includes the nature of the organization, purpose, method of functioning, and membership policy.
> c.   To have elected officers, which includes president, vice president, secretary, and treasurer.
> d.   To not establish dues at this time. [24]

An interesting off-shoot of CODA's discussion about accreditation standards, the field, and the future is represented in this next entry in 1978 summary notes. Issues of CODA's internal formalization and the organizational environment for dance were of increasing concern. The move toward internal formalization was necessary for CODA to be recognized and to solidify its place in the field. A strategic assessment of where CODA stood in relation to like organizations, with the realization that inter-organizational dialogues were important for all groups to succeed, is an interesting predictor for the evolution of the organizational environment for dance education:

> V.   Relationships Among Dance Organizations
>   1.   [W]e discussed the need for some kind of organized national effort on the part of dance people, individuals and groups.

....[I]t seems most unlikely that the various dance organizations can or will become one professional group. Each organization seems to have a particular thrust to its work and a way of functioning. Perhaps, though, it might be possible for us to clarify and recognize the specific nature and purpose of each group. Could we then form a kind of "alliance" that would give a unified national front and yet let each group pursue its own specific goals?

...[T]he main thrust of different organizations seems to be as follows:

National Dance Association	Concerned with dance in education, all levels. Quality of programs, teaching and research
[American] Dance Guild	Concerns are similar to those of NDA. Membership includes professional studio people as well as educators
C.O.R.D. [Congress on Research in Dance]	Concerned with research in dance, especially history, ethnology and anthropology
American Dance Festival	Concerned with dance as a performing art and furthering the quality of the experience.
C.O.D.A.	Concerned with shaping dance departments and developing quality major programs.

If an "alliance" type structure would be feasible, we could develop a united front on legislative matters as well as funding, avoid duplication in our professional work, and have a stronger base to work on issues such as accreditation.

....[W]e should explore this kind of possibility with the presidents of the four dance organizations. Alma was asked to make contact with the presidents to see if they would be interested in a spring meeting that would allow us to explore the possibility of an alliance structure. [25]

Unfortunately 1979 CODA summary notes indicate that CODA's efforts in coalescing the energies of other groups in the organizational field were not successful. Following their attempt at generating cooperative relationships between dance organizations with a stake in dance in the university, Council attention was shifted back to the matter of accreditation:

Item X Accreditation:
Winter '79 meeting of dance organizations in New York to discuss possibility of alliance of such organizations to be responsible for accreditation of college dance major programs was unproductive....Sam Hope and Washington Office of Education may be approached to get information on accreditation to bring to May meeting. Alma agreed to do this.

Item XI CODA Organization:
We agreed to be an unincorporated organization concerned with:
a. Development of guidelines for the shaping of dance major programs
b. Improving and maintaining the quality of dance major programs.
c. Identifying problems and current needs.
d. Sharing ideas and ways of working as administrators.
We are a process oriented group. Discussion topics emerge from current concerns of the membership.

Item XI, goes on to describe how an institution could join CODA, and the desirability of inviting members who can, "...work together harmoniously. In general, however, it was agreed the memberships reside with institutions rather than with individuals." Charter members were allowed to retain their individual membership indefinitely. CODA membership would be limited to 20 institutions. Officers were elected for three year terms. A statement on the nature and purpose of CODA would be generated by Alma Hawkins for approval in May. [26]

In May of 1980, Council members were introduced to Samuel Hope, Executive Director of the Office of Arts Accreditation in Higher Education. Hope was invited to the Council's meeting to review the processes necessary for accreditation, and to discuss the agenda of the Joint Commission for Dance and Theater Accreditation (JCDTA).

Hope informed Council member's of the two types of accreditation in American education - 1) regional, institutional accreditation (for colleges, universities, research laboratories, and other institutions receiving federal monies), and 2) specialized accreditation for professions; accreditation agencies for programs within institutions. He explained that in 1980 two such Accreditation associations existed for the arts, the NASM and the NASAD. These accreditation agencies were approved and monitored by the Council on Post Secondary Accreditation (COPA), which was designed to manage accreditation so that it did not intrude on an individual institution's legitimate mission or function. The

COPA endeavored to control over-zealous activity on the part of accreditors, and maintained ethical standards. Accreditation agencies and councils were monitored in turn by the US Office of Education (changed to the Department of Education by President Jimmy Carter in 1980), which oversaw and evaluated all accreditation related activities.

During the meeting with CODA members, Hope carefully outlined the history of how the process of accreditation for dance was started, and the potential benefits of accreditation for CODA members. After discussing the organizations and agencies that had guided the accreditation process to date, Hope explained that accreditation was not envisioned as a means to standardize programs, but as a mechanism for reviewing program quality given each program's institutional goals. A hallmark of accreditation in American higher education is that it is a voluntary process embarked on by a profession to insure quality and to manage the process of review by competent peer-practitioners in the field. By conducting a voluntary, yet thorough, comprehensive, and federally recognized means of evaluation and accreditation, the practitioners of academic and professional disciplines manage their own houses.

The creation of the JCDTA was initiated by directors of non-degree granting, professional institutions with an educational program. The JCDTA would, hopefully, lead to regular accrediting agencies for dance and theatre. Each new agency would then have to be in existence for three years to be officially recognized and eligible for its own federal support. Hope reported that the JCDTA was managed by the Boards of Directors of the NASM and NASAD. In order to create a comprehensive accreditation agency for dance, one that could viably manage non-degree and degree granting programs alike, Hope outlined the following steps for CODA members:

1. Agreement among a core of schools, representing both degree and non degree granting institutions to incorporate as a National Association of Schools of Dance.

2. Develop a code of operations.

238

3. Develop standards for accreditation.

4. Agree on an administrative structure for the new organization.

5. Agree on procedural documents to include:

a. A "self study" outline for institutions to complete before their review.

b. Procedural instructions for on-site review teams.

c. Procedural policies for selection of the review team.

The CODA's summary notes go on to outline the anticipated costs of institutional membership and the costs and timelines of institutional reviews. Hope considered the Council the most appropriate organization to assist in bringing degree granting programs into discussion with the non-degree institutions already working with the JCDTA:

> If we wish to proceed in the direction of accreditation as suggested....[W]e need to elect three people to attend a meeting in October to help establish documents preliminary to forming our own accrediting organization. Also we must decide whether we want joint professional school and institutional accreditation. Other disciplines have seemed to make this work. It is economically sound. (Art has a commission of 6 to deal with both. Music has two commissions.) Whatever we decide, we must accredit total disciplines rather than specialization's within the discipline (i.e. dance therapy). If we wish to work with the present commission, it could provide us with commission documents for study and evaluation. [27]

Alma Hawkins, Elizabeth Hayes, and Helen Alkire, with Nancy Smith acting as alternate (CODA's "Big Four"; a term of respect that dated back to Bennington days when Graham, Humphrey, Weidman, and Holm held the same distinction), were chosen to represent the interests of academic programs in dance at the October meeting of the JCDTA.

The creation of a National Association of Schools of Dance (NASD), one that would represent professional and academic programs in dance, is an important milestone in the history of dance in the American university. The Council of Dance Administrators grafted the needs and objectives of academic programs in dance into the working documents of the JCDTA. In October of

239

1980, Samuel Hope met with JCDTA members to begin their work. In 1981, the JCDTA was ready to agree on organizational bylaws, codes, and standards. At this meeting the NASD was formalized and voted into existence. NASD rules allowed for the acceptance of Charter memberships until June of 1982. Ten professional studio schools and 38 colleges and universities filed for charter status at this time, and in 1983 the NASD was officially recognized by the US Department of Education as the accreditation agency for dance:

> The major activities of the National Association of Schools of Dance are the accreditation of educational programs in dance and the establishment of curricular standards and guidelines. NASD is recognized by the United States Department of Education as the accrediting agency covering the field of dance. The Association is comprised of over forty member institutions, including public and private colleges, universities, and independent, professional training institutions. All NASD member institutions meet the standards and uphold the code of ethics of the Association as stated in the NASD Handbook....
> Broadly stated, the aims and objectives of the National Association of Schools of Dance are as follows:
> 1. To establish a national forum to stimulate the understanding and acceptance of the educational disciplines inherent in the creative arts in higher education in the United States.
> 2. To establish reasonable standards where quantitative measurements have validity, as in matters of budget, faculty qualifications, faculty-student ratios, library and physical facilities.
> 3. To foster the development of instruction of the highest quality while simultaneously encouraging varied and experimental approaches to the teaching of dance.
> 4. To evaluate, through the processes of accreditation, schools of dance and programs of dance instruction in terms of their quality and the results they achieve, as judged by experienced examiners.
> 5. To assure students and parents that accredited dance programs provide competent teachers, adequate physical plant and equipment, and sound curricula, and are capable of attaining their stated objectives.
> 6. To counsel and assist schools in developing their programs and to encourage self - evaluation and continuing self - improvement.
> 7. To invite and encourage cooperation of professional dance groups and individuals of reputation in the field of dance in the formulation of appropriate curricula and standards.
> 8. To maintain a national voice to be heard in matters pertaining to dance and particularly as they would affect member schools and their stated objectives. [28]

The creation of the NASD caused the Council to reflect on their place and reason for being in the organizational environment. The Council's mission was clear enough during its first ten years of function 1970 - 1980; it was a forum for participants to discuss the state of dance as an academic discipline and to discuss the role of Council members as managers of major programs in dance. But, now that a federally recognized accreditation agency existed, what was the purpose of CODA? In response to the creation of the new organization, Council members sought to clarify the group's internal sense of mission by inviting new institutional members to join, and by offering new services to dance administrators.

The Council's function throughout the 1970's was oriented toward developing and articulating standards for dance major programs. No federal agency or organization asked CODA's members to do this, they took it upon themselves to focus their work on these matters. CODA purposefully remained a "small, informal group of like minded individuals" throughout this period, taking on a self described persona in the field as the "dance mafia." [29] Although Council member's may have perceived themselves in this light, a humorous yet apt description of an organization perceived as a powerful family, the Council's activities were not universally known or recognized. In the late 1980's, in the context of a discussion I had with a dance administrator, who, according to his understanding "chaired the largest undergraduate dance program in America throughout the 1970's," I was surprised to learn he had never heard of the Council. He assured me at the time that he had no idea such an organization existed, nor was he aware of CODA during his tenure as chair. The culture of the Council, especially in the years 1970 - 1988 when CODA was led by the late Alma Hawkins, was strong, and internally focused. Following the creation of the NASD, Council member's questioned their mission and goals. Membership was expanded, and the Council began to think of how they might otherwise serve the environment. One positive initiative was CODA's 1985 "Conference on Dance Administration: Themes and Directions" at the University of Illinois at Urbana-Champaign. [30]

For some of CODA's members the group's organizational meaning came into doubt with the creation of the NASD. With CODA's commitment to participate with the JCDTA, there was discussion about the future of both organizations. But, matters of academic survival for dance, that threatened the discipline throughout the 1980's, may have delayed a true discussion on CODA's future. During an observation of the group in session in 1988, I witnessed what one founding member subsequently referred to as "our first real discussion about the future." Group members were in discussion when one Council participant raised her hand and commented "I just covered this topic at NASD last month, why am I here talking about it again?" The question was honest and very straight forward. As an observer it was interesting to note the ease with which the members of the Council turned their attention to the larger issue: why are we here? 31

The answer to this question was partially addressed in a subsequent free-flowing, and very open conversation. Council members considered the intellectual and practical overlap of their work with that of NASD, yet they also found clear ways to contextualize the unique aspects of CODA's process: a free-flowing and intuitive process of dialogue; a small, intimate group setting; a strong cultural history; no pressure to produce or comply. The Council continued to address the "why are we here?" question over the next few years, and continues to reassess its value to its members. Perhaps this is a unique attribute of an organization founded solely on shared interest; the Council's members are women and men committed to the quality and success of dance as a vital part of the American university.

For dance in higher education, the 1970's ended on a much less promising note than was presaged by the optimism of the beginning and middle years of the decade. By 1978 the nation's economy was pointed toward dramatic change. Throughout the latter 1970's, inflation ran high, and well paid, stable jobs were increasingly hard to find. International economics and global markets were undermining the lingering post-war American economic and manufacturing hegemony of the 1950's and 1960's. Corporate America was looking over its shoulder at the industrial and banking powerhouses of the Asian economies. Politically, America was finishing a period of upheaval that followed its engagement in Vietnam and the Watergate scandal of the Nixon Presidency, and turning much more toward conservative values. While American conservatism had clothed itself in economic policy, a very important part of their agenda was social, and empowered by a politically active Christian Coalition. An explicit goal of this new American conservatism was a refocusing and reclaiming of American morality and values. The man who came to symbolize this period in America history was Ronald Reagan.

CHAPTER 11

From "Boom" to "Bust": The Struggle for Survival in the Corporate University, 1980 - 1990.

Following the drama of the Iran Hostage crises and the political triumph of a resurgent Republican party in November 1980, former Hollywood actor - turned post-Goldwater conservative icon - Ronald Reagan, was elected the 40th President of the United States. The cultural mood in America had changed markedly in just a few short years. The liberal optimism that seemed to characterize Jimmy Carter's 1976 post-Watergate election was really the last breeze of a waning '60's social-political activism. By the time Carter was inaugurated, conservative groups with a far-right agenda were already at work, moving quickly to the center of Republican politics. With the election of Reagan in 1980, the conservative wing of the party gained control of the Oval Office and began to turn America around on issues as diverse as reproductive rights, fiscal policy, military spending, equal rights for women, welfare reform, and school prayer. The list was long and the effect on all aspects of American culture was profound: The "Reagan Revolution" had arrived.

At the end of the 1970's, American political and corporate leaders declared the nation suffering from a serious malaise. While politicians tried to address a perceived decline in American social values, they also raised fears that America's economic, cultural, and military vitality was at risk. Their fears were referenced internally and externally. Internally, fear was cast in terms of social-intellectual and moral decay; and, externally concern was referenced to economic decline and failure to contain communist militarism. Corporate leaders found themselves facing the rapid globalization of product-service markets and stiff foreign competition for market share. American businesses and industries would have to re-tool and "downsize" if they were to continue to reap the profits to which they had become accustomed. Downsizing, and cut-backs in budgets, services, jobs, and operations became the guiding principles for government and industry. Largely dependent on state, federal, and corporate funding, higher education followed suit and began its own season of downsizing, or, in academic parlance, "retrenchment."

Reagan's Revolution, like Franklin Roosevelt's New Deal, began in his first 100 days in office. Tax cuts, social legislation, increased military spending, government restructuring; the topics of the conservative agenda, moved quickly through House and Senate. [1] Corporate downsizing took on a sudden and sharp edge, with little fear a socially conscious federal government would brake the process or soften the blow. State legislatures caught in the tightening federal funding vice, looked for fat to trim from their budgets. Higher education became a prime target for their fiscal attention. University Chancellors and Presidents were called on to justify current expenses and anticipated budgets. Individual schools and programs were carefully assessed and evaluated for their contribution to the university's fiscal health. The "corporate university" became the model for action. Faculty did not take the turn toward a business oriented academy lying down; they did their best to retain programs, faculty lines, and faculty-governance privileges.

One must contextualize higher education as part of the larger culture to understand the dynamic of the problems the university faced in the 1980's. Traditionally, the university's place in society was 'above' and 'outside' the gritty, daily reality of political-corporate-social America. With the creation of large, state-managed systems of higher education the academy's interdependence with the myriad organizations and agencies managing American finance and culture began to shape the function and process of higher education. Soon even private colleges and universities found themselves inextricably tied to the organizational-

246

economic environment. As an organized system however, the university did not deem itself product driven, nor was it able, or willing, to adapt quickly and readily to the fast pace of change characteristic of the corporate world. Yet, this was exactly what was asked of higher education as it was forced by fiscal and social contingency to assume the character of a corporate-consumer university. Thus the university was provided a rude awakening to the consequences of attending more and more to the pressures and contingencies of vocational-professionalism.

Predicting the imperative of the university's response to cultural and political change, authors Stewart and Dickason (1979), discuss the impact of change on the university:

> At least one demographic impact will be positive. Institutions will be compelled to become more introspective and analytical, to undertake long range planning, something they did not have to do in good times. They will be forced to set priorities and develop strategies, overcome institutional inertia and make long overdue choices - for example, to identify areas of growing student interest and create new programs to replace those for which demand may have fallen off. A consumer orientation will benefit higher education.
> 2

Accountability and the consumer-student were new issues for higher education. Both were cause for alarm among academics comfortable with the tradition of the university existing outside the common concerns of corporate-consumer culture. Meanwhile at the periphery of the university's curriculum, overshadowed by its sister arts, and just recently independent of sports and leisure activities, was dance.

Dance began the decade looking over its academic shoulder. Enrollments had shown great promise in the early 1970's, and because many programs had made such a good start, their faculty, budget, and facilities issues were, for the most part, tolerable. There were problems; an over-worked faculty, studio space that was not designed for the needs of dance, limited production budgets, and support staff that was hard to find and harder still to fund. All things considered though, dance had established itself as an academic discipline and was moving forward. Yet, just as the young, unproven discipline was becoming more stable, the world around it was becoming more fluid, uncertain, and volatile.

Enrollment issues and the vicissitudes of downsizing were aggravated by an increasingly aggressive, student vocationalism in higher education. By 1980 a humanistic interest in finding a meaningful, life affirming, vocation following college was gone for the most part. The number of students entering higher education was in decline. The baby-boom generation no longer dominated the traditional 18 - 24 year old college population. Not only were there far fewer students to go around, many did not choose to attend college opting instead for professional development programs offered by business and industry. The limited numbers of students who were interested in a college education were selective in choosing where to go and what they would study. The corporate climate in America situated many of life's choices around income and the negative incentive of this generation possibly not having as much as the preceding generation. Issues of diversity were also impacting enrollments. African-American, Asian, and Latin-American student populations sought a higher education for divers purposes. The community college offered a cheaper, less time consuming, vocational alternative to the 4 year undergraduate curriculum. For other's, the specific, job-related professional academic program, became the education of choice. Enrollments in the liberals arts, humanities, and other non-vocational academic programs declined drastically.

In a predictive article for the *Journal of Higher Education* (1980), author Lyman A. Glenny discusses the nature of change and future trends for the university in "Demographic and Related Issues for Higher Education in the 1980's." [3] Glenny predicted the following seven assumptions in a section of the paper titled "Diversity and Enrollment in the Future":

1.   The downturn in the number of college-age youth will have immediate and by 1988 fairly substantial, if not drastic, effects on most of the higher education in the nation.

The College age population had flattened out, although women were expected to continue to enroll at greater rates than men. Minority youth would increase and be pragmatic, taking job-oriented majors, primarily in the community colleges. Women would increasingly enter occupational and professional fields and therefore tend to maintain enrollments at community colleges and professional schools.

2.   The several types of colleges and universities will be differentially affected by enrollment decline.

The large, state flagship universities, and the prestigious four-year colleges would be least affected by declines in enrollment. Community colleges would continue to offer attractive options to local citizens in short term occupational courses. Denominationally oriented private colleges and public four year colleges would be most affected by enrollment declines. Many of these would cease to operate or be forced to dramatically change their mission and goals. Private colleges would be more at risk than public institutions.

3.   Starting about 1985 to 1988, young people will begin to see the potential shortage of specialists in several major fields of academic and scientific interest.

By 1985 the tail end of the baby boom generation would be ready to graduate. Enrollment decline would be steady until at least 1998. Those who were enrolling would seek out prestige programs and universities. Specialization's with projected labor shortages would attract the limited applicant pool. Labor gaps would not be filled by retrained professionals but by young, technologically aware applicants.

4.   Adults entering college will not make up for the loss in the 18 - 24 year-old age group.

The number of adults returning to higher education was unlikely to increase as more retraining programs were offered by business, industry, and government. Distance learning would increase. Adults learners would take specific courses and be less likely to pursue degree programs to their conclusion. The percentage of adult males entering higher education would remain stagnant. Activity courses and vocation-specific courses would continue to attract the adult leaner.

5.   The most rapidly growing set of post-high school educational opportunities, aside from the advent of the community colleges, is that composed of social, religious, civic, and nonprofit organizations and of business, industry and government.

The numbers of people in professional development programs outside the colleges would increase. Industry and business would offer programs on this premise. Some colleges would be forced to offer educational services to business and industry.

6.   Other complications for colleges and universities will arise out of social factors unrelated to enrollment decline.

The college degree would be less recognized as competency certification. Business, industry, and government would increasingly do their own licensing. The degree would mean less as people become more vocationally specific. State governments would cease to rely on college certification for entry level employees. The inertia of the college system would make major changes toward the vocational university difficult if not impossible. Competition between colleges for top-rated students would become more rapacious.

7. Those institutions of higher education that do survive until 1995 will have stronger programs, more distinguished faculties, and better senses of mission and goals. [4]

Glenny's article outlines the tone and direction of thought on the future of higher education circa 1980. Much of what was foretold came to pass. And, from the perspective of 1999, much is still transpiring. Small, private, liberal arts colleges continue to struggle to attract sufficient numbers of students. Public, four year colleges and universities continue to experiment with ways to attract vocationally inclined undergraduates. University faculty, alarmed at an ill-prepared, complacent, and materially inclined youth reinforce academic pre-requisites and general education curricula. The focus on higher education as consumer oriented-vocational preparation continues.

In the 1980's, CODA programs represented some of the nation's strongest departments and strong academic programs in dance made up the bulk of NASD's initial university affiliates. Documents from CODA and NASD in the 1980's portray issues dance administrators and programs were facing in the corporate university. These papers provide an excellent contemporaneous record of the concerns of university dance educators during this period. Administrative issues are revealed in the narrative of CODA summary accounts. NASD documents include the NASD handbook, "Report to Members" newsletters, position papers on related topics, and the Higher Education Arts Data Service (HEADS):

The handbook, published biennially, includes NASD Standards for educational programs in dance as well as the Association's constitution, bylaws, code of ethics, and rules of practice and procedure.
NASD is a participating organization in the Higher Education Arts Data Service (HEADS) Project. The project includes an annual publication of statistical information about dance programs entitled NASD HEADS Data Summaries. This document provides comparative information about enrollment, degrees awarded, admission,

graduation, faculty, administration, budgetary matters, credit hour production, scholarships, faculty teaching loads, and student demographics, organized by size and type of institution. HEADS also allows participating institutions to develop special statistical comparisons with institutions of similar size and scope.

During the academic year, NASD publishes a Report to Members which is sent to dance executives of member institutions and to individual members. The NASD Report to Members includes information about the Association, descriptions of activities of interest to dance executives, and discussions of national arts policy issues. [5]

NASD position papers were and are printed for distribution. The range and focus of CODA and NASD positions papers, summary documents, and reports, like the articles of the 1930's reviewed in Chapter Five, lend context to the internal and external issues for 1980's dance in higher education.

In 1979, the Council's first agenda item for discussion dealt with the publication and distribution of the *Standards for Dance Majors* and the field's positive response to their efforts. The second and third agenda items considered "Retrenchment in Higher Education," and "Budget." Discussing "The Changing role of the University," CODA summary notes for 1979 reflect on the nature and range of the issues faced:

> Fewer people are going to universities. There are alternate forms of education such as those provided by the business world (large corporations) and professional world. The role of the universities is changing as a result of our change in populations....[A]nd ultimate goals of individuals. Students are job oriented and not Liberal Arts oriented. How do we address ourselves to these changes? Should we be job oriented or should we, in contrast to conservatories, continue to be humanistic? Our recent effort has been to work toward small numbers and high quality. We may need to take a different look and perhaps take a few less talented students to keep enrollments up. Perhaps we should look to the possibility of alternative dance jobs to those in performance. We need to develop a broader base of support for dance at all levels to open up these possibilities and to educate the American public.... [6]

Recruitment strategies were discussed with the goal of finding ways to insure a consistent enrollment base. Budget concerns focused on program cuts and the decline in real dollar.

In 1980 CODA met twice, in May and again in November. CODA's May meetings were devoted to the administrative role of the department chair. In November, items on the agenda focused on the decrease in undergraduate enrollments, maintaining standards in the face of declining numbers, and a decreasing MA and MFA applicant pool. By 1981 CODA members focused on strategies for survival and how "a small and relatively young department can defend itself against being eliminated in times of financial stress." [7] Summary notes outline a number of steps including faculty getting out of the studio and into the decision making process, and contacting sympathetic legislators, parents of major students, and other university faculty and administration. Meetings in 1982 were devoted to the same issues but with a self-assuring moment of reflection on how far the field had come in thirty years. Subsequent discussion related back to the wide range of issues dance educators were facing in their work: budgets, teacher training courses, changing cultural values, the job market, creative development of students who come into higher education with no preparation to work artistically, and creative career opportunities for dance majors who are not talented in choreography or performance. Summary notes for 1983 provide the following description of the "Current Situation":

A.　Enrollment Trends.
There seems to be a decline in numbers of students auditioning
1) lack of financial aid 2) students looking to other majors with dance minor.
B.　Job Placement of Graduates.
Small percentage are actually being placed but most work 1) many create their own jobs dancing and teaching 2) many work non-dance jobs 3) there are many small companies for performance and choreographic experience. It was suggested that NASD Research Committee do survey to track dance graduates.
C.　Undergraduate Deficiencies of Graduate Students.
It is important not to weaken the graduate program. CODA standards suggest 60% of course work at the graduate level open only to graduate students. The professional performer returning to school may need special options. a) senior level course outside the major, b) competency tests, c) reading lists for proficiency, are acceptable. We must be able to individualize program, make exceptions yet protect standards.

Alma Hawkins then addressed issues of teacher education. Her comments, transcribed by CODA secretary Beth Lessard, relate some concerns:

We talk about the difficulty of finding teachers for education courses--especially graduate courses. Why is this so? What can be done about the situation?
Dance is in transition--not only because of economic/social issues but also because our leadership is in transition. Many people who pioneered the programs (1950 - 1980) have retired or will soon leave. This also applies to faculty who have assumed responsibility for preparation of teachers.

When we were establishing the dance major program and justifying its place in higher education, we were careful to build a curriculum i.e. body of knowledge and not application of... [missing text, although "styles" of dance was most likely what were referred to], this was a necessary step. However, as our programs developed we were slow in realizing that we had a responsibility to prepare teachers who could carry on what we were creating.

Certainly a basic prerequisite is a strong background in dance as a performing art. But is that enough? The role of teacher involves more than technique and choreography - for example - methods of effective presentation, knowledge about the learning process, characteristics of the learner (child, adolescent), developmental aspects of learning, understanding of creativity as a process, and inter-personal relations as a factor of growth.

Many of us in the earlier period had courses in education, psychology, curriculum development, group process, creativity etc. Dance majors today do not get these courses - and probably won't because of time restraints and interest. The questions are: 1) How do we help prospective teachers acquire these related knowledge's? 2) How do we help current faculty expand understandings in related fields? 3) What should be the framework for graduate courses? In our discussions we said that we must value teaching: find ways to develop (i.e. workshops, summer session programs, sabbatical -- time to retool, reach out on own).... **8**

"Valuing teaching" and preparing the teachers of tomorrow was not only a practical issue, it was a philosophical issue about the discipline of dance. How had the field wandered so far from its origins in education? Had the desire to not be attached to physical education, and be recognized as arts-based, come to equate teacher training with that which 'had been' and, perhaps, was 'less than?' How had these leaders in dance *education* (author's emphasis) come to the point where they admitted: "we were slow in realizing that we had a responsibility to prepare teachers who could carry on what we were creating?" Were they so busy separating from physical education and establishing the field as arts-related that they forgot to address the future and function of its success? Was this a simple problem of absent-mindedness? Or, had the fruits of their turn toward the values and preoccupation's of the professional world, predicted earlier by their academic colleagues in physical education, come to be realized?

John Wilson, Professor of Dance at the University of Arizona delivered a paper to NASD members at their 1983 conference titled, "Education and Training Issues: Curricular and Institutional Practices." Wilson's intent was to "present some frameworks - systematic, historical, and philosophical - by which to view, assess, and approach our problems as reasonably and constructively as possible."[9]   Addressing these issues in the context of dance in the public university, Wilson asks his audience seven questions:

> What products in terms of post-degree citizenship should reasonably be expected of those who complete the studies of a dance program?
> What products in terms of scholarship and new knowledge should be expected of a dance program?
> What shall constitute the qualification of instructors to be appointed to a dance faculty?
> What professional and administrative relationships should be built between a dance program and other academic units and structures?
> What shall comprise the core curriculum of a dance program, and what shall be the plan for progression through studies?
> What shall be the standards and procedures for evaluation of student work and progress?
> What shall be the standards and procedures for evaluation of faculty work? [10]

Wilson goes on to provide a set of historical contexts, dividing the history of dance in higher education into three periods: 1926 - 1966, "the period of foundation to proliferation"; 1967 - 1981, "the period of evaluation to accreditation"; and 1982..., prophetically titled "the period of sustainment to autonomy."   According to Wilson, the first period was characterized by the dominance of Margaret H'Doubler's humanistic educational philosophy for dance, "natural to the goals of a liberal education," yet fertile ground for the growth of the idea that dance was an art form.   Between 1926 and 1966 the numbers of educational programs in dance increased from 1 to 277. [11] Wilson states that the reason for this proliferation, while facilitated by post-War economics and the baby boom, was H'Doubler's educational philosophy.   Meanwhile an encroaching professionalism, fostered at Bennington, was making significant inroads into the instructional practices of dance educators in higher education:

> By 1966 two factors were pressing hard on the old educational philosophy. Rampant proliferation of dance programs, many of which were not intelligently founded but were merely coat tailing on the pioneering of the older programs, was threatening to weaken the respect and integrity of dance in academe nationally.   Simultaneously, professionalism was rapidly becoming the standard for technique and production or choreography. Students and many faculty were increasingly vociferous in their insistence on "intensive professional training." [12]

255

Wilson then addresses the shortness of the second phase, "the period of evaluation to accreditation," attributing its brevity to a decline in the college age population, a severe national recession, and educational conservatism:

> We are all painfully aware of the reports of the decline and fall of higher education....[T]he 20% reduction of Michigan State University's operating budget and the accompanying elimination of salary lines; the closure of the University of Washington's prestigious kinesiology department; the loss of faculty lines from some of our leading "solid" dance departments....[A]n unknown number of dance programs are not represented here simply because their faculty do not receive travel monies for conferences....Hopefully the practice we will get through sustainment will gain for us autonomous stature. It will include: a demonstrated ability to attract and gather independent money; the creation of new kinds of jobs for our students; the pruning of weaker parts of our programs; and the containment of productions to the amount and level that local psychology can support. [13]

Wilson's concluding statement is a practical prescription for success - an ability to attract and create independent support, new kinds of jobs for students, a retooling of the curriculum, and a considered relationship between what the dance program offers and the needs of the community it serves. This was a realistic set of endeavors that could contribute greatly to the field's success. However, it is a prescription that may be easier said than done, and it has yet to be constructively implemented by leaders in dance education. Perhaps Wilson's original list of seven questions might have been augmented by consideration of questions related to his hope that getting "through sustainment" would lead toward newly demonstrated abilities of personnel:

'How do we attract independent monies, and for what purposes?'

This act in itself would go a long way toward justifying the continuation and sustainment of dance programs in higher education. The problem was (and is), what kinds of monies: Donor monies? Endowed Chairs in dance? Major capital donations? Research monies? Project driven monies? What organizational structure exists to help dance faculty conceptualize and articulate the need and use of independent monies and raise the dollars?

'What new kinds of jobs can we realistically expect our programs to help train our students for?'

Individual programs began to craft their own answers to this issue later in the decade, but the field has never really come together on accepting vocationalism in dance outside the implied post-graduate vocations of performance, choreography, and teaching.

'What component parts of our academic programs could possibly be retooled?'

Generally speaking, the discipline of dance is centered around six areas of study; dance technique, choreography, performance, history, education, and science. Technology has recently been added to the curriculum in some institutions. Is retooling and re-conceptualizing a curriculum in part contingent on the focus of other dance programs in a state system or region? Is it dependent on the expertise of long-term or newly hired faculty? Should this process happen quickly, or slowly?

'What considerations must be borne in mind to better fit the dance program with the amount and level of a local psychology?'

The containment of productions to a level appropriate to the sophistication of local populations is, at face value, a remarkably level headed suggestion. 'I didn't get it...What am I supposed to feel?'; these are comments are commonplace from audiences not acclimated to modern art ideas. However, containment of art expression flies off the track when it collides with artistic vision and personal taste, and the strong tradition in modern dance and art to experiment. Obviously Wilson is calling for a balance in this regard, but perhaps an ongoing effort at local taste development and artistic education would also be warranted. Wilson's article concludes with a section of "Questions and Answers." Here, he discusses his thoughts on the matters of student preparedness, the training of artists in the academy, inter-institutional replication of programs, and realistic vocational training and post-degree expectations.

In 1984, CODA members returned to their ongoing discussion on curricular matters. The curriculum was closely looked at in terms of enrollment trends, freshman attrition, recruitment, the encroachment of new liberal arts requirements on the BFA degree, minimum standards for graduate students, summer sessions, doctoral programs, and the differences between university trained and professionally trained dancers. Topics related to administration were also considered with special attention paid to a growing trend in student litigation. Enrollment figures revealed a leveling off, following the decline characteristic of the first three years of the 1980's. In the categories of undergraduate and graduate enrollments, the following statistics were reported:

Over the past several years there has been a drop in student enrollment that seems to be leveling off. Among the institutions represented by CODA, enrollment trends for 1984 - 1985 were as follows:

	Undergraduate	Graduate
Holding Steady	8 departments	7 departments
Decreasing	5 departments	2 departments
Increasing	1 department	3 departments

Causes for the leveling off or decrease in student enrollment can be attributed to complex factors including:
    a. student and parent vocational concerns - future employment.
    b. decrease in financial aid.
    c. increase in out - of - state tuition.
Out of state auditions do not seem to be paying off. A majority of freshman now seem to be coming from in-state.
We need to do a better job of convincing people of the importance of dance as a profession - parents, as well as students. [14]

Concerning the "Differences between University Trained and Professionally Trained Dancer[s]," summary documents report:

University trained dancers have an increased breadth of liberal arts experience. An "education" environment inclines to nurture the student and allow him/her to progress at a rate appropriate to the individual. It allows for an understanding of dance in a broader sense than just performance and dance students who wish to become teachers are better able to adjust to the expectations of academe if they have been trained in such an educational environment. [15]

One might think that this topic would have provided a context for exploring the substance of Alma Hawkins's previously cited 1983 summary comments, but it seems that it did not. The importance of the liberal arts experience, and a development of a broader appreciation for dance outside performance needed more than just recognition for its merit, it needed recognition for its worth. Conceptual and behavioral range and understanding needed to be valued and perceived as the basis for the training of "those who would follow." However, this issue took on another character in 1985 during the Council's discussion of graduate preparation in dance.

Before moving on in the history of the decade, a paper presentation to NASD in 1984 deserves attention because it brings to light a cultural issue that has a long history in dance, and subsequently aggravated the matter of acceding to the wishes of the consumer-student: Muriel Topaz visits the question "How does a broad based curriculum influence a dancer's career?" in an untitled address to the NASD in September of 1984. [16]

The important issue Topaz addresses in her paper is encapsulated in what she refers to as 'the deadly quip of the general manager of one of our most respected companies: "She can't be a good dancer - she reads at rehearsal." [17] In making her case for a broad curriculum, Topaz rejects the cultural notion of the "dumb dancer," and anti-intellectualism. Without directly confronting this matter, Topaz asks the field to consider the benefits of cognitive studies in dance:

> The field itself can only benefit from dancers with broader backgrounds and greater understanding of their art. As we become more articulate, we are slowly winning the increased respect of our fellow artists in allied fields. It has not been an easy path to respectability, nor should it have been considering our own insistence on negation of the dancer's intellectual powers. [18]

Implicit references to anti-intellectualism, and the benefits of correcting this state, are woven throughout Topaz's article as she discusses the importance of considering the value of cognitive understanding in dance notation, choreography, educating the "non-dancer," and in relations between the professional and the academic educator:

> It is of deep concern that we are on the brink of the same schism that exists in the other arts: the schism between the practitioner and the academic. If we insist on training our teachers solely in an academic setting, with no reference to the professional world, we will, in fact, increasingly distance one wing of the profession from the other. It seems to me essential, if we are to avoid that breach, that every teacher have some professional credential to enrich his or her preparation to teach. [19]

Recalling Erdman's and Limón's comments on this matter to participants of the 1966 - 1967 Developmental Conference on Dance, one might also ask that the professional entering the academy obtain some credential in pedagogy; a criteria for teaching rarely raised or discussed. Again, we see the conflict within the field regarding what appears to be an academic inferiority complex for dance in higher education. An intellectualism is needed for the discipline to advance, yet development of an intellectualism, in teaching, in art making, and in studying dance, is not to be confused with the transcendent, subjective, art experience of performance. Addressing the ineffable nature and act of dance confronts the educator. Avoiding the issue, the discipline accepts what I would argue is the easy way out; the act of having done the dance somehow instills the doer with the credential and license to teach. Somewhere in the schism that Topaz talks about may be a point of intersection: a place where thinking and doing are considered of equal share.

Dance in the Corporate University: 1985 - 1990

Most quality dance programs weathered the early years of the corporate university. Others dropped by the wayside as a result of budget cuts and declining enrollments. CODA documents for 1985 - 1989 illustrate the struggle to survive covering matters of enrollment and parental pressure to choose jobs related to a college major. The double major was a difficult alternative, often forcing students to take 5 years to complete their undergraduate degree(s). One interesting 1985 entry addresses the new corporate mind set:

Administrators are now management trained people rather than coming from the arts/education.

Reports are in the form of computer printouts with statistical information. Additional support staff is needed as the chair has limited time for involvement with such reports. The chair's time should be spent with developing a "vision" for the future of the department. Can we change the direction the university is taking as a corporation?

More information is coming from the top to the bottom rather than involving consultation. There is diminishing democracy in education.

We're dealing with business questions rather than artistic questions. **20**

Concerning long range planning, CODA members addressed related matters of who will lead, student vocations, and what were students getting from their dance education:

Who will want to be the department chairs for the next five years? Earlier chairs had more autonomy, now there are orders from the top. Its a different world and a different job now. It takes one kind of person to build a dance department from zero and a different kind of person to take over an established department. It requires a different set of values.

...The chair's position is both management and artistic vision. It is necessary to clarify for the central administration that it is counter-productive to have a chair who is a business manager who does not know dance.

It used to be prestigious to be in line to be department chair. Now its like the plague!

...[W]e need to get department representatives on power committees. Otherwise, we are wasting time re-establishing dance on campus.
Reasonable planning must consider limitations put on the university.

Part of long range planning is considering whether we're training students for what they are really going to do. Few will perform so we should be planning ahead on curriculum and look at what we are actually training them for.

We don't know what they are really getting from our programs. The first dance programs were not intended to put performers in the....Is it a problem that now many departments are concerned with perfecting technical skill, assuming all students want to enter the professional world? We could emphasize making better human beings whatever they do with the rest of their lives. Students now are more job oriented. They may be inspired by the wrong values. However, when we show through our teaching that our concern is for making them educated people, they begin to give that importance.

....[W]e can't have the same expectations for all students. The curriculum must allow for many options, not clones. All students may pursue a BFA degree but they have individual talents and we can help them toward a variety of goals. Faculty have to know they can't be all things to all students and students cannot have such expectations of faculty.... **21**

The Council revisited the value of a university education in dance through the lens of graduate preparation in 1985. In the mid-1980's the culture of dance in higher education continued to value the artist over the theorist. Scholarship in dance was looked at rather cautiously, partly because doctoral programs were in early stages of development, and partly because CODA's members, like many of their non-member peers, were enamored of the practicing artist:

> Some campuses offer both the MA and MFA. They are accepted into the graduate program, not to the degree. A preliminary choreographic project is completed in the first year which determines eligibility for the MFA. It is a combination of ability in performance or choreography as well as student choice.
> Most MFA's are two or three years. The trend is toward three years. MA's are one year. Length of the program should be comparable to the other arts.
> The MA is in history or research. Opinion was that we need to be positive about the MA and not have it be discards from the MFA. Production dollars go to the MFA and the MFA students are much more visible. This can make second class citizens of the MA students. We need to protect both the BA and MA with scheduling and resources. [22]

The consistent and regular attention paid the MFA student seems to conflict with the concerns Alma Hawkins raised in her 1983 comments regarding the need for education specialists. In hind sight, these comments, while honest and clearly self-critical, also seem to be curiously self-defeating. Where were the teachers of tomorrow to come from? In what mood would prospective scholars and teachers, the 'MA's,' come out of a program that implicitly cast them as "second class citizens?" These are questions that are hard to attribute to one, or even several traits and beliefs. A number of deeply rooted and conflicting cultural and educational factors had come together to make second class citizens of those who would choose a theoretical path in dance; the reference to Topaz's NASD paper above illustrates an aspect of this. In the next chapter I will review some contemporary thought on the nature of graduate preparation and education in dance.

But for now; back to the 1985 CODA summary notes, where the discussion has turned to the broad question of dance studies in an academic setting:

> Dance in the University
> In large urban areas there are a range of dance teachers and dance experiences available to the potential university dance major. The bulk of the country is rural and small town where television and movies are the role model. They come to the university from a background of drill team, baton twirling, and being voted best dancer in their high schools. They expect to be stars, overnight. They have to learn how to take class,

what's expected of them. That takes the whole first year as they come from an experience of learning a series of steps and putting them together, of selling themselves in mass-media hype. They don't know the difference between artistic and commercial dance.

...The question was raised whether modern dance is over or is it just living in the colleges? Our students go to New York and there's no modern dance. They end up in ballet or a floor barre and exercise class. The response to this was that modern dance is not over. It is always changing. We're going through a transitional pattern. The one thing that is durable is an understanding of movement. We need a balance of teaching conceptual movement and classical techniques.... [23]

CODA documents in the middle years of the 1980's attempt to contextualize the factors negatively influencing dance in the university. This was not meant to be an exercise in catharsis, but rather a rational assessment of what the practical issues were so that change could be considered. Enrollments continued to be a diagnostic measure of the health of dance programs and the discipline. External realities, such as student vocationalism or the degree to which students were prepared for the college dance experience, seemed outside their control. But, it was precisely such matters that had to be addressed if the discipline was not to shrivel on the vine and ultimately disappear. CODA raised the problems, but who would act on them? In the early 1980's there was no means for a strategic, and nationally organized, advocacy. While NASD members might wax philosophic on issues of advocacy, NASD was not an externally focused advocacy group. Its mission clearly prohibited these types of endeavors. The National Dance Association attempted to play the advocate's role but its affiliation with, and subordination to, the dominate structure of AAHPERD and the discipline of physical education, negatively impacted its effectiveness in national advocacy for dance-arts education.

Again, in November of 1986 CODA members came back to the issue of declining enrollments:

Current undergraduate enrollments show about 1/3 declining, 1/3 increasing and 1/3 remaining stable. Reasons for declining enrollments include parent's wanting secure jobs for their children after graduation, limited dance programs in public schools at the age when values are formed resulting in dance not being valued, and the influence of a high tech society. [24]

Subsequent CODA documents note the stability of graduate enrollments and the growing phenomenon of professionals returning to graduate school. One reason cited for this trend was the closing of many of the smaller modern dance studios and companies in New York. On curricular matters, members report a hard time getting courses in dance recognized as part of the general education component. University faculty had strengthened the general education component of the undergraduate curriculum in response to student vocationalism. Expanding general education requirements impacted the schedules of students pursuing professionally focused degrees such as the BFA. And, now that many dance programs were housed in divisions or colleges of fine and performing arts, dance curricula suffered the stigma of being outside the humanities, and were estranged from the curricula from which much of the general education requirement was drawn:

> A dean of fine arts was quoted as saying that on that campus the arts are not perceived as central to the university, technology is the future and the arts are peripheral. This attitude makes it difficult to hold one's own much less move forward. In some cases where national reports support the arts, "the arts" does not mean dance. It is up to us to be sure dance is included.... [25]

As the 1980's began to wind to a close university administrators and educators took stock of their part in enabling the academy's reactive period of response to the corporate university, rampant student vocationalism, and shrinking budgets. As if waking from a dream, educational theorists began to question and speak out against the harsh, new, and utilitarian persona higher education had acquired. Once again the arts were being freshly considered as an important part of human expression and learning.

Like the "Red Scare" of the 1950's and 1960's which resulted in American educational systems turning sharply toward requiring skill in the hard subjects, the 1980's represent a period when education reacted to the American public's fears. The effects of this turn of events are still in evidence as some colleges and universities close their doors, re-focus mission's, or develop new educational combinations in the hopes that their latest effort will bring in the numbers of students, and kinds of faculty, needed for survival.

Fear has always played a central role in cultural-political responses to historical events perceived as threatening. In terms of the role higher education was asked to play in vocational preparation in the 1980's, this fear emanated from the popular notion that America was rapidly, and perhaps irretrievably, losing ground to an Asian culture of academic discipline, work, and industry. The literature of organizational sociology and administrative science, a discourse from which the decision making processes for institutions both in and outside of business and industry was framed, was rife with studies and comparative analyses of American versus Japanese-Asian work related cultures. [26]

By the latter years of the 1980's the literature had evolved to be less alarmist, less explicitly racist, and more reasoned. Fears diminished as a result of a positive corporate response to competition in better products and streamlined budgets. A new temperance was also initiated in the university. There emerged a sensibility that America's diversity and broadly focused educational environment was not an indicator of cultural weakness, but was a resource and sign of cultural strength. From political and sociological research emerged the value of diversity and support for an end to intellectual, cultural, and economic colonialism. From the fear-based introspection and retrenchment of the early 1980's emerged a new valuing of cultural-intellectual flexibility, diversity, uniqueness, individuality, and personal initiative. Even though social and administrative scientists still raised concerns about a technologically illiterate work force, changes in living standards, and a growing number of unemployed, the halcyon days of rampant doubt, finger pointing, and unbridled downsizing were no longer so draconian and reactive. Still, retrenchment in higher education, as predicted by Glenny, and cited at the beginning of this chapter, was very much the order of the day.

CODA's members finished the decade's meetings hopeful that some relief and change had come and with it a better environment for dance in higher education:

Although there was a considerable variation from institution to institution, the overall picture regarding enrollment revealed that, for the most part, enrollment was up on the undergraduate level and either holding or slightly up on the graduate level.

It seemed clear that science was considered to be 'high priority' by the administration on many campuses. At the same time, however, there seemed to be a re-emphasis being put on liberal education and there was evidence that the arts and humanities were being given a clearer focus.

It appeared that more institutions were now equating creative activity with research, and that adding the word "creative" to grant requests was helpful in terms of getting funding. [27]

The picture was becoming somewhat more balanced and realistic. Undergraduate and graduates students in dance were being more practical about their expectations regarding careers. Many were staying in the local area creatively pulling work opportunities together. University jobs continued to be highly sought after and the applicant pool was usually large. CODA members noted a trend for position announcements to confuse necessary credentials and to ask for a great range of applicant skill. Ph.D.'s and MFA's found themselves competing for jobs that asked for a host of applicant skills. Again, members commented on the problem of MFA graduates lacking conceptual bases and understandings.

The Council's in-depth topic for 1987 concerned graduate degrees. Looking at national trends in dance, Council members commented on the growing notion of the MA as an intermediary degree between the BA/BS and Ph.D. Members recognized discrepancies between graduate programs. Some universities blended MA and MFA degree requirements, yet awarded the MA. This practice was hard to rectify in public institutions as the degree title was awarded by the state:

Distinction between the MA/MFA in terms of body of knowledge:
There seems to be a "core" requirement which is applicable to both MA and MFA programs on most campuses. The number of courses and types of courses described as "core" seemed to vary considerably between campuses, however, and the diversity of the curriculum beyond the core appeared to be extremely variable.

It was agreed that there should be a breadth of knowledge that goes beyond the undergraduate program at the master's level, as well as specialization (emphasis) within the degree programs.

The problem of confusion on the part of the public regarding the MA vs. the MFA was discussed. Although it was agreed that the two degrees are intended to serve different needs, it was clear that it would take a long time to educate the public. Unfortunately, ads for dance openings exacerbate the situation by stating "MA or MFA" or "MFA or Ph.D." as job requisites. The local demands of the institution for certain degree titles are sometimes the cause of the problem. **28**

Following discussion of the MA/MFA, CODA members discussed the need for doctoral programs. The demand for doctoral programs was increasing and it was felt that the focus of these programs should be toward training people to make an original contribution to the field. Council members plotted out paths for students in their pursuit of degrees, and Alma Hawkins summarized their discussions as follows:

General Conclusion: there should be a basic core for the doctoral program, an individually tailored specialization, and a concluding dissertation which would contribute to the body of knowledge. It should be a matter of "transmission of knowledge" rather than simply the "acquisition of knowledge...." The true purpose of the Ph.D. is both to "preserve knowledge" and to "contribute new knowledge" to the field.

...It was agreed that it was important to consider what the Ph.D. stands for in other areas, and to have some sort of similar standards. Our guidelines should be as rigorous and as relevant to the specific specialization (focus) of the degree as possible.

SUMMARY: Alma Hawkins. This session was concluded with a summary, by Alma, of the two paths that dance in higher education might take in the future...what she described as "a matter of dreaming...." Although there was agreement about this as a model, it was also noted that flexibility was important in terms of "crossovers" when students' wished to change the focus of their study.

Path #1:

BA degree (@ 4 years). This degree program would provide a broad foundation in the body of knowledge (e.g. include courses in theory, history, kinesiology, philosophy etc.) plus a studio component of technique, choreography and performance. It would allow for some flexibility for the individuals' particular interests.

MA degree: (@ 2 years). This degree would build upon the BA, and would entail continued breadth in the study of knowledge while allowing for in-depth study in individual areas such as history, notation, kinesiology etc. The program would end with some sort of creative work, either choreographic or research and could/should conclude with a thesis or its equivalent.

Ph.D. degree (@ 2+ additional years). On top of the MA, which has given both breadth and depth in individualized programs, we would build a doctoral program. This program would require greater depth of understanding in the discipline, perspective, research, scholarly work, new knowledge etc. The goal here would be preparing individuals for leadership roles as scholars, teachers, or administrators etc.

Path #2:

BFA degree (@ 4 years). This degree would still require a broad base in the body of knowledge, but more emphasis would be placed on the studio component in terms of curriculum. (It is the emphasis that is important here. Some institutions would still require the degree title to be BA: see NASD standards)

MFA degree (@ 3 years). This degree would be considered a terminal degree. It would still involve continued study in the body of knowledge with the study of production, creativity, aesthetics etc....[B]ut there would be greater emphasis in professionally oriented work such as performance, choreography, production....

Summary and Challenges for the Future: Alma Hawkins

...[W]e are trying to envision the full development of our discipline in dance. In the '60's we worked hard to establish criteria and standards for the undergraduate major. We identified the body of knowledge, with many long hours of effort, and we projected a graduate program....In the 1970's we worked at implementing the undergraduate major and also beginning graduate programs. In the '80's we are beginning to project terminal degrees, which would be doctorate in nature or MFA's in nature. Institutions in the last few years have had to adapt to practical situations....The challenge today is to clarify and implement the full development of the discipline in relation to each institution....This morning we identified a projected flow from the broad experience in the discipline to specialization's...in doing this [examining the two paths], we should...remind ourselves what the role of higher education is in this country. I think the general agreement would be that it is to preserve knowledge....[T]o create and add new knowledge....[A]nd to educate the human being for effective functioning in our particular society. We should have awareness of the needs and job opportunities, and be aware of that when building curriculum. But probably we should remember that the primary goal of higher education is not job preparation...[T]hat it is education. [29]

Hawkins continued to act as the leveling and mediating conscience of CODA. A masterful facilitator, Hawkins was adept at summarizing disparate and fractious discussions, bringing the conversation back to perspective and focus and situating its next direction. In 1988 Hawkins announced that she would retire as CODA's President at the end of their fall meetings. She was replaced by Nancy Smith-Fichter, a CODA founding member and gifted leader in dance education. Smith-Fichter had helped organize the "Dance as a Discipline" and "Developmental Conferences" of the 1960's, and played a central role in helping facilitate the development of NASD in the early 1980's.

Concluding this part of the chapter on CODA's decade of work addressing the upheaval of the Reagan '80's and the corporate university, the Council's 1989 summary notes include a section titled "Our Vision - Dance in the 21st Century":

Our vision of dance in the next decade?
Dance trends in the '90's? How will dance meet the students needs?
What are the positives? Are we returning to a holistic humanistic approach? We need to develop an artist with a global conscience who realizes that the body is the tool or metaphor for the new technologies.
Find new ways of saying the same thing. Try to stay enthusiastic. Students come in with their own values and the result of their education. We are put in a position of establishing their values and getting them to value the art form. K-12 is very vital.

Hopefully it will help them value other cultures and see dance as a viable means of expression for all people, not just dancers. We should hope for a rise in moral consciousness, and less interest in the self. There can be more use of dance in a variety of therapies.

There may be more of a blending of art forms together and also a melting [*sic*] of science with arts and cross disciplines while maintaining integrity and taste. This is vital to a spiritual and ethical life. Let's look for continued migration of dance into the regions....

Alma: Larger general ideas have merged as opposed to departmental ones. This morning was focused on all that is wrong. Back in the '50's and '60's there was little money, space, faculty, staff, and limited performance opportunities. But there was a vision-dance became a recognized academic pursuit with degree programs leading to a gain in all the above. This happened only because there was a vision. Today: there is a changing world with constant pressures. We must know where we are going and must always be interpreting what is happening. Yesterday we implied a need to get back to our roots, anthropology, movement versus styles. Help students to make honest efforts. Indirectly, this all impacts on having a commitment in something, be self directed, self forming. In curriculums we need new concepts in integrating values/ethics into classrooms. We need awareness of global factors. This has implications for leadership. Day to day paperwork should not be consuming. We must address faculty morale as part of the vision. Another aspect is the role of the leader in keeping the human element dominant, not objects. We must listen, care, support and build a sense of community. This is the heart of the program. Part campus and community. Once established, do not assume that things will stay. The more difficult task now to hold on to is to incorporate these concepts and see that they are put into action with students and faculty. The bottom line is not to get carried away with paperwork. Keep the larger vision in mind.
30

Throughout a 20 year period (1968 - 1988), Alma Hawkins led the Council of Dance Administrators and consistently tried to inspire its members to keep two central perspectives in mind - 1) always consider the larger role dance plays as a part of education and, 2) keep your eye and process on the clarity and realization of individual and field-based vision.

CODA documents of 1979 - 1989, clearly illustrate a wide range of issues and concerns faced by dance administrators. Yet these very challenges forced the Council's membership to critique and refine much of their vision, to clarify much of their intent, to critically assess much of their perceived success; and ultimately to come out on the other side of the decade stronger for having done so.

The Reagan 80's, began on a note of panic and fear; the American sky was falling and government had to let the brutal yet cleansing tidal forces of an unfettered market economy sweep clean the landscape of American business and industry. Self-perceived as occupying higher ground, higher education found itself on the flood plane, and as vulnerable as any other business or commodity to the vicissitudes of the corporate-consumer culture. Interestingly, the corresponding righteous tone of attending to Christian-family-American values was manifested in a narcissistic cultural turn toward attending to material matters, and taking care of number one. This was seen in the consumer-vocationalism that framed the thinking of students preparing for a higher education. Admittedly, self-serving narcissism had its origins in the 1960's and 1970's. Popular catch phrases of the 1960's, such as "Drop Out, Tune In, Turn On," "I'm OK, You're OK," and "Do Your Own Thing" helped amplify and prepare the way for the unfettered materialism associated with 1980's.

In the case of dance the oft asked question from students and parents throughout the decade was "can I (she/he) get a job following graduation?" The honest answer - after perhaps a bit of hemming and hawing - was "probably not." One could scarcely anticipate finishing a college dance major and having the opportunity of joining a company that paid its dancers regularly. Likewise, the possibility of acquiring a teaching position in higher education after graduation was not a realistic option. One had to expect to go on to graduate school and then perhaps a stint in the professional world before proving truly competitive for this limited, and tight market. Opening a private dance school was an option, yet statistics regularly tell us new businesses have a high failure rate and the economic rewards are hard to come by. The real problem, the real issue, was the lack of dance in elementary and secondary ('K-12') education. Dance educators knew that having dance accepted as sequential, curriculum-based subject matter was the disciplines' answer to its employment questions. In the 1970's and 1980's the issues surrounding certification for elementary and secondary dance educators were alternately a promising and yet elusive set of topics. These issues would take on a new life and focus in the 1990's. However, before turning to that chapter of this story, other aspects of the evolving story of dance in higher education must be discussed. In the 1980's, besides matters of curriculum, vocationalism and university cutbacks, the theoretical side of dance was steadily growing, especially in areas of scholarly inquiry, attention to multi-cultural perspectives in the curriculum, and refined specialization.

CHAPTER 12

Dance Scholarship in Transition: A Post-Modern Aesthetic

Taking a moment to consider changes in the ways in which dance was socially related and theoretically conceptualized, events in this arena helped the discipline reinforce its internal sense of academic integrity and substance. The development of dance scholarship has had an important and beneficial impact on dance as a discipline; both in terms of the field's sense of identity and in terms of increased academic recognition and relevance. Yet, scholarly activity in dance has also been a development fraught with the fears of the influence of the non-dancer, because as one may recall, serious dancers don't read.

The intellectual discourse on dance during its separation from physical education primarily addressed history, educational philosophy, and practical issues of identity. Over the years there have been a number of periodicals, other than physical education journals, that have included some information and commentary on dance in higher education. Many of these publications have come and gone, among them: *American Dancer, Dance and Dancers, Dance and the Arts,* and *Ballet News. Dance Magazine* has enjoyed a long history and played an important role in informing students about programs in higher education. *Dance Magazine* continues to be the most popular of dance related periodicals. Contemporary periodicals also include *Dance Teacher* and *Dance Spirit;* both of which include regular feature articles on faculty and university based dance programs.

Throughout the middle decades of the century 1934 - 1964, Louis Horst's *Dance Observer* was the official journal (some might say apologist) for the modern dance. *Dance Observer* included regular features on college dance, although most of these were calendars of events, features articles on dance teachers, histories, or art-opinion articles. Dance academics with an interest in research and writing referred their work to journals published by affiliated arts or to the *Research Quarterly* and the *Journal of Physical Education and Recreation* , official journals of the American Association for Health, Physical Education, and Recreation's (AAHPER). Scholarly inquiry in these journals focused on the practical matters of dance education or on dance as it was related to motor development, kinesiology, and exercise physiology. Theoretical consideration of what dance means, in culture, to people, or as artifact, developed slowly and did not substantively appear in the literature until the 1950's.

In the 1950's, *Impulse* helped shepherd the field's development of an identity, as dancers and dance theorists began to consider their subject in broad new contexts. *Dance Perspectives*, begun in 1959 and issued quarterly, was another important early journal devoted exclusively to dance. With Selma Jeanne Cohen and A.J. Pischl as editors, *Dance Perspectives* broke new ground in dance research in that its contents were historically focused and international in scope. Like *Impulse*, each issue of *Dance Perspectives* was devoted to a special topic, e.g. "Dances of Anatolian Turkey," which, according to the introduction for this issue, was the first comprehensive study in English of dance in Turkey. [1] A central purpose of *Dance Perspectives* was in developing comprehensive indexes of historical reference material. At the end of each year, an index was provided for materials that had appeared in each issue, along with a "Current Bibliography for Dance":

> This supplement to the regular, quarterly issues of "Dance Perspectives" has been compiled as a service to our subscribers. The usefulness of the Index is self-evident. The Bibliography represents a venture not yet undertaken by any other dance publication, though workers in the other arts have long recognized its value. This listing, by virtue of its international scope, indicates the widespread attention paid dance at the present time. [2]

Editor Selma Jeanne Cohen made a major contribution to the field of dance research by pointing to dance history as a largely untapped area for scholarly inquiry. Outside of *Impulse* and *Dance Perspectives*, between 1926 and 1965, the majority of theoretical research in dance was conducted under the rubric of dance as part of physical education.

In the late 1950's government educational initiatives, stemming out of the Sputnik scare and other precursors to the social-activist political agendas of Presidents Kennedy and Johnson, helped create an environment for change. The Elementary and Secondary Education Act, Education Professions Development Act, and other federal and state sponsored legislation provided funding for educators with an idea toward implementing educational policy or developing curriculum. [3]

While such contributions were important, especially as government funded projects were exposing more and more students to dance, they were not focused on theoretically situated or empirically based research. The idea of quantitative research in dance, e.g. testing an hypothesis and concluding its validity was, and still is, a very difficult task in aesthetic movement. Isolation of variables and securing a regular test population present enormous challenges. Qualitative research in dance anthropology, ethnology, sociology, therapy, and other topics suitable for discursive exposition emerged fully in the 1960's, with individual contributions appearing earlier. In part, research in dance was slow in its development because it had to wait for a critical mass of graduate students, faculty, and academic programs to begin this endeavor in the university.

Throughout the early and middle decades of the 20th century, individual scholars investigated the nature of dance from a number of theoretical perspectives. Anthropologists recognized the importance of dance as symbolic rite, and as expression of culture, although most glossed over dance because they either weren't comfortable with its form, or not able to discuss its function. In, *To Dance is Human* (1979), author Judith Lynne Hanna discusses some of the conceptual barriers that confronted early anthropological and cultural scholarship in dance:

> The comparatively lagging state of dance studies has several explanations. Scholars generally have a limited view of dance, although it is a nearly universal and complex behavior. "Then they danced" is the common remark. Ethnocentrism reigns to such an extent that scholars call dances which differ from their ballet or jig a "lewd ambling" or "imitative fornication" - there has been little awareness that some dances involve body parts other than the limbs. Scholars' notions about dance in their own cultures influence their views of dances in other cultures: false dichotomies are drawn between "primitive" and "non primitive," and they both often have comparable complexity in their movements and meanings, and in the rules for combining these.
> Scholars often fail to distinguish dance from similar motor behaviors. Franz Boas set a precedent in anthropology: dance to him was "the rhythmic movements of any part of the body, swinging of the arms, movement of the trunk or head, or movements of the legs and feet" (Boas 1955: 344): The problem here is that we can apply this description to many work activities. Dance as emotional behavior is overemphasized (R. Marett 1914: Langer 1953), and Curtis Carter (1976), calls the conceptual plague besetting the understanding of dance a misguided separation of dance from intelligence. The history of the mind/body division can be traced from the writings of the Greeks to current critics. Viewing dance as a primarily conditioned phenomenon (cf. Alan Lomax 1968) perpetuates this problematic conceptualization. [4]

In the field of dance and ethnology Gertrude Prokosch Kurath was an early scholar whose work influenced the field. Kurath was honored at the 1972 Conference on Research in Dance, sponsored by the Committee on Research in Dance. Introducing Kurath to conference participants, Shirley Wimmer includes some biographical information on her subject:

> Gertrude's undergraduate and graduate studies at Bryn Mawr (1928) and Yale were in Art History, Music, and Drama. She also had a rich and varied background in Modern Dance, having worked with the leading artists-teachers in Europe and the United States from 1923 on....
> We actually met for the first time during the summer of 1951....William Fenton was visiting her at the time, and they were celebrating the release of their Bureau of American Ethnology Bulletin on the Iroquois, which had just been published....
> ...I believe 1946 was a turning point for Gertrude, because then her deepening study of dance ethnology began. From 1949 on, she was busily recording her field work on film, tape, and in articles for the various Folklore Journals - American Folklore, Midwest and Western Folklore; for Music Quarterly, Dance Magazine, American Anthropologist, Southwestern Journal of Anthropology, Scientific Monthly, etc.... [5]

Other scholars investigated aesthetic inquiry and dance. In a letter dated November 6, 1979, Gertrude Lippincott recalls the early days of research in dance aesthetics and provides some historical background on the development of a community of dance scholars. Lippincott had completed her Master's of Arts thesis at New York University under the direction of Martha Hill in 1943. Titled: "Aesthetics and the Dance: A Study of Some Problems in Dance Theory Presented for the Dancer," Lippincott's thesis was popular among dance educators seeking to clarify theoretical problems in dance:

> In response to some recent inquires as to the availability of my Master's degree thesis in Dance, written at New York University in 1942 - 43, I have decide to have the manuscript copied and to send it the various friends and colleagues who have asked for it....
> So many changes and developments have occurred since 1943 in the area of dance literature, research and scholarship, in dance publications of all types, in related arts, in libraries devoted to dance, in organizations interested in promoting the welfare of dance, in the art of dance itself, in its wide acceptance by the general public, and in the financial support of the dance by the federal government, foundations, corporations, etc....
> One cannot help but be amazed at the tremendous increase in dance literature in the past thirty-five years. In dance aesthetics nowadays, one can look at Collingwood, Langer, Feibleman, Ames, Sheets-Johnston, and many other for materials. Quite a few aestheticians have turned their attention to the dance field with the result that the august American Society of Aesthetics devoted a program at its 1970 conference in Boulder [Colorado], to the performing arts, and included a three-part dance session with Juana de Laban, Selma Jeanne Cohen, and yours truly taking part. At the 1968 conference in Austin [Texas], both Juana Laban and I presented papers on dance. [6]

While dance criticism was an early scholarly endeavor, critical analysis of contemporary works did not truly rise to the criteria of research in dance. In addition to the scholarly writings of Kurath and Lippincott, other scholars were beginning to investigate dance from a number of perspectives, among them Suzzane Langer whose *Feeling and Form: A Theory of Art Developed from Philosophy in a New Key* (1953), and *Philosophy in a New Key: A Study of Symbolism of Reason, Rite, and Art* (1957), helped dance scholars investigate a phenomenological approach to dance. However, it was in organized activity in dance; the journal devoted to dance, the group of scholars with a theoretical interest in dance, and the output of graduate students in theses and dissertations, that were a catalyst for change in dance research in the 1960's and early 1970's.

DanceScope: Exploring Dance as an Aesthetic Discipline

The National Dance Guild began publishing *Dance Scope* in 1965. The first issue included articles on dance criticism: "To Be a Critic," by Walter Sorell; the previously mentioned article on current issues in dance and American culture, "A Bright Future for the Arts," by Gertrude Lippincott; "Far Beyond the Far Out: Some Experimental Choreographers," a report on the beginnings of what would later be termed post-modern dance, by Cecily Dell, and the kind of facility dancer's dreamed about in "An Ideal Dance Theatre," by Thomas Watson. [7] Marcia B. Siegel was the first editor for *Dance Scope*. In her opening statement Seigel pays homage to Louis Horst, and frames the tone of the journal's purpose:

> ...[O]ur purpose, then, is to explore the scope of dance as a theatre art and as an aesthetic discipline. Rather than fill the rest of the space with noble aspirations, I am inclined to let the magazine speak for itself. We begin modestly but, I think, with a character of our own that does not need explaining.
> ...[W]e owe a great deal to the spirit of the late Louis Horst. Teacher, composer, critic and editor, Louis Horst gave an aesthetic rationale to modern dance in a way that no dancer or choreographer could have done....
> We cannot hope to fill the place left by the Observer, but we do hope to take up the banner. We will not always say things Louis Horst would approve, but we will be mindful of his devoted and inquiring spirit. So it is, we hope without too much presumption, that we affectionately dedicate ourselves to the memory of Louis Horst and "Dance Observer." [8]

In subsequent issues, *Dance Scope* provided the field with a palette of writings and feature articles that touched on the range of matters pertinent to dance. Editorial choice ranged from criticism to anthropological inquiry. Social commentary on the nature of racism in the arts, dance pedagogy and the history of educational dance, and gender and dance were just a few of the topics dealt with in its pages. In its 16 year history (1965 - 1981), *Dance Scope* expanded the range and focus of dance related research and commentary, and supported the development of scholarship and critical inquiry.

The Committee on Research in Dance: Organized Action for Dance Research

Clearly focused and organized research activity in the realm of dance got off the ground in 1965 with the founding of the Committee on Research in Dance

(CORD). CORD began as an ad hoc committee of interested individuals who came together at the 1964 National Council on Arts in Education (NCAE) Conference at Oberlin College. Following the 1964 NCAE meeting, an expanded group met again in the spring of 1965 in conjunction with the National Dance Teachers Guild's annual conference to continue to manage and steer the course for CORD's future.

Following its inception in 1964 - 65, CORD Membership was opened to the general public in 1967, and in 1969 the first issue of *CORD News*, a bulletin for the membership that included current developments in dance research, was published. In this issue, CORD Chair Bonnie Bird reviewed the formation of the Committee in a report to CORD's members:

> The Committee on Research in Dance would not be in existence today if it had not been for the meeting of the National Council on Arts in Education at Oberlin College in 1964. At this time, Catherine Bloom, Head of the Arts and Humanities Division of the United States Office of Education, brought with her Dr. Esther Jackson, Theater Specialist in the Office, to the conference. Fortunately, Dr. Jackson and Miss Bloom realized the implications of this meeting for the field of dance - with emphasis upon research in the area of dance....[T]he possibility of a future meeting of dance educators in New York City, with both Miss Bloom and Dr. Jackson in attendance, was discussed. The National Dance Guild [American Dance Guild] had already scheduled its annual convention to be held in October in New York City; Lucile [Nathanson: NDG member]...very kindly made arrangements for the Young Men's Hebrew Association to be available for an evening session. I assisted her in making contacts with various persons in dance, those in dance education, and those who are administrators in charge of programs in schools and colleges and who, therefore, would have a serious concern for the possibilities of research in the dance field
>
> As a result of this meeting, which I found enormously stimulating, we discovered from a research standpoint that we did not know a great deal about our field nor very much about related fields. This fact provided us with a stimulus to continue to meet as a kind of ad hoc committee to consider the ways in which the field of dance might be enriched or benefited if information about the possibilities for research and support for various kinds of field activities might be developed. Thus, CORD evolved from the ad hoc committee which had now grown to approximately 70 persons who have expressed real interest in this kind of endeavor. The first meeting was held in the Spring of 1965 and some wheels began to turn. Dissemination of information about the government's interest in receiving proposals for research stimulated the submission of a number of proposals.
>
> The fact that funds were given for several projects stimulated a way of looking at the field of dance that has, I think, helped to upgrade our own professionalism and to stimulate dialogue in the field which, to my knowledge, was on a new level. Most encouraging has been the involvement of dancers not only within the colleges but also within the professional field as well. I would add...that some important ideas have been set in motion. We have learned how to organize our ideas and to state our goals as a

result of trying to write a proposal. We, or at least I, have been forced to think in a more orderly fashion and in larger contexts than formerly. [9]

Dr. Jackson was followed as Head of the Office of Education Division of Arts and Humanities by Jack Morrison, who played such a helpful role in facilitating Alma Hawkins's plans for the 1966 - 1967 Developmental Conference on Dance. By 1968 Morrison had been replaced by Dr. Irving Brown, who, by 1969 had left his position with the Office of Education to become Director of Fine Arts at the University of Maryland. Brown was invited to address the 1969 CORD membership meeting and to share his thoughts on funding and directions for dance research. Brown references the Education Professions Development Act (EPDA), which supported teacher education and the development of the profession. At the time of Brown's speech:

> ...[T]hey [the administrators of the EPDA] have no money at this time; they simply have the fragments of funds which are left over from the individual programs they have now absorbed. The National Foundation for the Arts and Humanities Act, Title 13, provides them with approximately $100,000.00 a year....[W]hen they have money, it appears to me...that they will be open to all kinds of research proposals....[10]

Brown goes on to discuss the potential for dance to employ the benefits of the International Education Act (IEA) - an (then) un-funded initiative to implement the exchange of ideas in education - and the Vocational Education Act (VEA), for state managed funding for the education of professionals; although the wording of the act was interpreted to exclude artists. To get around this, Brown suggested that monies could be used to educate those in dance who work in allied fields, e.g. administration, technology, and design. There was also supportive provision for facilities, for student loans, for faculty members, and for research in training. [11] Brown's address was followed by a question and answer period where the definition of the term professional was discussed. The turn from federal management and funding of projects to the states was also debated. State arts agencies were a growing phenomenon:

The State Arts Councils of Illinois and New York are known for their tremendous support of dance. The fact that the National Endowment Act provided matching funds for - well, outright grants - and then, in addition, matching funds for the establishment of State Arts Councils, got a lot more going than we had ever experienced before. Some of them are moving ahead actively and strongly, and some of them are pattering along behind, dragging their feet in a sense. [12]

At CORD's 1969 meetings, Chairman Patricia Rowe introduced discussion on the topic of dance research in an editorial written for *CORD News*. Four types of research were differentiated; descriptive, experimental, historical, and philosophical. Within these, perspectives of aesthetic, philosophic, and historical inquiry seemed to dominate the fields interest:

> ...[A]s we know, a research problem in dance or any other discipline falls within at least one of four types of research. Whether a study is to be descriptive, experimental, historical, or philosophical research determines the nature of its data, the manner of collecting it, and the means of treating that data within the context of the specific research problem. Recently there has been evidence of a possible trend to identify, separately, aesthetic research from philosophical research. At the same time, there is a move toward combining philosophical with historical research designs. Regardless of the outcome of these trends, emphasis on the aesthetic aspects of philosophy provides sharper distinctions for studying the dance that are decidedly different from the prevalent problems in movement curriculum development, teaching, and dance studies of an analytical, chronological, and cultural level. (Incidentally, CEMRAL - Central Midwestern Regional Laboratory - will soon complete its survey of the published empirical aesthetic inquiry of the past 70 years, including approximately 5,000 studies in all areas of aesthetics and 149 in dance).
>
> Undoubtedly one of the major stumbling blocks to the part time researcher is the unknown status and seeming inaccessibility of previous research findings. One possible remedy to this problem is to conduct a regular systematic review of periodicals which include as a matter of editorial practice reports on dance related topics and studies. This kind of periodic review of resource materials can benefit the researcher in three ways:
>
> 1.   In the discovery of knowledge that may be useful in itself or in the conduct of research.
> 2.   In the disclosure of potential topics for research study.
> 3.   In the location of whole or partial models for designing one's own research procedures. [13]

In this article Rowe reviews other potentials and roadblocks impacting the recognition and potential for dance related research. *Dissertation Abstracts International,* the index for doctoral dissertations, had no category for dance. Dissertations were grafted into listings for whichever field seemed most closely related to the writer's topic. The development of intelligently organized and accessible databases was needed to assist the scholar with an interest in dance.

Dance notation sources were being consolidated in New York at the newly formed Dance Notation Bureau, and out of Columbus, Ohio, via the Bureau's Extension program with the Ohio State University.

Following the lead of Selma Jeanne Cohen's *Dance Perspectives*, an important early function of *CORD News*, was to list extensive bibliographic sources. Commentary in early issues of *Cord News* , makes it clear that these dance scholars were really having to start from scratch:

> For the first two years CORD maintained the same membership, met informally identifying and formulating genuine needs which could be met by the organization - needs that did not seem to be answered by any other research groups or committees. CORD's content and its duration were one and the same. Conference topics, speakers, the dates and meeting sites were more frequently intuitively than logically decided upon....Numerous operational meetings were devoted to agreeing upon a definition for research, pinpointing the multiple unknowns, isolating and agreeing upon the most crucial research needs of the directors and officers of CORD. As so frequently had been done in the past, university situated CORD members determined the needs for non-member graduate students.... [14]

In a continuing effort to clarify their activities, CORD's Board of Directors accepted and passed a resolution submitted by Allegra Fuller Snyder at the Director's March 6, 1971 meeting in Columbus, Ohio. Snyder's resolution is another example of the kind of foundation laying that CORD had to do to shape thinking about the new endeavor of dance research - both within and outside of the discipline:

> RESOLUTION
>   Be it resolved that one of the goals of the Committee on Research in Dance is to bring to the attention of the academic community, and encourage its active recognition of, the fact that research has now become an acknowledged area of concentration and necessary to many aspects of the teaching of dance at the college and university level; that the teaching of dance may no longer be looked upon merely as an activity - with the number of teaching hours that is considered a legitimate work load for a person involved in the teaching of dance based merely on classroom hours; that a number of faculty members in the field of dance are involved in lecture classes and teaching in such areas as dance history, dance ethnology, dance therapy, aesthetics, philosophy etc., and need an accepted and acknowledged work load which is commensurate with equivalent loads of other members of the academic community, a work load that acknowledges the necessity of continuing enrichment of one's own awareness in his fields of interest through research and investigation and the documentation and publication of these findings for the further growth and development of the field as a whole. [15]

CORD News acted as a clearinghouse for information and as a forum for CORD member's to frame the subject matter of research in dance. CORD conferences were presented from a particular point of view, e.g. "New Dimensions in Dance Research: Anthropology and Dance: The American Indian" (1972), and "Dance and Anthropology, Psychology and Ethnomusicology" (1974). In 1974 *CORD News* evolved into *Dance Research Journal,* and in 1978 the Committee on Research in Dance changed its name to the "Congress on Research in Dance," a moniker that remains with the organization today.

The importance of the creation of CORD cannot be underestimated. It was within this organization that the field clarified the nature and breadth of dance related research in the academy, thus giving the discipline not only increased exposure, but also an agreed upon theoretical foundation. In 1978 CORD members with an interest in dance history broke off from the group to form another important organization; the Society of Dance History Scholars (SDHS), which was incorporated in 1983. The official journal of SDHS, *Studies in Dance History,* is a monograph series on the history of dance and related disciplines. Today, both CORD and SDHS sponsor annual conferences that draw international audiences. National conferences, and regional special topics conferences, provide a forum for expansion in the field of research on dance. *Dance Research Journal* has grown into the field's premiere academic journal, published biannually. The current missions for CORD and SDHS state:

The Congress on Research in Dance (CORD) is an interdisciplinary organization with an open, international membership. Its purposes are 1) to encourage research in all aspects of dance, including its related fields; 2) to foster the exchange of ideas, resources, and methodology through publications, international and regional conferences, and workshops; 3) to promote the accessibility of research materials. [16]

The Society of Dance History Scholars is a not-for-profit organization dedicated to promoting study, research, discussion, performance, and publication in dance history and related fields....SDHS defines dance history in the broadest possible terms. The field encompasses the tradition of Western theatrical dance from renaissance and Baroque court entertainment's to postmodern dance theatre: the dance traditions of non-Western cultures; and a range of theatrical and participatory dance forms constitutive of popular culture - from country dancing and the waltz to the·tango and MTV. [17]

Academic Research in Dance

The Dance Division of AAHPER (now the National Dance Association), began compiling graduate theses and dissertation citations in reference volumes titled *Research in Dance*, in 1968. [18] *Research in Dance III*, compiled by Mary Alice Brennan in 1982, provides data for the number of theses and dissertations completed in the periods 1901 - 1964; 1964 - 1967; 1967 - 1970; and 1971 - 1981. Looking at selected totals for alphabetized categories provides a sense of development of scholarship in dance and the degree of interest in certain subject areas:

Table 2: Development of Scholarship in Dance-Selected Categories: 1901 – 1981.

		Volume			
		Research 1	Research 2	Research 3	
Subject	1901 - 64	1964 - 67	1967 - 70	1971 - 81	Total
Anthropology	0	0	0	27	27
Ballet	18	5	13	72	108
Careers	0	6	2	1	9
Choreography	103	111	124	419	759
Fitness	1	0	0	14	15
History	74	28	33	114	249
Kinesiology	0	0	0	40	40
Modern	4	43	53	103	203
Therapy	16	9	13	168	206

19

The figures illustrate the suddenness of the dance boom after 1970. For the subject of careers, the totals provide a clue as to the dynamic of the topic for dancers. A few studies were done in the early days for dance in higher education of the mid-'60's (six in the three year period 1964 - 1967), but the numbers fall off thereafter. The simple fact was that in terms of careers for dance the opportunities were limited. The increase in therapy in the period 1971 - 1981, suggests a growing interest in vocational preparation and an application of art ideas to rehabilitation and healing; again, perhaps indicative of the baby boom generation's search for a humanism and personal fulfillment in a career track. Brennan cites 990 master's theses and 256 doctor's degrees awarded in the period 1971 - 1981:

The acceleration in production in research is the result of the great number of persons now engaged in dance; the large number of educational institutions which currently offer majors and minors in dance; and increased understanding of the nature, purposes, and values of research; and competent training in research design. As dance has moved forward the need for an appreciation of its research has grown. We have learned that research itself can contribute to the body of knowledge of this field, as well as, for example, to improved pedagogy, understanding and development of creativity. More sophisticated bases for judging artistic products, deepened appreciation for the tradition of art, and clarification of the student dancer-teacher dynamic. [20]

Research in Dance IV: 1900 - 1990, published in 1992, is exclusively devoted to bibliographic and abstract information on doctoral research. The development of computer data bases permitted the inclusion of abstract information, and provided a means to search for this data without having to visit card catalogues, or review individual dissertation abstract volumes by hand. The title for *Research in Dance IV: 1900 - 1990* suggests doctoral theses in dance were completed in the early decades of the 20th century. The earliest citation in *Research in Dance IV* is William Fenton's "The Seneca Dance; A Study of Personality Expression in Ritual," Yale University, completed in 1937. Unfortunately Fenton's abstract is not included in the text. Abstract entries that are provided however illustrate the substance of early doctoral research:

Gladys Andrews: Ed.D., New York University, 1952:

> "A Study to Describe and Relate Experiences for the use of Teachers Interested in Guiding Children in Creative Rhythmic Experiences": This study relates and describes experiences in creative rhythmic movement as a medium of expression. It further deals with the nature of creative expression. It consists of two parts: the first is concerned with the needs and characteristics of children in early and middle childhood and the second part is a manual about the contributions of creative rhythmic movement to the development of children in the elementary school. In this study, creative rhythmic movement is not considered as an activity in itself, but as one means of contributing to the total development of the child. [21]

Lisa Lekas: Ph.D., Florida University, 1956:

> "The Origin and Development of Ethnic Caribbean Dance and Music": This study traces the historical development of the ethnic dance and music of the Caribbean Islands and examines their importance and significance from a sociological and anthropological point of view. The function of dance as an integral part of the life of the people is used to demonstrate how culture may be studied through the artistic manifestations of dance and music. The influences of the original Indians, the Africans, and the colonizing Europeans are discussed

and included is (*sic*) a survey of dance and music in the individual islands of the Caribbean. [22]

Patricia Sparrow: Ph.D., New York University, 1963:

> "The Choreographic Devices: Their Nature and Function as Related to the Principle of Opposition": A description of the devices which can be utilized in choreography and a demonstration of how they relate to the principle of opposition. A survey of selected professional dance teachers reveals devices they use in choreography. These findings serve as a basis for choreographic work titled "Forms and Versions" which explores opposition factors. [23]

Maxine Sheets: Ph.D., University of Wisconsin- Madison, 1963:

> "The Phenomenology of Dance": This descriptive study questions "what is dance?" and leads to implications for education based on phenomenological analysis. It explicates the nature of the illusion of force created by dance and includes the isolation and explanation of the phenomenological structures of time and space, the qualities of movement, the symbolic expressions, and the motions of abstraction and dynamics. [24]

The majority of doctoral work listed in *Research in Dance IV: 1900 - 1990* was written after 1960. According to data illustrated in a graph for the document, "Dissertations by Decade," the horizontal bar representing time lies flat until the 1930's when an increase is detected. By 1960, 30 dissertations had been completed. In the following decade this number shoots to 190, and by the time computer based data were analyzed, 600 titles were obtained. [25] Providing the academic setting for doctoral research in dance were the "Top 10" universities; ranked in order of their respective number of dissertations: New York University, Texas Women's University, University of Wisconsin-Madison, Columbia University, University of North Carolina, Ohio State University, Temple University, University of Southern California, Indiana University, and the University of Michigan. Since 1990, a change has occurred in Top 10 ranking. The University of Wisconsin no longer offers a doctoral program and moving to the top of the list is the new Ph.D. program in dance at the University of California-Riverside. Riverside's Ph.D. is the nation's first doctoral program created specifically for dance. Emerging out of the University of California's

286

cooperative graduate program in dance history, the Ph.D. program at Riverside focuses on advanced studies in dance history and theory.

The number of abstracts in *Research in Dance IV* devoted to ballet is worth noting. An explanation for the dominance of ballet in doctoral research, particularly in the period 1971 - 1990, may reside in a number of factors. The histories of music and ballet are intertwined, the history of criticism in the ballet is extensive, the cultural history of ballet is long and fairly well documented, professional positions in ballet are more common than in modern dance, its movement vocabulary is codified, and individual movements of this vocabulary, such as the *plie* (a bending of the knee), and *grande battement* (literally, "big kick"), are easily isolated for the purposes of scientific analysis. As a qualifier in doctoral research modern dance was less frequently identified in the statistics due to the ready use of comparable terms such as creative dance, or dance education, that suggest a modern approach to movement. The expansion of dance research in the colleges points us toward an important change in dance scholarship that evolved in the late 1970's and early 1980's: the rise of post-modern dance, and an accompanying widening of the scope and application of scholarship in the literature on dance.

Dance Scholarship and Pedagogy in Transition: A "Post-Modern Aesthetic"

In the first decade for dance in higher education, 1926 - 1936, the focus and development of dance programs was concerned with creative, modern dance of Euro-American origin, conceptualized in the behaviorist, creative, scientific, and liberal-humanist perspective of Margaret H'Doubler. In subsequent decades, 1936 - 1966, college dance struggled with issues of identity in its sibling rivalry with physical education. While retaining essential elements of H'Doubler's philosophy in the rationale for dance in the academy, almost surreptitiously, within the day to day experience in the classroom and in the studio, college dance began to assume the cultural characteristics of the professional field. The ensuing conflict between

287

liberal and professional orientations gathered strength during this period. In the 1960's, matters of identity for dance in the academic world were not only impacted by the academic struggle to get out from under physical education, but also by a professionally resurgent ballet; symbolized by the success of George Balanchine's coup in acquiring access to the resources of the Ford Motor Company, and a new vision for modern dance as the professional field turned toward a post-modern aesthetic, symbolized in the work of the Judson Church choreographers. The efforts of dance educators to separate from physical education was manifest in ways that have been discussed; the conferences of the 1960's and the creation of independent dance departments. The influence of post-modernism was slower to accumulate and its real impact in the academy was felt many years after the presentation of new choreographies at the Judson Church.

A hallmark of post-modernism was an end to artistic borders and traditional constructs for making and doing dance. In 1965, The *Drama Review* noticed the arrival of post-modernism, and revisited the topic in 1975. In introductory comments to the March, 1975 issue of *The Drama Review* , editor Michael Kirby explains the rationale for a second look at post-modern dance:

> The New Dance has been one of the most radical innovations in the performing arts in our time. Yet what we have been calling the New Dance is no longer new, it began around 1962....[P]erhaps it would be better to use a term that already has had some usage and refer to this recent work as "post-modern dance." This at least has the advantage of making a historical point: "post-modern dance" is that which has followed modern dance.
> In "The Rise and Fall and Rise of Modern Dance," Don McDonagh tries to avoid this kind of thinking by juxtaposing discussions of the work of people such as Merce Cunningham, Alwin Nikolais, Meredith Monk, and Yvonne Rainer under the single rubric "modern dance." (He does refer to work from the nineteen-thirties as "historic modern dance") What, however, are the characteristics that make certain contemporary work so different from modern dance, as it is generally known?....
> ...[I]n the theory of post-modern dance, the choreographer does not apply visual standards to the work. The view is an interior one: movement is not preselected for its characteristics but results from certain decisions, goals, plans, schemes, rules, concepts, or problems. Whatever actual movement occurs during the performances is acceptable as long as the limiting and controlling principles are adhered to.
> This rejects the musicalization of movement that typifies modern dance. Although Cunningham separated movement from the actual movement accompaniment, a "melodic" flow and a musical phrasing of his movements kept the music internalized in the behavior of the dancers. Post-modern dance ceases to think of movement in terms of music

288

> In the discussion of their work, the post-modern dancers do not mention such things as meaning, characterization, mood, or atmosphere....[T]heir work, unlike almost all modern dance, is not about anything. Dance is not used to convey messages or make statements. The dancers are merely themselves, they do not personify individuals, types, forces, and so forth. This means, among other things, that they use costume only in formal and functional ways. Their clothing does not send messages or represent. Unlike Merce Cunningham in a piece such as "Winterbranch," they never use lighting to suggest an imaginary place or to invoke a particular scenic atmosphere. Lighting functions only as illumination, not in terms of mood or effect, and many of the post-modern dance pieces are done outdoors in natural light. [26]

The non-traditional nature of the post-modern aesthetic caused repercussions in college dance. Academic dance was confronted with a new, largely indeterminate message from the artistic, professional world. Indeterminate in the sense that while the rules for making dances were changing, they were not changing toward a new set of 'rules.' The evolution of dance in the professional world presented collegiate dance with a charge: to contextualize what could, conceivably, degenerate into a post-modern indeterminate, and sectarian relativism, into a new approach that would be cohesive and purposeful in educationally viable terms.

The term ineffable has been used by some to describe the subjective, aesthetic nature of the dance experience: "Why is our syllabus for a studio technique class often only a half-page? Because dancing has such a density of content, of being, of implicit power that it is, thank God, ineffable." [27] Post-modernism in dance pushed the notion of the ineffable out of the technique class and into the composition class; where techniques for craft and composition were the theoretical foundation of choreographic pedagogy. Post-modernism also stimulated a reconsideration of what was transpiring in the classroom, where the traditional canons of modern dance history, aesthetic criticism, pedagogy, and philosophy could be challenged by post-modern theoretical perspectives; whether feminist, critical, positivist, or deconstructivist. As new ways of viewing dance found a place in academic programs, the processes of change initially promoted a certain sectarianism. Tradition and experiment; diversity and change, were topics that confronted dance faculty in new, and often conflicting ways.

If, as Kirby states above, in post-modern dance, "Dance is not used to convey messages or make statements. The dancers are merely themselves, they do not personify individuals, types, forces, and so forth"; and, "...In the theory of post-modern dance, the choreographer does not apply visual standards to the work", it was not a great conceptual leap toward thinking that the dominate theoretical-aesthetic-cultural paradigms for dance were likewise outdated and in need of revision. How was one to come to an aesthetic or intellectual judgment if everything in art-dance was up for discussion, and interpretation and standards were negotiable? The conceptual moorings for art-dance in higher education were coming loose. In the midst of a struggle to survive in the corporate university, dance education was having to retool its focus and purpose to include a much broader conceptualization of the meaning and place of dance in art and culture. In an article written for the *Journal of Physical Education, Recreation and Dance* (1990), titled "Educating for the Future: A Post-Modern Paradigm for Dance Education," author Penelope Hanstein comments on some of the issues a post-modern aesthetic posed for dance art and education:

> ...Occupying the minds of curriculum theorists who concern themselves with such issues is the emergence of a new post-modern paradigm which has its roots in the scientific discoveries derived from a post-modern view of the universe. As William Doll (1989) points out, "We see our vision of the universe turning from the single, stable, eternal one of Newtonian modernism to the complex, chaotic, finite one of post-modernism (p. 243). Post-modernism as a paradigm, a kind of foundation or architectural design which posits certain assumptions about reality, is by definition somewhat elusive. Toulmin (1982) explains that we are in the midst of a post-modern world "that has not yet discovered how to define itself in terms of what is, but only in terms of *what has just ceased to be* (p. 254) [author's emphasis]. **28**

As in science, in dance, a post-modern perspective was more in tune with what had been than with what would be. The post-modern world for dance was not only tied to a post-modern world for science, it was also tied to the discoveries derived from a post-modern view of the art. While reflecting the environment in which they exist, dance programs, like other disciplines in the arts, sciences, and humanities, shifted with the intellectual-aesthetic landscape, but with the added element of its own unique development of an artistic post-modernism, as a vital, and stimulating ingredient for change.

Shifts in the landscape for dance came at a time when re-invention was in the air in all of higher education, and dance, like other disciplines, was embarking on an expansive journey of redefinition. Post-modernism, multiculturalism, and diversity were the terms of a new engagement for dance in education. Academic interest in matters of diversity and multiculturalism in the arts prompted curricular attention to dance forms outside the Euro-American concert dance reference; the form and style that had dominated the curriculum for decades. African and Afro-Caribbean forms, the dances of the Pacific islands, and other newly labeled world-forms made inroads into the curriculum as faculty made an effort, albeit often a cursory one, to respond to the need for diversity in the dance program. In conjunction with change on a broad disciplinary scale, a new breed of dance educator/artist/scholar (or permutation thereof), came to the fore to help lead the way. The discipline is still in the processes of change. Recent evolutionary contributions toward change will be referenced in the next chapter of the story of dance in the American university.

Another environmental impact on the culture of modern dance in the universities was that, by the early 1980's, modern dance was falling on hard times in the professional world. The strains of surviving in a conservative art culture, retrenchment in government and corporate funding for the arts, shrinking university budgets for company residencies (a term used to describe a visit to a campus by a dance company usually consisting of a number of master classes and a performance), coupled with the high cost of salaries, studio space, and production, culled many modern dance groups out of existence. A new breed of student began to show up at the door, the returning professional.

In the colleges, modern dance was losing its dominate position as the curriculum was expanding to include ballet and other dance forms outside the modern tradition in technique, coupled with an increasingly broad perspective on theoretical studies in dance. Multicultural-professional-educational-technical-choreographic-historical-feminist-deconstructivist-political? What was the dance program supposed to do? How could any one program serve so many interests, and do this well? The ascendancy of styles other than modern in dance education was an attempt to keep up with the professional world as it was expanding its notion of what dance was, and a response to higher education's interest in a discourse that rejected marginalization, intellectual colonialism, and cultural disenfranchisement. Evolution in the cultural and artistic worlds of dance stimulated evolution in the academic.

Scholarship and critical inquiry within dance education had come a long way since the insecure and ill-defined days of the late 1950's. From first efforts in determining a field for research in dance, beginning in the areas of anthropology, ethnology, and criticism, had emerged a new scope and range of research in dance. New scholarship emerged out of feminist studies, out of a revisited history, new political theories of art and dance, dance science and medicine, the sociology of dance, and, even from technology for dance. [29] The theoretical perspective with which one chose to view dance impacted the scope and consequence of scholarly findings - ranging from deeply layered, theoretical wanderings that largely remain the intellectual province of an elite few, to new, and practical viewpoints and applications. Expansion in the discourse has been beneficial. Change has come to the discipline as a result of new paradigms for considering the world. Post-modern change and evolution has helped dance acquire academic stature as an important and provocative corporeal-artistic-cultural representation of human nature.

With all the changes that were experienced by dance programs in the 1970's and 1980's, one area of inquiry that did not rise to new levels of scholarly refinement was the area of research in dance education. Considered investigation into the effects of dance in education has remained largely anecdotal. Outside the anatomical, physiologic, and medicinal, research in dance education remains a realm of case studies. This is a terrain strewn with the remnants of fitful half-starts; projects begun and research paradigms unrealized. The reasons for this are fairly simple: time, human subjects, money, and refined research hypotheses.

For years dance educators have been making claims regarding the benefits of a dance-arts education. Again I refer to the 1940 comments by Walter Terry in Chapter 6, comments that Terry attributes to Elizabeth Hartshorn, director of dance at Connecticut College for Women regarding the benefits of curricular studies in dance:

> ...[B]ut at Connecticut College for Women Elizabeth Hartshorn, dance director, finds that the contemporary dance stimulates desire for activity, integrates the body and the mind, leads to appreciation and acquisition of beauty in human movement, increases sensitivity to environment, develops interest in the other arts as well as the dance, develops poise and self assurance and accuracy. [30]

Such claims are not uncommon today. Speaking from personal experience as a dance educator, I know that focused study in dance enhances the student's physical self-image and expressive capacity in use of the body. Bringing art ideas to expression through the body enhances skill in non-verbal communication, and practicing dance technique enhances skill in complex neuromuscular patterning: the list goes on. But, in pursuit of validating any of these notions I have no access to empirical proof. There is nothing in the literature to quantitatively prove that dance, dancing, or dance making does anything to help people be better educated, be better citizens, or be better prepared intellectually or kinesthetically for life's challenges. I sense that experience in dance does truly, educate. I think that it does, but I do not *know* that dance does anything for anybody. The fact that little has been empirically proven about the educational benefits of dance does much to prevent the discipline from taking a full and broadly recognized place at all levels of education. Only in the very recent past, in the last few years, has the issue of knowing what the arts do for students begun to be explored scientifically. Critically considered, quantitatively referenced, empirically based research in the area of dance education is the next great challenge for the discipline.

The Discipline Revisited: Multiculturalism and Changing Demographics

Having survived the first shock waves of university retrenchment and declines in enrollment, dance in higher education was on to new and broader horizons. New ways of looking at dance, and in appreciating the range and scope of dance world wide - perspectives that had been accumulating in their strength and persuasiveness over the previous two decades - led to new ideas for the curriculum and a new appeal for dance to students. The academy was in the vanguard of organized education's recognition that the future involved working toward an end to intellectual, gender-based, racial, and social marginalization. At the end of the 1980's the new perspective was multicultural, as common sense and demographics indicated a profound change in American society, and as diverse groupings within the population demanded equal access to the benefits of American life and education. Social activism, intellectual revision, and state and federal legislation designed to ensure public rights and access to fair treatment stimulated academic attention to matters of diversity, broad representation, and an expanded world view. As noted above, dance educators responded to change in a number of ways. Curricula were expanded to include world dance forms; what had previously been labeled primitive was re-termed primal, what had previously been viewed as foreign was attended to in a new light as diverse, vocational preparation was actively considered, technology was brought into the studio and into the classroom; the field was expanding. Change has been met with varying degrees of welcome acceptance, fitful recognition, and, in some cases derision and scorn. The culture of dance in America, especially in performance, is deeply felt by its practitioners and advocates, and is propagated by the cross currents of cultural trends, many styles, and dominate forms. Post-modernism has led to an abandoned delight in blending styles and forms, yet still: ballet remains at the cultural center; modern dance remains at the academic center and pulls classical dance in new, aesthetically challenging directions; jazz dance evolves toward popular tastes; dance in musical theatre takes notions from each to satisfy the demands of storyline, the producer's desire, and public interest; world forms expand the vision for dance yet largely remain corporeal artifacts. Tradition and experiment collide on the stage and in the classroom; the field's movement toward change is not without friction and uncertainty.

Through its official *JOPERD* journal, the American Alliance for Health, Physical Education, Recreation, and Dance has sponsored a bi-annual issue devoted to topics in dance titled "Dance Dynamics." Issues of "Dance Dynamics" were organized by the National Dance Association (NDA). As the official association for dance within the larger alliance, the NDA was, throughout the 1980's, the preeminent national organization representing the interests and concerns of dance educators in the schools and in the colleges. At the turn of the decade, a 1990 issue of Dance Dynamics was a forward looking edition titled "Dance, 1990 and Beyond - Future Trends", and was edited by Dianne Howe.

In the context of "Dance, 1990 and Beyond", author Janice D. LaPointe-Crump, addresses her concerns for dance in "The Future is Now - An Imperative for Dance Education":

> One of the legacies of post-modernism is an awakening to the cross-cultural linkages binding nations and peoples. Unheralded political events in eastern Europe during the waning weeks of 1989 point to the dawning of broad-based interchange and harmony. On the downside, the post-modern era has been characterized by a fatal attraction to micro-bits of cultural data and intellectual fragmentation. Images seem to bombard themselves, like colliding electrons....[T]his kind of thought pattern has threatened to empty arts education of valued, rich content.
>
> ....[W]arnings about the juxtaposition of the so-called trivial with the significant and the acceptance of a pluralistic cultural arena are valid. Connecting this argument to the development of a core of dance knowledge, if the arena of dance study is to be enlarged to accommodate pluralistic views of dance, will serious, thorough enterprises be compromised? Will the rigor of present dance curricula be undermined by instituting sweeping changes to create a new scenario for dance within arts, humanities, and physical education? I think not.
>
> ...[B]roadening the base of dance studies does not necessarily result in negative fragmentation. Instead, a framework for illuminating the essential properties of dance, thereby deepening our understanding of it as a component of basic education, can emerge. **31**

LaPointe-Crump goes on to discuss the importance of the conferences of the 1960's, specifically referencing the 1961 Conference on Movement and the 1965 Dance as a Discipline Conference for their contributions to a vision for the breadth and substance of dance as an academic program. She laments the fact that, following these conferences, the field turned toward "the notion that dance education is foremost a preparation of the performer-artist-teacher..." [32] arguing that this is " an imbalanced, narrow diet with little context to guide an understanding of dance within the broad matrix of American and world culture." [33] LaPointe-Crump further questions the wisdom of favoring a non-verbal educational experience in dance, and a prevailing patronizing attitude toward "ethnic, folk, liturgical, social, jazz, and tap dance...considered inferior, unpolished, unimportant, and unwelcome." [34]

LaPointe-Crump's article is fresh air in a discourse that had, by this time, become conflicted. Post-modernism in dance education was not universally met with open arms and an accepting spirit; substantive change hardly ever is. Post-modern dance led to both curricular change and cultural resentment: classes in world forms and other non-traditional techniques were added, but in many cases, were not mainstreamed into the curriculum or counted toward degree requirements. These classes were taught by adjunct faculty, and were rarely presented with pride as a product of the dance program, and, as LaPointe-Crump writes, were patronized.

In making her case for a reconsidered dance curriculum, LaPointe-Crump writes:

> Leaving the audience unattended, providing a narrow range of dance experience, and ignoring the native roots of dance has been costly. Dance is now admired but not understood; enjoyed but not advocated. With few discernible links to the real-life issues, dance has no discerning, committed public.
> It has taken nearly 25 years for us to recognize that socialization, happiness and well - being are byproducts, and not the cardinal points, of an education in the arts. Those early visions of dance education in America, etched in the 1960's, are today largely unfulfilled.
> ...[W]e urgently need to determine what constitutes vital knowledge by which the individual can know and easily represent the facets of the dance experience. Clean thought and expression are encouraged when there is a commonality of symbols. A goal centered vision for dance as a discipline must embrace a path of learning that is not only cohesive and progressive but also consistent and rigorous. The beauty of improved vision can radiate from clarifying the totality of dance as a richly symbolic and ritual-laden language. [35]

LaPointe-Crump's article is a very good place to end this chapter, as she concludes her thesis that, in fact, a pluralistic study of dance is not a travesty, using the metaphor of multiple languages in dance:

> Integrating dance as a lived experience, expressed through a comprehensive language, is the door to the future of dance in American education. Calling together a full range of creative and contemplative tendencies, a core of knowledge about dance must be shared first within the profession and then advocated in professional and public forums.
> Finally, authorizing a core of dance knowledge neither disenfranchises an individual scheme nor negates the radical nature of the issues out of which conflicting types of art arise" (Beiswanger, 1981, pp. 282 - 283). Studied from a variety of educational contexts, dance can achieve status as a central agent of American culture. [36]

CHAPTER 13

Experiments with Change in the Dance Program

As the 1990's began dance in higher education continued to struggle with the issues referenced in the previous chapter. Programmatic survival in a corporate-educational climate was still of central concern. Budget cutbacks seemed never-ending and funds for program development and capital expense were competitive and hard to come by. For many dance programs, even those with long standing reputations, enrollments remained flat or were in decline. The field was in need of new contexts for dance in education. Other issues that impacted the university dance program included realizing and activating curricular attention to multiculturalism, rapidly expanding opportunities in the interaction between the arts and technology, and developments in dance related scholarship which provided new paradigms for considering dance in art and culture. The practical matter of attending to planning for dance led a number of programs to consider radical shifts in their missions and curricula. Such change is well illustrated by the example of events that transpired for the first program for dance in higher education in the early 1990's, at the University of Wisconsin-Madison.

By the middle years of the 1980's, the dance program at Wisconsin had fallen on hard times. Unlike most dance programs in peer institutions, dance at Wisconsin continued to be academically affiliated with physical education in a Department of Physical Education and Dance. Reflecting developments in other departments located in the nation's major research universities, Wisconsin's physical education program, which dominated the department in terms of faculty and resources, had turned away from movement education and toward the physiology of human movement and issues related to sport. The dance program's relationship with the physical education program was plagued by the implicit and explicit cultural differences that had evolved between the fields over time, differences that have been outlined in the context of this book. New faculty had not joined the dance program in a number of years, and the faculty that were present were unable to come to agreement on a vision for the future of dance at the university. By 1985 enrollments in undergraduate (BS and BA), graduate (MS, MA, and MFA), and the doctoral program (Ph.D.), were in decline and the college Dean, unable to prod faculty toward substantive change, was threatening suspension of the degree programs in dance.

In 1987 - 1988 the Dean's threat was carried out when it was announced that the dance program at Wisconsin, the first in higher education, was no longer accepting majors. To reinvigorate the dynamic for dance at Wisconsin, a group of faculty in dance and the related arts conceived of a new program titled Interarts and Technology, or IATECH. Based on similar programs at other major research universities, including ACCAD (Advanced Computing Center for the Arts and Design) at The Ohio State University, and the University of Michigan's CPAT (Center for Performing Arts and Technology), Wisconsin's IATECH program was designed to, "educate students in an integrated arts curriculum consisting of the arts of sound, movement, and the visual arts primarily through the utilization of computer and video based technologies." [1]   Within two years of the 1991 acceptance of a degree program in Interarts and Technology, the numbers of undergraduates enrolled had increased to a sustainable margin. The administration at Wisconsin maintained its interest in reinstating the dance major, partially as a result of the success of the IATECH program, and partially as a result of openings in faculty lines brought about by retirement. The undergraduate major in dance was reinstated in 1993 - 1994, and plans are in motion for the return of the MFA degree program in the near future. [2]

Another example of change is illustrated by events that transpired at the University of California-Los Angeles, where the first independent, arts-affiliated dance department at a research university was formed by Alma Hawkins in 1962. In this case, change came about in the direction of muticulturalism. In 1995, UCLA's department of dance was absorbed into a new Department of World Arts and Cultures, within the School of Arts and Architecture Change for dance at UCLA met with concern from leaders in the field, in part because of the legacy of leadership in dance education that had been pioneered by Alma Hawkins. Losing an independent dance program of the stature of UCLA's was a blow to the field's struggle to maintain the integrity of other dance programs threatened by a decade of retrenchment and educational downsizing in the university. But the evolution of dance at UCLA may also be viewed as an experiment with the future in that UCLA's was the first major program in dance to attempt substantial revision toward institutionalizing muticulturalism in the arts. Within the department of World Arts and Cultures the dance program continues to offer graduate degrees (MA and MFA) in dance. The World Arts and Cultures department's mission statement, as it appears in the text of UCLA's current website reads as follows:

> UCLA's newest academic department is at the forefront of innovative interdisciplinary and cross-cultural study of the arts. The Department of World Arts and Cultures was launched in July of 1995 to help dancers, performing artists and scholars develop new responses to the complex issues facing the arts today. Developed through the consolidation of the Department of Dance and the World Arts and Cultures Interdepartmental Program, it is housed within the School of the Arts and Architecture.
> The new academic unit combines the most compelling features of both programs: the Dance department's commitment to integrating theory and practice from a global perspective, and World Arts and Cultures' unique emphasis on cross-cultural study. The resulting department focuses on the creation, critical analysis and cultural study of arts practice throughout the world. With an emphasis on the diverse populations of the United States, the curriculum integrates performance practice, studies in cultural and performance theory, and applied forms of knowledge. [3]

Technology and multiculturalism have been two important areas for change for dance in the 1990's. Yet implementing technological or multicultural approaches to dance has generated concern in the field as educators grapple with the issues each presents the discipline. Technological applications for dance have made great strides in the past two decades. In 1989 the National Dance Association published a monograph titled *Dance Technology: Current*

301

Applications and Future Trends. In this volume, editor Judith A. Gray discusses the origins of interest in employing technology to facilitate dance education:

> ...[O]f all the arts, dance would seem the least likely to accede to the vagaries of rapid change and the relentless advances of this modern technology. Dance, the art of human movement, on the surface appears non technologically inclined. It is the self-sufficient art. Indeed, dance education pioneer Margaret H' Doubler believed that dancers were their own teachers, students, textbooks, and laboratories. She would have no doubt included computers in that list had she been aware of their existence and function...
>
> The first attempts to consider the possible collaboration between computer and dance occurred in the 1960's at the University of Pittsburgh. Under the direction of Jeanne Beaman, the choreographic process was gingerly codified and manipulated using a computer and a comparatively remarkable memory capacity - although sadly, the results of this collaboration were neither published or performed. In the 1970's a few dance researchers devised a methodology to computerize Labanotation - the symbolic "scoring" system for coding and recording dances....It wasn't long before computerized dance notation systems incorporated graphics and sound so that notated dances could be reproduced symbolically on a monitor along with synthesized sound effects. [4]

At Simon Fraser University in British Columbia, a prototype computer image of the human figure was created by Lynne Weber and S. W. Smoliar that they termed "Sausage Man." Weber and Smoliar's model lacked a versatile range of motion. "Bubble Man" was the next model for exploring computer generated human movement, developed by Colin Emmett at England's Royal College of Art. "Bubble Man" was able to cast shadows and provided more realistic joint movements and elevations of limbs. [5]

Developments have continued throughout the decade, and conferences on dance and technology (the first of which was held at the University of Wisconsin in 1992), have demonstrated the latest applications; from more sophisticated programs in body images, some of which allow multiple figures to engage in three dimensional, virtual choreography, to programs that permit the simultaneous presentation of text, filmed or virtual performance, and notation on one screen. Yet, technology challenges dance education in a number of ways. In an article for *Dance Research Journal* (1998), author Richard Povall discusses the matter of the ubiquitous nature of technology and technological change, as such matters impact dance and dance education:

Technology is with us - its part of our daily life and culture, and while some fear and decry the technocrats, we also revel in their works and indulge their perceived control over us...

...There is a received wisdom amongst the dance community that technology is a dangerous thing - that to use technology as an integral element is to detract from the body, from the choreography and design, from the core of what is dance. We don't discuss the dangers of using increasingly high-tech lighting systems; we don't question that computers can at some level be used to help choreographers make work; we don't doubt that computers can help us refine and develop notation systems, and that video cameras are at least partially successful in their ability to capture work for later retrieval and analysis. [6]

Povall continues to outline the pro's and con's of actively engaging technology for the purposes of dance. There is the matter of access to technological apparatus, and the time necessary to develop sufficient skills in managing these systems, time spent away from the actual doing and making of dance. There is also the degree of control one must relinquish - in terms of developing performance that is removed from human participatory experience - and the degree to which the technology mandates the kinds of spaces in which one may create. The conventional isolation of the choreographer's creative experience, as she or he works alone in a studio with their dancers, is also impacted by interaction with technology. Choreographers using technology to generate new compositions are restrained by the sophistication of the program used, and by their own skill in ensuring that the dance is not superseded by the facility and glamour of the technology. No doubt technology will continue to move forward and take us with it. Its potential in dance has caused great fear, excited anticipation, and ambiguous indifference. Quite certainly technological developments in dance, as in all areas of our lives, will continue to grow and evolve; challenging our sensibilities, confronting our tastes, awakening our fears, and delighting our infatuation with the new.

Multiculturalism in dance also presents the field with challenges and opportunities. While the idea of experiencing and viewing dance in multicultural contexts has evoked the dance educator's inherent interest in the expressive potential of human movement, in many cases interest and subsequent engagement have collided with the field's essentially conservative sensibility. Consider, for example, this anecdotal story of one person's experience with multiculturalism as a graduate student in dance at UCLA.

In a conversation with this student I asked, "What was your experience like at UCLA, in learning and using multicultural dance forms in technique and choreography?" Paraphrased, her response was; "Well, while we had the opportunity to study dance forms other than modern and ballet, like Javanese and Korean dance, we weren't permitted to count credits earned in these classes toward our degree. The more important issue was in choreography. I spoke with the faculty about using some of the techniques I had learned in Indonesian dance and music in creating a new work in contemporary choreography and my request was met with silence, as if by asking this, I had violated some unspoken rule of appropriate behavior." [7] Admittedly one student's experience, this story does point to two of the central issues the field has to address in its pursuit of multiculturalism: what role do multiple forms play in the acquisition of technique and, how are traditional forms referenced in the creation of new works of art?

For many in dance education, allegiance to a sense of tradition confronts us as it arrives at, and intersects with, diversity expressed through multiculturalism. Anthropologist Joann Kealiinohomoku asked her colleagues to consider ballet as a form of ethnic dance 30 years ago; many then were startled at this idea. [8] The field has expanded its thinking since Kealiinohomoku's admonition, but I still wonder about our actions. For many, world forms are non-western dance forms that are learned and presented as a kind of corporal tradition; as cultural artifact of and by the body. In this context these forms are replicate and presentational, but are not evolutionary, nor are they meant to be creatively stimulating. I am left to ask, in teaching and practicing world forms, do we clearly and fully understand the goal of including these in an educational curriculum? An educational rationale for the inclusion of a cultural form (or any dance form) in a curricular plan might be that the student practices the form while simultaneously studying the cultural and physical geography and history of the region from which the form evolved. If a unified approach isn't applied to all forms students are exposed to, including modern and ballet forms, then the frame of reference for 'not-modern,' 'not-ballet,' is that of 'other,' and of being of and about, 'other.'

Beyond thinking about diversity as it is manifested through performance and the acquisition of movement techniques, other questions come to mind in considering the inclusion of multicultural forms in the curriculum: how else must we rethink the curriculum to actually go about diversifying dance as an academic discipline? What is the effect of diversity on artistic-choreographic experiment? Does attention to diversity, and the accompanying important considerations of appropriation, authenticity, acculturation, and transculturation, stifle or augment artistic invention? How comfortable are contemporary dance educators in discussing and deconstructing non-western dance forms for the purposes of cultural understanding, movement analysis, or for stimulating new directions in choreography? Is everything up for grabs, or are some things sacred? Do we know the difference?

Another set of questions arises if we consider recent attention to diversity as a result of the influence of the corporate university. Are matters of diversity in the curriculum, at least in part, being promoted because this enhances the educational program as commodity? Education is more a product-driven business than many of us are willing to admit. Why? Because diversity makes good business sense. Like shopping at *WalMart*, the "superstore," success in education today is in providing the greatest range of attractive products under one roof. Are we embracing diversity, at least in part, for similar reasons?

How have we framed diversity in practical terms in the curriculum? Is our attention to providing the movement experiences of a multicultural perspective diverting our attention from the long term place the substance of diversity will have in the curriculum? And, outside considering non-western dance forms, the question remains; how *do* we fit musical theater and jazz dance forms into an educational dance curriculum? These are questions for the present and for the future. In many ways, dance education in the 1990's, like the post-modern aesthetic discussed in the last chapter, is unaware of what it has, or wants to become.

Organized Activity: New Specialization in the Field

Like other disciplines, dance in higher education has benefited from a refinement in the field of organizations that serve its constituents. Over time the field has expanded to presently include over 40 professional-service organizations that attract both national and international membership. The evolution of the organizational field for dance education in the past two decades is important to the history of dance in the university. This is an evolution that has been marked by change. Organizations such as the "Dance Critics Association," "Black College Dance Exchange," "Dance and the Child International," the "International Association for Dance Medicine and Science," and the "International Association of Blacks in Dance," have joined and enriched the organizational field for dance and dance education, a field that, in the early 1970's was made up by a handful of groups. In the summer of 2000, many of the national-international organizations for dance education will collaborate for the first time at an international conference titled "Dancing in the Millennium," scheduled for July 19 - 23, 2000 in Washington D.C. The Dancing in the Millennium Conference is a joint conference of:

> Congress on Research in Dance
> Dance Critics Association
> National Dance Association
> Society of Dance History Scholars

With the participation of:

> American Dance Guild
> American Dance Therapy Association
> Country Dance and Song Society
> Dance and the Child International /USA Chapter
> Dance Films Association
> Dance Heritage Association
> Dance Librarians Committee/American Library Association
> Dance Notation Bureau
> Dance USA

International Association of Blacks in Dance
International Association for Dance Medicine and Science
Laban/ Bartenieff Institute of Movement Studies
National Dance Education Organization
Preserve, Inc. **9**

The National Dance Association evolved out of the National Section on Dancing (1931 - 1963), and the Dance Division of the American Association for Health, Physical Education, and Recreation (DD of AAHPER: 1963 - 1974). With the creation of an Alliance structure in 1974, AAHPER consisted of the National Associations (with various titles and interests in the broad areas of sport, physical education, recreation and leisure, health, and dance), the Districts (regional associations of similar range and focus), and the States (affiliated, but independent state versions of the larger Alliance). Even with the creation of a national association for dance, Alliance leaders resisted adding a 'D' to the organization's moniker. Adding the 'D' took four more years of campaigning to implement. In 1978 the Alliance's name was changed to the American Alliance for Health, Physical Education, Recreation, and Dance - AAHPERD.

Since the founding of the Dancing Section in 1931, dance educators in the Alliance had worked hard and long for organizational recognition. Governance issues for dance as it existed within the Alliance had been a major concern to NDA leaders for decades. In financial, cooperative venture, and operational terms, the support provided dance by the Alliance was often meager and conflicted by what seemed to be arcane and self-defeating policy turns. [10] By the late 1980's the national associations were feeling the effects of an outmoded governance structure. To address the needs of the organization at the national level, Alliance leaders met in 1991 to look at alternative governance structures. The Alliance Board of Governors considered four models for change: "Models I - IV." Ranging from a tight coupling of Associations (I), to a loosely-knit federation (IV) of independent organizations, Models I - IV focused on the degree to which Alliance structures would be affiliated financially and in terms of shared management and mission. Model III, just to the left of center in terms of formal relations between Alliance

Association's, was chosen and presented to AAHPERD's membership for consideration in 1992.

Under Model III, National Associations were permitted a new and much greater autonomy in their individual pursuit of resources, inter-organizational contacts, and membership development. However, despite the best efforts of the NDA leadership to access the benefits of Model III, by 1994 the National Dance Association was in danger of bankruptcy. To study options for saving the NDA, Association President and Interim Executive Director Jane Bonbright appointed a Future Directions Task Force in 1995. As Co-Chair of this group (1995 - 1998), I reported to the members of the Task Force and to the NDA Board of Directors. In my final report to NDA leaders in 1998, I summarized the events that had transpired between 1995 and 1998, events which subsequently led to the creation of the new organization, the National Dance Education Association:

> Four years ago the current manifestation of the NDA Future Directions Task Force was organized by Jane Bonbright to help the NDA Board of Directors envision and implement plans for the NDA's future. The FDTF has been sustained in its activity by NDA Presidents Lynnette Overby [1995 - 1996] and Sara Lee Gibb [1997 - 1998].
>
> Over these past four years we have met and worked to insure the success of NDA in response to a variety of events, issues, and concerns. After our first meetings [of the Future Directions Task Force] in St. Louis, which coincided with the Fall 1995 [Alliance] BOG [Board of Governors] meetings, the immediate fiscal need of NDA was addressed when a loan was secured from the Alliance that helped NDA get back on its financial feet. The autonomy permitted Associations under Model III was used to our benefit and in 1995 - 1996 NDA became more financially sound. The degree of autonomy NDA enjoyed in producing goods, securing external support, and working with other groups in the environment helped NDA become more stable and active in the field. However, Model III also illustrated the fact that for a National Dance Association to really thrive separate 501(c)3 status was necessary. Unfortunately separate non-profit status is not possible for the NDA as an Association under AAHPERD.
>
> In the Fall of 1997, at the AAHPERD Board of Governors meetings, the Alliance leadership withdrew its commitment to Model III. Model III was perceived as being the source of an increasing lack of cohesion within the Alliance, as Associations were acting independently in the environment. AAHPERD leaders, sensing the need for an overarching mission that would tie the Associations, Districts, and States more closely together, brought forward a series of motions and votes that would serve to end Model III, reassert central control of Associations under AAHPERD management, and shape the endeavors of Associations by having their actions relate to a unified mission of promoting "Healthy, Active Lifestyles."
>
> To be sure, there were some tense moments during and following the Fall 1997 BOG meetings. The NDA Board left Reston [Virginia, location of the Alliance Headquarters] feeling a bit like they had had the rug pulled out from under them. These feelings though, were just symptomatic of deeper issues that had been accumulating for many years: the environment was changing, organized efforts for arts education were

evolving, the need for a national organization aligned with the goals of dance as art-based education was apparent.

To these ends, and following the 1997 BOG meetings, the NDA Board decided to seek separation from AAHPERD. The time certainly seemed right, after all the Alliance was looking toward increased centralization and actions reflecting a specific mission that was not inclusive of the changing needs of dance education. Separation, while on the surface a dramatic event, was understood by many to be a rational response to the evolution of dance as a discipline. But separation also carried with it a number of other issues: If dance leaves the Alliance, what would stop other Associations from doing the same? How to untie a set of legal, fiscal, and material cords that connected dance to AAHPERD? Active consideration of separation was a process that elicited deep felt responses from NDA members. [11]

As the winter of 1997 - 1998 came to a close, so too did the debate over NDA separation from AAHPERD. The legal and cultural ramifications of attempting to separate dance from the larger Alliance seemed too great. In March of 1998, NDA Board members and the Co-Chairs of the Future Directions Task Force met in Baltimore, Maryland to discuss the options that were available. Out of these discussions was raised the possibility of creating a new organization. With additional input from sources both in and outside of the NDA, the group decided that the best answer to all of our concerns was to simply initiate a separate and independent National Dance Education Association (NDEA; which, as a result of Alliance concern over the similarity in acronyms between NDA and NDEA, changed its title to the National Dance Education Organization [NDEO] in May of 1999), to pursue the goals of dance as a separate, arts-related, curriculum-based discipline. This allowed for the creation of an organization unfettered by the rules of alliance, one with independent legal status, and one, hopefully, that would allow the nation's dance educators to empower a future that was in the best interests of arts-related dance education. The NDA continues to exist as part of AAHPERD, left to pursue the interests of dance as these relate to promoting the Healthy-Active Lifestyles mission of the Alliance.

Recent developments for dance in K-12 education helped stimulate the creation of the new organization. Opportunity for positive change in dance education came about as a result of several federal initiatives in the early 1990's. In, "Dance Education 1999: Status, Challenges, and Recommendations" (1999), author Jane Bonbright writes:

In 1994, President Clinton and Congress signed into legislation [the] Goals 2000: Educate America Act, which aligned dance with arts in education and declared the arts equal to other core curricula (math, science, language arts and foreign languages, government and civics, and history). The National Endowment for the Arts (NEA), National Endowment for the Humanities, the USDOE [United States Department of Education] granted $1 million to support an initiative by the four national arts education associations [National Art Education Association, National Dance Association, Music Educators National Conference, and American Theater Education Association] to develop and write standards in the four arts disciplines - dance, music, visual arts and theater. The national standards for dance education identify content and achievement standards for what students should know and be able to do in dance at the benchmark grades of four, eight, and twelve. Of supreme importance to dance education [in elementary and secondary education], the *National Standards for Dance Education* accomplished several things:

1. It was among the first national documents to identify and describe dance as a creative art form in education.
2. It aligned dance with art education.
3. It validated dance as a discrete discipline and partner with core subjects in education.
4. It clearly described discrete content, skills, and knowledge to be learned in dance education.
5. It provided benchmarks at grades four, eight, and twelve.
6. It supported consistent and sequential learning taught by qualified dance educators.
7. It dramatically changed pedagogical content and process [for dance]. [12]

The development of dance education programs in American schools would help stabilize dance programs in higher education - both in terms of student preparation for advanced studies in dance and in vocational opportunity. Yet, while passage of the Educate America Act and the creation of the *National Standards for Dance Education* bodes well for dance in K-12 education, there is still much to be done to implement these goals and objectives. There is still disagreement in the field regarding the content of the Standards. Few school districts have institutionalized an arts-based curriculum in dance. State certification for dance educators is not common. Fortunately, however, the impetus is toward change and increased visibility for dance in K-12 education. The National Dance Education Organization is currently working with other national education organizations to address the future potential of dance in the schools.

Educating Tomorrow's Dancer: Some Thoughts from the Field

As the history revealed in this text approaches the present, the last concern I address, prior to making some projections for the future of dance in the American university, involves a discussion of educating tomorrow's dancer. I reference some current opinions of this topic in contemporary articles by leaders in the field.

In a series of articles reminiscent of its "College of Career" column of the 1960's, *Dance Magazine* addressed issues of dance in higher education in the 1990's. "Dancers in Cap and Gown" appeared in *Dance Magazine's* 1994 - 1996 issues. In each installment, leading educators were asked to respond to contemporary issues in a round-table format. For the September 1994 issue of *Dance Magazine*, "Leading members of the American College Dance Festival Association in the Southeast discuss the nature of multiculturalism, technique, and the place of repertory in college dance programs." [13] In this article, dance educators Patty Phillips, Lynda Davis, and Nancy Smith-Fichter (Florida State University), and Timothy Wilson and Gretchen Warren (University of South Florida), respond to six questions posed and moderated by Phillips:

What is the most important issue facing university dance programs today?

Fichter responds first, stating that the "isms" are of central concern. Attention to muticulturalism must be considered in conjunction with technological change, "changing age and changing demographics": "the challenge is to deal with these issues, not in a trendy or token way, but in a way that will help the student advance in his or her mission while addressing an increasingly changing world." [14] Wilson states that diversity needs to be at the center of the curriculum, to which Fichter responds: "I think we are afraid that we will lose some of the things for which we fought so long, such as providing professional training in the classical forms. There is the danger of becoming trendy and dilettante so that the refining isn't happening." [15]

311

Warren contributes the following statement that, while honest and forthcoming, raises the fearful sub-text of concerns many in dance education have regarding multicultural change:

> We have to remember that the majority of jobs out there are not in a bunch of peripheral ethnic dance forms. The majority of jobs still happen to be in classical ballet and modern dance. Very few of our undergraduates come to college to get an intellectual understanding of the dance world. They come in because they like to dance, and they hope they are going to become dancers. For me, the biggest issue is in changing the image of college dance as being outside the professional dance world. This just is not true anymore. The standards for the faculty in the last twenty years have gone way up. As the economic situation becomes worse, there are a lot of retiring dancers out there who want jobs, and the academic job market is becoming a very desirable one. The standards for hiring are going up and up.... [16]

Following Warren's assessment of the real world, and the need for students to learn to dance at professional levels if they hope to use their college experience in pursuing a vocation in dance, the conversation turns to:

How are we preparing our students and for what are we preparing them?

The gist of this part of the discussion has to do with the college experience in dance as a sort of apprentice preparation to dance, and make dances, professionally. Wilson raises the concern of the colleges becoming the sole resource in training for contemporary (modern) dance, but this issue is passed by to discuss the problem of what life for the dancer is like after college. In response to the next question:

What kinds of jobs are there for graduates of our programs? Are we preparing performers? Teachers?

Smith-Fichter: "Parents ask, What can we guarantee after four years? I say, "Nothing. If you choose to make your life in the arts there is no guarantee....What you can guarantee is that they will get an excellent education, both professionally and as humanistically as possible." [17]

Wilson: "One thing we can give them besides dance is a sense of self. They are investing their bodies and souls in this art, learning about who they are." [17]

Would that we knew that this latter statement was true. The rest of the group's discussion is in response to the following questions;

What is the place of repertory in our programs?
The majority of students in college dance programs are women - What is the place of young men in our programs?
How about department budgets: How are we surviving?

The discussion on these final three questions covers familiar territory; each participant says repertory is good, getting men into dance is hard because of cultural attitudes toward men and dancing, and comment on the lack of dance experiences in the elementary and secondary schools. Budget cutbacks for university dance programs are a harsh reality, with most cutbacks coming in allocations for performance and production. Fichter's closing comment sums up the central concern with retrenchment, "These cuts, without additional funding, would put us back to the way it used to be in the university: teaching people about dance, not actually *doing it .*" [19]

This roundtable discussion, like so many others, seems to spin in on itself as dance educators have no easy, or comfortable, answers or solutions to the issues that confront the discipline, or perhaps more importantly, about the culture from which the student emerges. The view is internally focused, about dance in isolation, about preparing for the art of dance with little concern about the issues that face the people being prepared. If, as we are reminded by the press and by our own understanding of educational demographics and statistics, 25% of students are seriously at risk of not reaching a productive adulthood, approximately another 25% are educationally disadvantaged, and about 30% of students in the schools are of Hispanic or African-American heritage, how do these figures and trends impact the nature and focus of our *educational* (author's emphasis) programs in dance? [20] Indirectly pressed to answer these questions in a popular magazine, perhaps the responses above are to be expected. But, where can one find discourse that confronts contemporary social-educational issues, the nature of positive change, or proposes answers for dance in the academy that are new and forward thinking? Oddly enough, some answers seem to arise in journals outside of dance. One example is an article titled "Educating Dance Educators - What Next?", published in the summer 1995 by the Council for Research in Music Education, and written by Luke Kahlich.

In this paper, Kahlich begins his text by asking: "Do we need a new breed of dance educator? What kind of breed do we have now, and what will be their future challenges? What does dance have to contribute to general education and how do dance educators relate to the curriculum, to the school, and to local, state and national educational goals?" [21] In the context of the real issues that face students, can dance afford not to take a moment to recontextualize the disciplines nature as part of an educational system? Kahlich thinks not, writing:

> In the world of dance training and education, most of the applied pedagogy has been based on historical modeling (i.e. teaching what and how you were taught). Although this may have served the western classical form well in terms of preservation, it is not pertinent to the current and increasingly diverse functions and demographics of our students, schools, society or our art form. As Sylvie Fortin (1992) writes, "The consequence of teaching as one has been taught fails to answer the new and changing demands of our western society (p. 37)." [22]

Kahlich asks provocative questions about the discipline. He questions the dance educator's role in preparing for the future skills any educator is expected to bring to their work, citing Cetron (1985), as stating, "The educator of the future will have extensive experience with such topics as brain development chemistry, learning environment alternatives, cognitive and psychosomatic evaluation and affective development." [23] Educators projecting the future overwhelmingly predict a much greater range of skills and competencies demanded for those who would enter the field. Kahlich rhetorically asks: "What are the implications for dance educators?" [24]

> I hear that students are unmotivated, lazy and inattentive. This approach, it seems to me, is like the doctor telling you, as you sit before him/her coughing and wheezing, that you are definitely "sick," and like many doctors, we have often attempted to name and "medicate" the symptoms of problems, rather than understand their root causes, which may include ourselves. In dance, we still tend to deliver information and skills with the philosophy and perspective of 19th century Swedish and German gymnastics where failure was seen as the fault of the student or teacher, and rarely (if ever) of the "system." In a recent faculty retreat, some of my colleagues lamented a lack of passion of their students. I wonder, however, how we can expect passion from a student who has just completed twelve years of "education" in a system that discourages and distrusts things such as "intuition," "feelings," or "passion" because they are difficult or impossible to measure and quantify. The vast majority of these students have not been taught or encouraged to seek, value or channel passion or feelings positively, except of course as extracurricular activities, emphasis on the "extra," with little or no attachment to the curriculum. [25]

Kahlich's article is an excellent call to the field to make the effort to project dance into the future, as educational medium and in preparing dance educators to meet the challenges that they will face in working with a diverse, often challenged, student population. There is a real and present need for the field of dance in education to continue to refine and clarify its artistic goals, its educational objectives, its relationship with other disciplines and content areas in education, and provide a realistic assessment of the benefits of the dance experience for students of all ages.

Projections for the Future

In ending this text, Luke Kahlich's cautions loom large in my thinking. The question of how dance educates people is still in need of clarification. To me it seems that this question has driven the work and thinking of every university dance educator: what are our students getting out of this thing we call a dance education? As I continue to educate *through* dance, I realize more and more the need for continued efforts toward clarification. I believe Kahlich is right when he says, "In dance, we still tend to deliver information and skills with the philosophy and perspective of 19th century Swedish and German gymnastics where failure was seen as the fault of the student or teacher, and rarely (if ever) of the system." [25] Exactly what the system is, is a question we have been very reluctant to address. A system implies a conceptual approach. Going back to the dictionary for meaning, as was done for dance at the beginning of this text, we find that 'system' is defined as a noun with the following primary meanings - "1. A group of interacting, interrelated, or interdependent elements forming a complex whole" and " 2. A functionally related group of elements." [26]

Some have tried to conceptualize a systematic approach to dance education. In Margaret H'Doubler's thinking the system was the considered process of revealing the "knowing subject-object known" relationship through science, philosophy, and the creative exploration of movement. To Martha Hill, the system was what professional artists said it was, as they prepared to perform abstract, technically challenging, and individualistic art statements that a Euro-American culture deemed professional. To contemporary educators working outside a Euro-American professional tradition, dance has become a poignant cultural symbol of individuation; a cultural ground against which life as it is experienced as "other" may be supported. This is not to suggest that people of European origin do not also engage in cultural dance to reinforce sense of self and individuation. The professional context of dance is what lends its meaning such a close connection to art, and art dance has come to symbolize dance in education.

Perhaps these perspectives only underline the problem in attempting to define and contextualize too broad a term (dance), too narrowly. Or, conversely, of attempting to define and contextualize too narrow a term (dance), too broadly. When the terms dance and education are joined at the metaphoric hip we must think both broadly and narrowly. We must come to a system that permits a dance experience for many different students, from many different backgrounds, and with many different interests. The system we envision must be an interrelation of complex elements forming a whole, for teachers and students alike. The future will be realized through the success (or lack thereof), of our collective efforts to analyze, assess, include, reject, and refine understanding of the useful elements that comprise the complexity of an interrelated system for dance education. To this end, dance educators must, at some level, reject the notion that dance is an ineffable act in education. Dance may continue to enjoy its complex, and one might argue, schizophrenic persona outside the academy. But within ivied walls, I would argue that our obligation is to try to *know* what it is our students are learning - as far as that is possible given our current knowledge of the body-mind, current social trends in culture and the arts, and educational theory. To be sure, we can never know that all that we intend in educating our students is working. But, this fact should not prevent us from continuing to try to clarify our educational goals, objectives, and projected outcomes.

In the course of writing this volume, one of the more interesting aspects of the culture of educational dance that I have come to more fully understand, is a great fear of intellectualizing dance. I think that we are fearful of relating the felt, and the objectively understood in the contexts of our dancing, dance making, reflecting on dance, and deconstructing its elements. We reject the notion of the dumb-dancer, yet perpetuate this notion through our refusal to engage in conceptually assessing the merit and worth of dance as art and in education. If we promote a culture of anti-intellectualism, and if we refuse to accept the imperative of a valued multiculturalism, we risk losing our connection to the future. If we turn away from the responsibilities that result from the current trend of systematized education being pushed into realms of learning and behavioral adaptation formally consigned to the family, and if we do not actively seek an inter-relatedness between learning through dance and learning through science, the humanities, the other arts, and through understanding basic tenets of ethical living, then our students will do no better than we when they replace us.

Another aspect of our future that I have learned to better appreciate in the process of writing this book was summed up by conference members of the · Developmental Conference on Dance when they stated:

The conference participants felt that it was important that professional and educational leaders in dance give consideration to standards of quality that should be used as a guide in the establishment of new dance curricula. They recognized that all major programs will not be the same. In fact, curricula will vary markedly because of the uniqueness of each situation. For example, one would not expect the dance major in a small liberal arts college to be the same as the program in a large university....Diversity among our institutions will give strength to the total effort in dance. But under girding all of the differences should exist the standard of quality. [28]

"...all major programs will not be the same." Has this been the case? In many regards it has not, as faculty lack the vision or resources and support to truly come to terms with what it is they can be. For dance in higher education the tendency has been to imitate standards, and not to address the unique traits and characteristics each combination of dedicated faculty may bring to bear in crafting an evolutionary model for dance education. The pressures against programmatic individuation do not only come from within, the desire to be like the other is institutionally embedded in higher education; everybody wants to be like Harvard. Not only is it conceptually easier to imitate, it is an easier sell to administrators and parents looking for a replica of the gold standard. It's human nature. It's a tough thing to overcome, especially in a world where so much can be learned about the envied other so quickly.

Being different is hard: to be the iconoclast, in a sea of programs all seeking to look like the same kind of fish; beautiful, yet strong and fearsome to predators. Perhaps in our zeal to not "be" physical education, but to "be" dance, we have forgotten that, in many ways, dance is as great (and yet much less culturally defined), a thing to champion in education as is the notion of a physical education. Physical education is currently a misnomer; in the universities physical education has become about refining the science of exercise physiology and strategies of sport, with satellite programs in recreation. In the schools physical education is about athletic education.

For dance in higher education, the discipline has come to be about art. The adaptation of the conservatory model was a way out from under physical education, and a way to identify with art. In dance art the end result of activity is performance. We have made performance the focus of dance in higher education, although this need not be so for all programs. We must help the faculty of each program bring to the fore that which makes their cooperative effort substantial. We must also help the field expand its notion of the merit and worth of dance related pedagogy, developed multicultural appreciation, and theoretical inquiry. Excellence in dance education must be referenced not only to professional art standards, but also to individual creativity, to cultural understanding, to theoretical appreciation, and to intellectual and kinesthetic development. The dance program should reference the desire dance faculty have to collectively and individually excel, and the community in which it resides. But, ultimately, and perhaps most importantly, dance in higher education must attend to the charge of the academy: to push back the boundaries of knowledge, to forward the cultural legacy, and to contribute to society.

Acknowledging this charge, I leave this text to those who will revisit and refine this history in the future. Weeks before the turn to a new millennium, I reflect on the nature and history of higher education. This story started with a moral, socially responsible community of scholars almost one thousand years ago. The seed was planted then that learning is part of realizing our humanity, and is preparation for our contribution to civilization. This has framed the subsequent development of all disciplines; it has been no different for dance. Our roots as dance educators lie in our conviction that dance may contribute to connecting us: to our bodies; our vessels in life, to our inherent creativity; that which opens the door of the future, and to our shared humanity; our empathy for others. In doing so, dance may help prepare those who will follow us, for their future. This is the legacy for dance; that something which passes through us, is in us, and is us; is passed on. The future for dance in the American university is in realizing this vision with ever increasing clarity and commitment.

NOTES

- Introduction -

The term higher education references instruction within a college or university. The terms college and university are different manifestations of the same organized activity and refer to post-secondary institutions for advanced learning. As an independent unit the college is usually limited in its size, scope, and focus. The college traditionally awards the bachelors degree in the liberal arts or sciences. Today, colleges may also award masters and doctorate degrees. The University has traditionally been a center for teaching and research offering undergraduate, graduate (masters and doctorate), and professional (e.g. medicine, law, architecture, engineering),degree programs. Universities offer many kinds of academic programs and may consist of several colleges. These terms may at times be used interchangeably within the narrative of this manuscript. They are differentiated when circumstances regarding the independent aspects of their development in academic history require.

1.   American Heritage Dictionary 2nd College ed., *s.v.* "dance."
2.   Cicero. *Marcus Tullius Cicero: Orationes.* 1908: "Pro L. Murena" 6(15).
3.   Wagner. *Adversaries of Dance: From the Puritans to the Present,* 1997.

- Chapter 1 -

1.   Durkheim. *The Evolution of Educational Thought,* 1969.
2.   Ibid: 22.
3.   Abelson. *The Seven Liberal Arts: A Study in Medieval Culture,* 1906.
4.   Durkheim. *The Evolution of...,*1969: 47.
5.   Ibid: 31.
6.   Rashdall. *The Universities of Europe in the Middle Ages, Vol. 1 and 2,* 1895: 8 - 9.
7.   Schachner. *The Medieval Universities,* 1938: 45.
8.   Durkheim. *.The Evolution of...,* 1969: 68.
9.   Ibid: 84.
10.   Schachner. *The Medieval Universities, 1938:* 47.
11.   Rashdall. *Universities of Europe...,* 1895: 7.
12.   Paulsen. *The German Universities: Their Character and Historical Development,* 1895:18.
13.   Duryea. "Evolution of the University," 1973.
14.   Baird. *Rise of the Huguenots of France,* 1900.
15.   Mallett. *A History of the University of Oxford: Vol. 1, The Medieval University and the Colleges Founded in the Middle Ages,* 1924.
16.   Conrad and Wyer. "Liberal Education in Transition," 1980.
17.   Lee. *A History of Physical Education and Sports in the U.S.A.,* 1983: 17 - 18.
18.   Conrad and Wyer. "Liberal Education..."1980.
19.   According to Jack Morrison, writing in *The Rise of the Arts on the American Campus* (1973), dance was banned altogether on the campus of the newly founded University of North Carolina while just to the north Thomas Jefferson suggested that dance be included in the curriculum of the University of Virginia. (Morrison 1973: 13) The fitful inclusion of dance in colonial and post revolutionary college curricula was largely the result of individual interest and implementation. Wide-scale consideration of dance in academic programs came about in the late decades of the 19th century as an activities course for women (Morrison, Jack. *The Rise of the Arts on the American Campus.* New York: McGraw-Hill Book Company, 1973).
20.   Rudolph. *Curriculum: A History of the American Undergraduate Course of Study Since 1636,* 1977.
21.   Ibid:1.
22.   Hofstadter and Smith. *American Higher Education: A Documentary History,* 1961.

23.   Ibid.; Sloan. "Harmony, Chaos, and Consensus: The American College Curriculum, 1971; and Conrad and Wyer. "Liberal Education...," 1980.
24.   Gates. *Dictionary of American History,* 1940: 27.
25.   Blum (et. al). *The National Experience...* , 1989.
26.   Ibid.
27.   Rice. *A Brief History of Physical Education,* 1926:162.
28.   Blum (et. al). *The National Experience...,* 1989: 447.
29.   Paulson 1895. *The German Universities...,* and Conrad and Wyer. "Liberal Education...," 1980.
30.   Lee. *History of Physical Education...* , 1983.
31.   Williams and Brownell. *The Administration of Health and Physical Education,* 1934.
32.   Ibid; and Rice. *A Brief History...* 1926.
33.   Williams and Brownell. *The Administratio of...,* 1934.
34.   Rice. *A Brief History...* 1926: 162.
35.   Vesey. "Stability and Experiment in the American Undergradute Curriculum, 1973; and Jencks and Riesman. *The Academic Revolution,* 1968.
36.   Blum (et. al). *The National Experience...,* 1989.
37.   Ibid.
38.   Ibid.
39.   Ibid. *The National Experience...,* 448.

- Chapter 2 -

1.   Morrison. *The Rise of the Arts on the American Campus,* 1973:12 - 13.
2.   Ibid: 13.
3.   Marks. *The Mathers on Dancing. Including: An Arrow Against Profane and Promiscuous Dancing Drawn out of the Quiver of the Scriptures, by Increase Mather,* 1975.
4.   Ibid: 31.
5.   Ruyter. *American Visionaries...,* 1979.
6.   Wilkinson. *The Dance of Modern Society,* 1884: 6-7.
7.   Marks. *The Mathers on Dancing.,* 1975.
8.   Wagner. *Adversaries of Dance.,* 1997: xii.
9.   Blum (et. al). *The National Experience...,* 1989.
10.   Stebbins. *Delsarte System of Expression,* 1902: 391.
11.   Ibid: 386 - 387.
12.   Ruyter. *American Visionaries...,* 1979.
13.   Ibid.
14.   Stebbins. *Delsarte System...,* 1902.
15.   Ruyter. *American Visionaries...,* 1979: 21.
16.   Ibid.
17.   Findlay. "Dalcroze: The Nature of Rhythm," 1962: 8.
18.   Ibid.
19.   Lee. *History of Physical Education...,* 1983: 91.
20.   Blum (et. al). *The National Experience...,* 1989.
21.   Haley. *The Healthy Body and Victorian Culture,* 1978: 92.
22.   Ruyter. *American Visionaries..,* 1979; and Lee. *History of Physical Education...,* 1983.
23.   Cremin. *The Transformation of the School: Progressivism in American Education 1876 - 1957,* 1961: 104.
24.   Hall's attention to practice in the biomechanical-anatomical possibilities of movement presages the point of view Margaret H'Doubler would later develop when she set out to define a basis for the study in dance at the University of Wisconsin. (Hall, G. Stanley. *Educational Problems.* New York: Appleton, 1911).
25.   Hall. *Educational Problems,* 1911: 42 - 43.
26.   Lee. *History of Physical Education...,* 1983.
27.   Ibid: 102.

28. Blum (et. al). *The National Experience...*, 1989: 515.
29. Ibid: 506.
30. Dewey. *Dewey on Education,* 1959: 1-2.
31. Ibid; Lee. *History of Physical Education...*, 1983; and Ruyter. *American Visionaries..,* 1979.
32. Williams and Brownell. *The Administration of...*, 1934: 31-32.
33. Dewey. "Experience and Education," 1938, in: Conrad. *ASHE Reader on Academic Programs in Colleges and Universities,* 1987: 113 - 119.
34. Ibid.
35. Vesey. "Stability and Experiment...," "1973: 11.
36. Marks. *The Mathers on Dancing...,*1975: 31.
37. Stanley and Lowrey. *Manual of Gymnastic Dancing,* 1920.
38. Lee. *History of Physical Education...,* 1983.
39. Ibid.
40. Ruyter. *American Visionaries...,* 1979.
41. Lee. *History of Physical Education...,*1983: 200.
42. Anderson, Sargent, and Gulick also recognized the need for an academic society for physical educators and were prominent in founding the first professional organization for physical and health educators, the American Association for the Advancement of Physical Education (AAAPE) in 1885. Rice (1926), states: "...Anderson was largely responsible for the organization of the association and was a teacher of physical education in Brooklyn at this time" (Rice 1926: 227). In 1931 (by this date the AAAPE had evolved into the American Physical Education Association [APEA]), the APEA sponsored the first national, professional organization for dance educators.(Rice, Emmett, A.   *A Brief History of Physical Education.* New York: A.S. Barnes and Company, 1926).
43. Lee. *History of Physical Education...*, 1983; Murray. "The Dance in Physical Education," 1937; and Ruyter. *American Visionaries...,* 1979.
44. Prevots. *American Pageantry: A Movement for Art and Democracy,* 1987: 1.
45. Ibid., and Prevots. "University Courses in Pageantry and American Dance: 1911 - 1925," 1988.
46. Interestingly, 20 years later dancers in professional education found themselves in a similar predicament having to "untie" themselves from German affiliations.   Martha Graham rejected an offer from the National Socialist (Nazi) Party to perform at the 1936 Olympics, largely as a result of Nazi anti-semitism. Hanya Holm had to disavow her connection with the German modern dancer Mary Wigman for similar reasons of identification with a militaristic and intolerant society. (deMille, Agnes. *Martha: The Life and Work of Martha Graham, A Biography.* New York: Random House, 1991; and Sorrell, Walter. *Hanya Holm: The Biography of an Artist.* Middletown, Connecticut: Wesleyan University Press, 1969).
47. Lee. *History of Physical Education...,* 1983: 170.

- Chapter 3 -

1. Kendall. *Where She Danced,* 1979.
2. Ibid; and Ruyter. *American Visionaries...,* 1979.
3. Ibid.
4. Duncan. *The Art of the Dance,* 1928: 63.
5. Colby. *Natural Rhythms and Dances,* 1922.
6. Ruyter. *American Visionaries...,* 1979: 57.
7. Kendall. *Where She Danced,* 1979.
8. Ibid: 51 - 52.
9. Ibid: 106.
10. Blum (et. al). *The National Experience...,* 1989.
11. Soares. *Louis Horst: Musician in a Dancers World,* 1992: 40.
12. Sherman. *The Drama of Denishawn,* 1979: 3.

13.   Louis H. Chalif trained in Europe in Russian Ballet techniques. In America, Chalif established himself as an early teacher of folk and national dances. Chalif's techniques melded ballet barre and position exercises with the rhythmic movement patterns of folk dance. The "Chalif Method" with Sargent's and Gilbert's "Aesthetic Dancing." Both were techniques for instruction in dance popular in women's physical education programs prior to the introduction of Colby's "Natural Dancing" and later, Margaret H'Doubler's method. (Chalif, Louis, H. *The Chalif Textbook of Dancing*, New York: Isaac Goldman Coy, 1916).

14.   Spiesman. "Dance Education Pioneers: Colby, Larson, H'Doubler," 1960.

15.   Margaret H'Doubler published her instructional manual for dance in higher education in *A Manual of Dancing* H'Doubler's text, and her other contributions to dance in American higher education are discussed in Chapter 4. Another early text, *The Dance in Education* (1924), was published by Agnes and Lucile Marsh. Agnes, a Teachers College faculty member and Lucile, who taught at Smith College, elaborated on Colby's earlier text and developed her concepts of Natural Dancing further. (H'Doubler, Margaret. *A Manual of Dancing*. Madison, Wisconsin: Tracy and Kilgour, 1921; and Marsh, Agnes and Lucile. *The Dance in Education*. New York: A.S. Barnes and Co., 1924).

16.   Ruyter. *American Visionaries...*, 1979: 111.

17.   Colby. *Natural Rhythms and Dances*, 1922: 7 - 10.

18.   Ibid: 13 - 14.

19.   Kirstein. *Dance: A Short History of Classic Theatrical Dancing*, 1974: 353.

20.   Gray and Howe. "Margaret H'Doubler: A Profile of her Formative Years 1898 - 1921," 1985a.

21.   Kirstein. *Dance: A Short History...*, 1974.

22.   H'Doubler. "Interview with Carl Gutknecht...,"1972a: 11.

- Chapter 4-

1.   Blum (et. al). *The National Experience...*, 1989.

2.   Nesbitt. *Wisconsin: A History*, 1973: 404.

3.   H'Doubler. "Personal Data Sheet," 1971; and Wilson. "The Thought of Margaret H'Doubler: A Critical Perspective," 1981.

4.   Gray and Howe. "Margaret H'Doubler: A Profile..., " 1985a.

5.   Hagood. "The Organizational Sociology of Dance: An Analysis, Comparison, and Environmental Description of Primary Organizations Advocating Dance in Higher Education," 1990.

6.   H'Doubler. "Interview with Mary Alice Brennan," 1972b: 2 - 4.

7.   Ibid. "Interview-Gutknecht," 1972a: 1 - 2.

8.   Ibid. "Interview-Brennan," 1972b: 11.

9.   Ibid. "Interview-Gutknecht," 1972a: 2.

10.   Ibid: "Interview-Gutknecht," 3.

11.   Ibid.

12.   H'Doubler. "Interview-Brennan," 1972b.

13.   Gray and Howe. "Margaret H'Doubler: A Profile...,"1985a.

14.   Moore. "A Recollection of Margaret H'Doubler's Class Procedure: An Environment for Learning," 1975; and Wilson. "The Thought of...," 1981.

15.   Glassow. "Interview with Laura Smail," 1976: 60.

16.   H'Doubler. "Interview-Brennan," 1972b.

17.   deVries. *Physiology of Exercise* , 1980: 84.

18.   Rose. *The Wisconsin Dance Idea* ,1950; 40.

19.   H'Doubler. "Interview-Brennan 1972b: 8.

20.   H'Doubler. "A Way of Thinking," 1948: 6 - 7.

21.   H'Doubler. "Interview-Brennan," 1972b: 19.

22.   Remley. "The Wisconsin Idea of Dance: A Decade of Progress 1917 - 1926," 1975: 186 - 187.

23.   Ibid: 192.

24.   Ibid; and Trilling. "History of Physical Education for Women at the University of Wisconsin 1898-1946," 1951.
25.   Ibid.
26.   H'Doubler. "Interview-Brennan," 1972b: 5.
27.   H'Doubler. "Interview-Gutknecht," 1972a: 2.
28.   H'Doubler. "Interview-Brennan," 1972b; Gray and Howe. "Margaret H'Doubler: A Profile...," 1985a; Gray and Howe. "The "H'Doubler Idea of Dance and its Effect on the Physical Education Curriculum 1919-1927," 1985b; Remley. "The Wisconsin Idea of Dance...," 1975; and Wilson. "The Thought of...," 1981.
29.   H'Doubler. "Interview-Brennan," 1972b: 20.
30.   Remley. "The Wisconsin Idea of Dance...," 1975: 182.
31.   Trilling. "History of Physical Education for Women...," 1951.
32.   H'Doubler. "Interview-Brennan," 1972b.
33.   H'Doubler. *A Manual of Dancing*, 1921: 7.
34.   Ibid.
35.   Ibid.
36.   Ibid.
37.   Ibid.
38.   Ibid. *A Manual...*, 8.
39.   Ibid: 9.
40.   Ibid. *A Manual...*, 11.
41.   Ibid: 12.
42.   Remley. "Wisconsin Idea of Dance ...," 1975: 190.
43.   H'Doubler. "Interview-Brennan," 1972b: 12.
44.   H'Doubler. *The Dance and its Place in Education,* 1925.
45.   Wisconsin. "College of Letters and Science Document # 33," 8 June, 1926 .

- Chapter 5 -

1.   Martin. *Introduction to the Dance,* 1939.
2.   Kendall. *Where She Danced,* 1979.
3.   deMille. *Martha: The Life and Work of Martha Graham, A Biography,* 1991; Kendall. *Where She Danced,* 1979; and McDonagh. *Martha Graham,* 1973.
4.   Siegel. *Days on Earth; The Dance of Doris Humphrey,* 1987: 108.
5.   Ibid.
6.   Ibid. *Days on Earth...,* 22.
7.   Ibid.
8.   Ibid. *Days on Earth...,* 29.
9.   Lloyd. *The Borzoi Book of Modern Dance,* 1949.
10.   Ibid: 316 - 317.
11.   As referenced in Chapter Two note [46]: In 1936 the name of the "Wigman School" was changed to the "Hanya Holm School." Holm requested the name change because the rise of the National Socialist Party in Germany was fanning anti-German sentiment in America and Holm felt that for the school to survive it must break its ties with its German founder.
12.   Russell. "John Martin on Audiences: A Conversation with Carroll Russell, "1962.
13.   Oddly, Tamiris, an early exponent of the modern aesthetic, successful in her choreographic work, favorably reviewed in the press by John Martin, and a driving force behind organized production activity in modern dance, was not invited to participate in the Bennington programs. This may have been due to the fact that while Tamiris was recognized as a performer and choreographer, she was not known for her theory and philosophy on dance in art or in education. Tamiris' husband, Daniel Nagrin, is quoted by Elizabeth Cooper (1997) as saying that the fact Tamiris was not invited to Bennington "...was a painful blow to her and in the perception of many writing and thinking about dance at the time and since, it seemed to prove something negative." Tamiris remained active in the field of concert dance well into the 1940's, and then turned

her attention to choreography for the musical theatre. Another reason Tamiris was not invited to participate in Bennington sessions may be due to the fact that she was simply not liked, especially by Martha Graham and Doris Humphrey. Agnes deMille (*Martha: The Life and Work ...*, 1991), a successful choreographer of the ballet, a confidant of the early modern dancers, and a member of the Dance Repertory Theatre, writes in her biography of Martha Graham of her distaste for Tamiris and suggests that Louis Horst, Martha Graham, and Doris Humphrey felt the same. Tamiris' ready acceptance of popular themes and styles for use in her choreography, attention to "Negro" themes in her early choreography, coupled with her dynamic personality, and flair for self-promotion, are possible reasons for this. Tamiris was widely known for her work with African influenced music as context for her choreography. Janet Soares, in her biography of Louis Horst (1992), writes that Horst liked Tamiris but was concerned that she used "low" art ideas (Soares. *Louis Horst: Musician...*, 1992: 65). In her biography of Doris Humphrey (*Days on Earth:...*, 1987), dance historian Marcia Siegel suggests that Tamiris's personality and flamboyant nature did not sit well with the more aesthetic personalities of Graham, Humphrey, and Horst. Whether or not any overt or latent racism played a role in Tamiris' exclusion from the " inner-circle," it was the dance artists Martha Graham, Doris Humphrey, Charles Weidman, Hanya Holm (representing the German school), composer Louis Horst, and critic John Martin that attracted the attention of Martha Hill and Mary Josephine Shelly. Certainly the subject of Tamiris' fall from grace is worthy of further research. (Cooper, Elizabeth. "Tamiris and the Federal Dance Theater 1936-1939: Socially Relevant Dance Amidst the Policies and Politics of the New Deal Era." *Dance Research Journal* 29, no. 2 [1997]: 44).

14. Kriegsman. *Modern Dance in America: The Bennington Years,* 1981.
15. Soares. "Barnard's 1932 and 1933 Dance Symposium: Bringing Dance to the University," 1997.
16. Kriegsman. *Modern Dance in America...*, 1981: 5 - 6.
17. Soares. "Barnard's 1932 and 1933 Symposium...," 1997.
18. Ibid: 193.
19. O'Donnell. "Martha Hill," 1936; and Kriegsman. *Modern Dance in America...*, 1981.
20. Soares. *Louis Horst: Musician....*, 1992: 61.
21. Soares. "Barnard's 1932 and 1933 Symposium...," 1997: 193.
22. Kriegsman. *Modern Dance in America...*, 1981: 7.
23. Ibid.
24. Soares. "Barnard's 1932 and 1933 Symposium...," 1997: 194.
25. Ibid: 194.
26. Sorrell. *Hanya Holm: The Biography of an Artist,* 1969: 57 - 58.
27. Lloyd. *The Borzoi Book...*, 1949: 317.
28. Kriegsman. *Modern Dance in America...*, 1981.
29. McDonagh. *Martha Graham,* 1973: 100.
30. Kriegsman. *Modern Dance in America...*, 1981: 29.
31. Siegel. *Days on Earth...*,1987.
32. Ibid: 145.
33. Soares. *Louis Horst: Musician...*, 1992: 135.
34. Kriegsman. *Modern Dance in America...*, 1981; and Anderson. *The American Dance Festival,* 1987.
35. The curriculum at Bennington was complete (technique, composition, history and criticism, pedagogy, music for dance, stagecraft) with the notable exception of course work in biomechanical foundations in dance. I have found no reference to any specific course work in kinesiology, or of a scientific approach to movement and dance, in references to aspects of the Bennington curriculum. Some limited references are found including: an article written by Barbara Page (1935). Page writes: "An attempt is made to give the student an understanding of basic laws of physics and kinesiology in terms of their relation to the human body, to present an analysis of rhythmic, temporal, and spatial possibilities, and then to guide the student into individual discovery of techniques" (Ibid: 12). In 1934 H'Doubler paid a visit to Bennington, performing a

demonstration on dance and showing a film about dance at the University of Wisconsin (Kriegsman. *Modern Dance in America: The Bennington Years,* 1981: 42). From this we may assume H'Doubler commented on the scientific aspects of her approach to dance training. Kriegsman also lists two other lectures that were related to a scientific approach to dance, one by Irma Dombois-Bartenieff and Irma Otto-Bentz on Rudolf von Laban's work in developing a system for dance notation (1936 [Ibid: 57]), and a lecture on "Thalamic Communication" given by Dr. Douglas Campbell of the University of Chicago, at the Bennington Summer Session at Mills College in 1939 (Ibid: 87). (Page, Barbara. "Contemporary Exponents of the Dance." *The Journal of Health and Physical Education* 4 no. 35 [1935]:11-14, 60).

36.   Kriegsman. *Modern Dance in America...,* 1981; and Anderson. *The American Dance Festival,* 1987.

37.   Heymann. "Dance in the Depression: The WPA Project," 1975; and Cooper. "Tamiris and the Federal Dance Theatre...," 1997.

38.   Heymann . "Dance in the Depression...," 1975.

39.   Cooper. "Tamiris and the Federal Dance Theater...,"1997.

40.   In *Black Dance: From 1619 to Today* (1988), Lynn Fauley Emery cites 1925 as the date for the first off-campus concert given by the Hampton Institute Creative Dance Group (Emery 1988: 244]. In citing this date Emery references an October 1938 article by Michael Lorant for the *Dancing Times*: "Hampton Institute: Negro's Unique Dancing Academy" (Ibid.). The 1925 seems to be a typographical error since Haskins [1990] reports Charles Williams' attendance at Bennington for choreographic study in the 1930's. At the beginning of her section on the Hampton Institute Creative Dance Group (Ibid: 244) Emery writes: "While Winfield, Guy, and Sawyer were dancing in New York City, another concert group was being developed at the all-black college, Hampton Institute, in Hampton, Virginia." The first performance by Winfield's "Negro Art Theatre Dance Group," which included Guy and Sawyer, was April 29, 1931 (Ibid: 242).   On page 245 of her text, Emery writes: "At the same time the Hampton Creative Dance Group was making its first appearance in New York City (November 1935]" (Ibid: 245) - 10 years after a 1925 formation.   The 1935 date for the Creative Dance Group's off-site concert given by Haskins is more plausible.   Charles Williams, writing for *Dance Observer* in 1937, states that: "The school year beginning 1937 - 38 marks the start of the fourth year's work of the Hampton Institute's Creative Dance Group which is making a special endeavor to discover and develop Negro and African folk dances." (Emery, Lynn Fauley. Dance Horizons. Princeton, New Jersey: Princeton Book Co., 1988; and Williams, Charles. "The Hampton Institute Creative Dance Group." *Dance Observer* 5, no. 8 [October 1937]: 98).

41.   Haskins. *Black Dance in America: A History Through its People,* 1990: 72 - 75.

42.   Williams. "The Hampton Institute...," 1937: 97 - 98.

- Chapter 6 -

1.   Soares. *Louis Horst: Musician...,* 1992.

2.   St. Denis and Bridge. "The Dance in Physical Education," 1932: 12.

3.   Marsh. "The New Dance Era," 1932: 23.

4.   Ibid.

5.   Beiswanger. "Physical Education and Modern Dance," 1936.

6.   Ibid: 413.

7.   Ibid.

8.   Shelly. "Art and Physical Education-An Educational Alliance," 1936: 476.

9.   Ibid.

10.   Ibid.

11.   Murray. "The Dance in Physical Education," 1937.

12.   Ibid: 10.

13.   Ibid: 11.

14.   Ibid: 12.

15.   Howe. "What Business Has the Modern Dance in Physical Education," 1937.
16.   Ibid: 131 - 132.
17.   Ibid: 132.
18.   Ibid.
19.   Today, the dance science and medicine community is growing and quite viable. However, the attention paid to the effects of ballet training far outweighs critical appraisal of the techniques modern dancers use in preparation for performance.
20.   Shelly. "Art and Physical Education...," 1940: 55.
21.   Ibid: 56.
22.   Ibid.
23.   Martin. *Introduction to the Dance,* 1939: 292.
24.   Ibid.
25.   Ibid: 300.
26.   Ibid: 300 - 301.
27.   Ibid: 303.
28.   H'Doubler. *Dance: A Creative Art Experience,* 1940: ix - xi.
29.   Ibid: 92.
30.   Wilson. "The Thought of Margaret H'Doubler: A Critical Perspective," 1981.
31.   Terry. *I was There,* 1978: 68.
32.   Ibid.
33.   Ibid: 68 - 69.

- Chapter 7 -

1.   Williams and Brownell. *The Administration of Health and Physical Education,* 1934: 43.
2.   In 1934 the Association's formal structures and affiliates included five committees, eleven sections, and nine affiliated organizations. For a complete list please see Appendix A. Ibid: 44.
3.   Hagood. "The Organizational Sociology of Dance: An Analysis, Comparison, and Environmental Description of Primary Organizations Advocating Dance in Higher Education," 1990.
4.   Lee. *A History of Physical Education and Sports in the U.S.A.,* 1973.
5.   Lee. "A Synopsis of the Development of the National Section on Dancing," 1973.
6.   Ibid.
7.   LaSalle. "The Organizing of the Section," 1969.
8.   O'Donnell. "Petition to the American Physical Education Association," 1932.
9.   Lee. "The Formation of a Committee to Report on Dancing at the 1931 American Physical Education Association Meeting," 1931.
10.   Murray. "Petition to Form a Dance Section in the American Physical Education Association," 1931.
11.   Lee. "A Synopsis...," 1973.
12.   Hagood. "The Organizational Sociology of...," 1990.
13.   Hawkins. *Modern Dance in Higher Education,* 1954.

- Chapter 8 -

1.   Hawkins. *Modern Dance in Higher Education* 1954: 1.
2.   Ibid: 2.
3.   Ibid: 17 - 18.
4.   Soares. "Barnard's 1932 and 1933 Dance Symposium: Bringing Dance to the University," 1997: 193.
5.   "New School Series." 1934: 6.
6.   Hawkins. *Modern Dance,* 1954: 110 - 111.
7.   Ibid: 1.

8. Hayes. "The Dance Teacher and the Physical Education Administrator," 1954; in: Lippincott. "Selected Articles from the Journal of Health, Physical Education, and Recreation," 1958: 26 - 28.
9. Ibid; and Hayes. "The Education, Training and Development of Dance Educators in Higher Education," 1978.
10. By the mid-1950's other organizations were coming into being to help articulate the goals of dance in education. Today's American Dance Guild (ADG), founded in 1956 as the National Dance Teachers Guild, was a New York based organization designed to meet the needs of creative dance educators nationwide. The ADG's mission was to improve instruction, develop community awareness, and to support progress for dance at community, state, and federal levels. From 1965 until 1981 the ADG published *DanceScope*, providing a forum for professional and academic commentary on dance. The ADG also acted as parent organization for the Committee on Research in Dance in 1965; today's Congress on Research in Dance (CORD]. CORD has come to play an internationally important role in furthering the substance and range of dance scholarship. For many dance educators in the south, mid-west, and west however, the ADG was viewed as an organization for those in America's northeast. Although its membership briefly grew to national levels during the Dance Boom of the 1970s, the ADG never fully assumed a recognized national leadership role as an organization with a direct impact on dance in higher education [Hagood. "The Organizational Sociology of Dance...," 1990].
11. Hayes. "The Dance Teacher and...," 1954.
12. In the 1950's, Murray Louis traveled to New York and began a long and fruitful relationship with modern dance choreographer Alwin Nikolis. In the 1960's and 70's Louis become a major figure in American modern dance through his solo career and partnership with Nikolais. Today, Louis directs the Louis-Nikolis dance company and school in New York City.
13. Van Tuyl. *Impulse*, 1951: ii.
14. Ibid: 10 - 11.
15. Prevots. *Dance for Export: Cultural Diplomacy and the Cold War*, 1998.
16. Ibid.
17. Vesey. "Stability and Experiment in the American Undergraduate Curriculum," 1973: 16.
18. Ibid.
19. Kraus, Hilsendager, and Dixon. *History of the Dance in Art and Education*, 1991.

- Chapter 9 -

1. Vesey. "Stability and Experiment in the American Undergraduate Curriculum," 1973: 16-17.
2. Joel. "The Kennedy's at the Ballet," 1961: 30.
3. In the 1930's a national agency for the arts was a dream of political followers of President Franklin Roosevelt. In 1936, the arts were subsidized by federal monies through the Works Progress Administration-Federal Theatre Project, a part of Roosevelt's "New Deal" program designed to put people back to work during the Great Depression. Throughout the 1930's many were hopeful that Congress would authorize a permanent arts agency. However, this was not to be the case as conservative forces in Congress stalled and eventually derailed the legislation that would have established a National Arts Agency in 1939 (Code, Grant. "Dance Theater of the Works Progress Administration: A Record of National Accomplishment." *Dance Observer* 7, no. 3 [March 1940]: 34-35).
4. Johnson. "Speech Announcing the Creation of the National Foundation for the Arts and Humanities," 1965.
5. Duncan. "PressTime News," 1964: 3.
6. Ibid: 4.
7. Joel. "Ford Foundation Controversy-Pros and Cons," 1964: 35.
8. Lippincott. "A Bright Future for Dance," 1965a: 9.
9. Ibid.
10. Dougherty. "Dance and Physical Education," 1967.

11. Wooten. *Focus on Dance II; An Interdisciplinary Search for Meaning in Movement,* 1962.

12. Moomaw. Personal correspondence re: 1961 Conference on Movement and 1965 Dance as a Discipline Conference, 1994.

13. Lippincott. "A Bright Future...,"1965a: 10 - 11.

14. Lippincott. "A Bright Future...," 1965a: 10.

15. Lippincott. "Report of the Arts," 1965b: 11.

16. The 1963 AAHPER convention meetings were important for planning the Dance as a Discipline conference and the NSD's petition for Divisional Status. The idea that dance was a discipline separate from physical education was not widely accepted by AAHPER members. The desire for a new organizational structure within AAHPER was tied up in the larger issue of academic individuation for dance. In her 1986 oral history for the NDA- AAHPERD Archives NSD member Esther Pease recalls the 1963 AAHPER General Assembly and NSD member Cathryn Allen's "take us or leave us" speech as swinging the assembly vote for division status for dance (Pease, Esther. "Oral History-1986." national Dance Association. Reston, VA: AAHPERD-Archives, 1986.) Division Status was granted following the National Convention in March of 1963. The new title was used during the period 1963 - 1964, with the first National Conference of the Dance Division in 1964. In a personal communication to the author NSD Past-President Virginia Moomaw recalled; "At the spring [1963] meeting of the National Board it was approved and we became a Division. This meeting must have been after the convention as I remember that nice Mary Fee [1963 - 64 DD of AAHPER Chair] sending me a telegram saying it had been approved and we were now a Dance Division" (Moomaw. Personal communication, 1994).

17. Terry. "New Spirit in the Colleges," 1965.

18. Smith. "Introduction: Dance as a Discipline," 1967: i.

19. Ibid: 15.

20. Hagood. "Studies in the Sociology of Dance: The Organization and Culture of the Wisconsin Dance Council," 1994b.

21. Maynard. "Eugene Loring Talks to Olga Maynard," 1966a; and "Eugene Loring Talks to Olga Maynard-Part II," 1966b.

22. Maynard. "College Controversy: The University of California at Irvine," 1966c.

23. deMille "Agnes deMille Speaks to Congress on the State of the Arts: Her Statement and Questions and Answers before the House Select Subcommittee on Education," 1970: 82.

24. Ibid: 62.

25. Maynard. "College Controversy...,"1966c: 62.

26. Ibid.

27. Ibid: 63.

28. Ibid.

29. Ibid. "College Controversy...," 63 - 64.

30. Ibid: 64.

31. Ibid: 65.

32. Hawkins. "Introduction." In: *Dance : A Projection for the Future,* 1968: v.

33. Hagood. "The Council of Dance Administrators: A Sociological Analysis of Group Culture," 1989: 57.

34. Van Tuyl. "Manifesto." In: *Dance: A Projection for the Future,* 1968a: 7.

35. Ibid: 129.

36. The University of Wisconsin-Madison, home of the world's first university dance major, maintained its dance program within the Department of Physical Education for Women until the effects of Title 9 and the Educational Opportunity Act prompted the joining of Men's and Women's Departments of Physical Education into a Department of Physical Education and Dance in 1976. Since then the Dance program has enjoyed a great deal of autonomy but still remains a program within the Department of Kinesiology in the School of Education.

37. Council of Dance Administrators (CODA). "Summary Documents," 1976.

38. Erdman. "Dance in Education-Statement I," In: *Dance; A Projection for the Future,* 1968: 65.
39. Ibid.
40. Ibid.
41. Ibid. "Dance in Education...," 66.
42. Ibid: 68.
43. Nikolais. "Dance in Education-Statement II." In: *Dance: A Projection for the Future,* 1968: 71.
44. Wilde. "Dance in Education-Statement III. In: *Dance: A Projection for the Future,* 1968: 75.
45. Limón. "Dance in Education-Statement IV. In: *Dance: A Projection for the Future* ,1968: 78.
46. Prevots. *Dance for Export...,* 1998.
47. Limón. "Dance in Education...," 1968: 80.
48. CODA. "Summary...," 1968. .
49. Martin. "Letter re: Developmental Conference on Dance," 1968.
50. Hills. "The Major Event of the Year," 1968: 1G.
51. Hill. "Report of the Committee on Percussion Accompaniment for Dance," 1934.
52. Ibid.
53. Hering. "The Peerless Princess Turns to Dance," 1968.
54. Ibid; and Gibb. Personal Communication re; American Dance Symposium, 1999.

- Chapter 10 -

1. Lippincott. ""Report of the Arts," *Impulse,* 1965b: 8.
2. Roemer states that vocationalism was more pronounced among women undergraduates during the period 1970 - 1978. He discusses gender differences from the perspective of enrollment numbers. Total numbers of undergraduate degrees for women increased 20.6% in the period 1970 - 71 through 1977 - 78, compared to figures for men of 3.3%. Occupational-social theory is used to explain the difference: e.g. increases in enrollments for women were not attributable to a concerted effort at liberating certain fields of study from a tradition of male dominance, variable statistics in women's interest in subjects generally accepted as male dominated are evidenced. However, it was found that women were more occupationally interested in pursuit of a higher education then were men. Roemer's data regarding gender are of interest to an analysis of dance, a discipline traditionally dominated by women students and women faculty (Roemer, Robert E. "Vocationalism in Higher Education: Explanation from Social Theory." *The Review of Higher Education* 23, no. 2 (Winter) 1981: 23-46. In: *ASHE Reader on Academic Programs in Colleges and Universities,* edited by Clifton F. Conrad, 155-169. Lexington, Massachusetts: Ginn Press, 1987).
3. Roemer. "Vocationalism in Higher Education...," 1981: 160.
     *There is a mathematical error in the original table as reported by Roemer. The percent change for women from 1970 - 1971 to 1977 - 1978 was listed as 188.3%. Actual number should have 288.3% in Table 3 on page 160 of the Roemer *(ASHE Reader)* text (see: citation in note #2: Conrad 1987).
4. The term "changing the world' is an apt descriptor for the tone of the thinking of many young dancers in the 1970's. I attended the State University of New York-College at Brockport as an undergraduate dance major in the mid to late 1970's. At that time the dance department at Brockport was one of the largest in the nation. It was a time of great potential. We felt we were on the brink of something very new. I clearly remember the feeling of great opportunity for us, as we prepared to bring dance to the people. Our conversations were full of hope and excited discovery. We really did think we could change the world with dance. It was a very heady time.
5. Roemer. "Vocationalism in Higher Education...," 1981: 157.
6. Swisher. "PressTime News," 1968: 3.
7. ACDFA . "Mission Statement," 1998.

8.   Baker. "Frisbees and Unicycles Versus The Politics of Paternalism," 1973: 62.
9.   Dell. "Far Beyond the Far Out," 1965: 18.
10.   Ibid: 63.
11.   Ibid. "Far Beyond the Far Out."
12.   In the popular consciousness of dance after the 1960's, Yvonne Rainer's "NO Manifesto" has come to represent the new aesthetic for dance termed "post-modern." Rainer was an early leader of the Judson Church. According to Banes (1980), Rainer "formulated a strategy for demystifying dance and making it objective. It was a strategy of denial: NO to spectacle no to virtuosity no to transformations and magic and make believe no to the glamour and transcendency of the star image no to the heroic no to the anti - heroic no to trash no to camp no to seduction no to involvement of performer or spectator no to style no to seduction of spectator by the wiles of the performer no to eccentricity no to moving or being moved" (Banes, Sally. *Terpsichore in Sneakers: Post-Modern Dance.* Boston: Houghton Mifflin Company, 1980: 43).
13.   ACDFA. "Mission Statement," 1998.
14.   Hawkins. "Letter to Dance Administrators Council," 1973.
15.   CODA . "Summary," 1972: 1.
16.   Ibid. 1976.
17.   Terry. "Collegiate Dance," 1940: 68.
18.   Van Tuyl. "Creative Dance Experience and Education, "1951; Hawkins. *Modern Dance in Higher Education,"* 1954; Hayes. "The Dance Teacher and the Physical Education Administrator,"1954; Wooten. *Focus on Dance II;   An Interdisciplinary Search for Meaning in Movement,* 1962, and Dougherty. "Dance and Physical Education," 1967.
19.   CODA . "Summary," 1976: 8 - 9.
20.   Ibid. "Summary," 1977a: 10 - 11.
21.   Ibid. 1977b: 1.
22.   This document is included in Appendix X.
23.   Hagood. "The Organizational Sociology of Dance..." 1990.
24.   CODA. "Summary," 1978: 2 - 3.
25.   Ibid: 6 - 7.
26.   Ibid. "Summary 1979: 9 - 10.
27.   Ibid. "Summary," 1980a: 1 - 3.
28.   NASD. "Brochure," 1985:1.
29.   Hagood. "The Council of Dance Administrators...," 1989.
30.   In 1985 the Council of Dance Administrators provided their first service conference to other dance administrators; the "Conference on Dance Administration: Themes and Directions," June 23 - 28, 1985, held at Allerton House, a residence of the University of Illinois, Urbana-Champaign in Monticello, Illinois.   The conference proceedings document, edited by Nancy Smith, is available from: The Ohio State University, Department of Dance, 1813 North High Street, Columbus, Ohio, 43210-7977.
31.   Hagood. "The Council of Dance Administrators...," 1989.

- Chapter 11 -

1.   Blum (et. al). *The National Experience: A History of the United States,* 1989.
2.   Stewart and Dickason. "Hard Times Ahead," 1971: 17.
3.   Glenny. "Demographic and Related Issues for Higher Education in the 1980's," 1980.
4.   Ibid: 374 - 378.
5.   NASD. "Brochure," 1985: 10 - 11.
6.   CODA . "Summary," 1979: 1.
7.   Ibid. "Summary," 1981: 3.
8.   Ibid. "Summary," 1983: 3.
9.   Wilson. "Education and Training Issues: Curricular and Instructional Practices," 1983: 1.
10.   Ibid: 1 - 2.
11.   AAHPER. *DANCE DIRECTORY,* 1966.
12.   Wilson. "Education and Training Issues...," 1983: 4.

13.   Ibid: 4 - 5.
14.   CODA. "Summary," 1984: 1.
15.   Ibid: 3 - 4.
16.   Topaz. "Untitled, National Association of Schools of Dance," 1984: 1.
17.   Ibid: 3.
18.   Ibid. "Untitled, National Association of Schools of Dance."
19.   Ibid: 9.
20.   CODA. "Summary," 1985: 2.
21.   Ibid: 3.
22.   Ibid.: 6.
23.   Ibid:. "Summary," 7 - 8.
24.   CODA . "Summary," 1986: 1.
25.   Ibid: 2.
26.   Child. "Culture, Contingency and Capitalism in the Cross-National Study of Organizations," 1981; Cole. *Work, Mobility and Participation: A Comparative Study of American and Japanese Industry,* 1979; Kamata . *Japan in the Passing Lane,* 1982; McMillan. *The Japanese Industrial System,* 1984; Ouchi. *Theory Z: How American Business Can Meet the Japanese Challenge,* 1981; Pascale and Athos. *The Art of Japanese Management,* 1981; and Sayle. "The Yellow Peril and the Red-Haired Devils," 1982.
27.   CODA. "Summary," 1987: 1.
28.   Ibid: 6.
29.   Ibid: 10 - 13.
30.   Ibid. "Summary," 1989: 10 - 11.

- Chapter 12 -

1.   And. *Dance Perspectives 3,* 1959.
2.   Cohen and Pischi. "Index to Dance Perspectives and Current Bibliography for Dance 1 959," 1960: i.
3.   Brown. "Report of Annual CORD Membership Meeting; Part 1," 1969: 4.
4.   Hanna. *To Dance is Human,* 1979: 8 - 9.
5.   Wimmer. "Gertrude Prokosch Kurath," 1974: 31 - 34.
6,   Lippincott. "Aesthetics and the Dance: A Study of Some Problems in Dance Theory Presented for the Dancer," 1943; and "Letter to the field re: developments in dance scholarship," 1979.
7.   Seigel, Introductory editorial for: *Dance Scope,* 1965.
8.   Ibid: 2.
9.   Bird. "Report of Annual CORD Membership Meeting," 1969: 1 - 2.
10.   Brown. "Report of Annual CORD...," 1969: 4.
11.   Ibid: 5.
12.   Ibid: 7. Besides contextualizing the opportunities dancer educators had in funding their projects, CORD members considered the question: what is dance research? Methodologies, perspectives, procedures for proposals; these concerns were new territory for many of the Committee's members. A first area of interest was in dance therapy, a field of study that had been explored by Bird Larson at Barnard College, and Margaret H'Doubler at the University of Wisconsin. Throughout the 1950's and 1960's interest in dance therapy grew. The field's important early leaders included Marian Chase, Blanche Evan, Mary Whitehouse, and Alma Hawkins. The American Dance Therapy Association (ADTA), was formed in 1966, and in 1968 CORD and the ADTA co-sponsored a "Workshop on Dance Therapy: Its Research Potentials." The first graduate program in dance therapy was initiated at Hunter College in New York City in 1971 (Levy, Fran J. *Dance Movement Therapy: A Healing Art.* Reston: Virginia: National Dance Association, 1988).
13.   Rowe. "Comments from the Chairman of CORD," 1970: 1.
14.   Rowe. "Comments from...,"1971: 4.

15.   Ibid: 5.
16.   CORD. "Mission Statement," 1999.
17.   SDHS. "Mission Statement," 1999.
18.   Gray. *Dance Technology: Current Applications and FutureTrends,* 1989.
19.   Brennan, Mary Alice (ed.) *Research in Dance III.* Reston, Virginia: National Dance Association (Stock # 243-26992). Available from: AAHPERD, 1900 Association Drive, Reston, VA. 20191.
20.   Brennan 1982: 1 - 13.
21.   Ibid: 21.
22.   Ibid: 41.
23.   Ibid: 18.
24.   Ibid. *Research in Dance III* 96 - 97.
25.   Ibid: viii.
26.   Kirby 1975: iii - iv.
27.   Smith-Fichter. "The Future of Dance in Higher Education," [?]: 6.
28.   Hanstein. "Educating for the Future: A Post-Modern Paradigm for Dance Education," 1990: 56.
29.   Intriguing, and to some, exciting new possibilities for dance have evolved out of the interaction between dance and technology. With the development of the personal computer in the early 1980's came advances in computer managed dance notation. "Laban Notation," the notation and documentary standard for most dance programs, was made computer friendly through the development of "Laban Writer," and electronic renderings of the body through such applications as "Life Forms" software. "Life Forms" is a product for the Macintosh computer created by Kinetic Effects, a Seattle based company, and has been used by such choreographers as Merce Cunningham, a leader in the use of computer technology and dance. Lucy Venable (the Ohio State University), and Tom Calvert (Simon Fraser University, Vancouver, Canada), were early leaders in exploring technological applications for dance. Venable has led the development of *Laban Writer* , and Calvert has published a number of articles on *Life Forms* and computer based dance animation. For additional background information see: *Dance Technology: Current Applications and Future Trends* , Judith A. Gray (ed.) Available from: National Dance Association, Reston, Virginia (1989); Calvert, T.W. "A Computer Based Language for Human Movement." *Computing and the Humanities* 20, no.2(1986) : 35 - 43; Badler, N. "Animating Human Figures: Perspectives and Directions," *Pro Graphics Interface,* (1986):115 - 120; Bruderlin, A . and T.W. Calvert. "Goal Directed Dynamic Animation of Human Walking." *Computer Graphics* 23, no. 3 (1989): 233 - 242; Herbison-Evans D. *A Human Movement Language for Computer Animation* In: Tobias, J. (ed.) *Language Design and Programming Methodology* New York: Springer, (1979) : 117 - 128. For current information on dance and tecnology see: Povall, Richard. "Dance and Technology: Technology is With Us"; "Wechsler, Robert. "Computers and Dance: Back to the Future"; Steggell, Amanda. "The Inverted Relay Race"; and Naugle, Lisa Marie. "Technique/Technology/Technique." in: *Dance Research Journal* 30, no. 1 (Spring 1998).
30.   Terry. *I Was There,* 1978:69.
31.   La Point-Crump. "The Future is Now-An Imperative for Dance Education," 1990: 51.
32.   Ibid: 52.
33.   Ibid. "The Future is Now...,".
34.   Ibid.
35.   Ibid.
36.   Ibid. "The Future is Now...," 53.

- Chapter 13 -

1.   Mission Statement, Interarts And Technology,1992.
2.   Brennan. Personal communication re: University of Wisconsin dance program, 1999.
3.   UCLA, Department of World Arts and Cultures "Mission Statement," 1999.

4.   Gray. *Dance Technology: Current Applications and Future Trends,* 1989.
5.   Ibid.
6.   Povall. "Dance and Technology: Technology is With Us," 1998: 2.
7.   Paprock. Personal Communication re: Developments at UCLA dance program 1999.
8.   Kealiinohomoku. *An Anthropologist Looks at Ballet as a Form of Ethnic Dance,* 1970.
9.   Marsh. Conference publicity: "Dancing in the Millennium-2000," 1999.
10. Hagood. "The Organizational Sociology of Dance...," 1990.
11. Hagood. "Report to the Future Directions Task Force: National Dance Association,"1998.
12. Bonbright. "Dance Education 1999: Status, Challenges, and Recommendations," 1999: 33 - 34.
13. Phillips. "The View from Florida: Dancers in Cap and Gown-Part Three," 1994.
14. Ibid : 58.
15. Ibid.
16. Ibid. "The View from Florida...," 58 - 59.
17. Ibid: 60.
18. Ibid: 60.
19. Ibid. "The View from Florida...," 61.
20. Kahlich. "Educating Dance Educators - What Next?" 1993.
21. Ibid.
22. Ibid.
23. Ibid. "Educating Dance Educators...," 22.
24. Ibid: 3.
25. Ibid: 5.
26. Ibid. "Educating Dance Educators...,"
27. American Heritage Dictionary 2nd College ed., s.v. "system."
28. See: note 35, chapter 9.

Appendix A
Curricular Plan for the First Specialized Major in Dancing - The University of Wisconsin-Madison, 1926

The following is a reproduction of the original document organized in chart form to illustrate the breadth and sequencing of the first major curriculum for dance. Reprinted with permission from the University of Wisconsin-Madison Archives

LETTERS AND SCIENCE DOCUMENT 33, JUNE 8, 1926

The Department of Physical Education recommends to the Faculty of the College of Letters and Science, the following course in Dancing to be offered as a specialized major within the Course in Physical Education for Women.

PHYSICAL EDUCATION MAJOR IN DANCING

I. SPECIFIC REQUIREMENTS
    A. Prerequisites
       1. Professional

Class	Credits
Physiology 1	4
Anatomy 120	6
P.E. 56 (Kinesiology)	3

       2. Non - Professional

Class	Credits
English 1, 33, or 30	10 or 12
History (freshman course)	6
Science (regular freshman course biology recommended)	10
Psychology 1	3
Philosophy 21 and 25 or substitute course	6
Art History 51, 52	6
Speech 1, 16, 18, 19, or substitute course	10 to 14
Music - Theory and History courses	5 to 10
Education 41, 90	5
Foreign Language	8 to 14

Major Requirements

Class	Credits
P.E. 60 (Rhythmic Form and Analysis)	1
P.E. 165 (Dance Composition)	2
P.E. 146 (Philosophy of Dancing)	1 to 3
P.E. 19 (Supervised Teaching)	4
P.E. 90 (Teaching and Adaptation)	2
P.E. 43 or 49 (Folk Dancing)	1 or 2
Thesis Requirement	4

Major Electives, from which students must select not less than 4 and not more than 10 credits.

Class	Credits
P.E. 42 (Plays and Games)	1
P.E. 45 (Swimming Technique)	1
P.E. 81 (Camp Leadership)	2
P.E. 43 or 49 (Folk Dancing)	2
P.E. 163 (Gymnastic Therapeutics)	4 (year)
P.E. 80 (Community Recreation)	2
P.E. 16 (First Aid)	1

II. GENERAL REQUIREMENTS

A. Total number of credits required for graduation shall be 124.

B. The degree conferred shall be B.S. in Physical Education.

C. Physical Education 20 is required throughout the four years, but receives no academic credit.

D. Students who present 2 units of foreign language, or less, are required to secure 14 credits in one language. Students who present 4 units are required to secure 8 credits in one language. Students must have at least 2 units in the same language in order to receive entrance credit. One unit in two or more different languages receives no credit. (One unit or year of high school language equals four university credits.)

E. Departmental (special techniques required) 4-10 credits and not more.

F. Electives to be chosen from Letters and Science courses carrying credit toward the B. A. degree.

PHYSICAL EDUCATION MAJOR IN DANCING

FRESHMAN YEAR

Semester I

English 1a	3
Foreign Language	4
Science* (Biology)	5
History	3
	1
	5

Semester II

English 1b	3
Foreign Language	4
Science* (Biology)	5
History	3
	1
	5

* recommended course

SOPHOMORE YEAR

Semester I

English 30 or 33	2 or 3
Physiology 1	4
Speech 1	3
Speech 18	1
PE 60 (Rhythmic Form & Analysis)	3 to 5
	14 to 16

Semester II

English 30 or 33	2 or 3
Speech 1	3
PE 120 (Anatomy)	6
Foreign Language, major or electives	3 to 5
	14 to 16

Suggested Major Studies

PE 49 (Folk Dancing)	1
Music 44 (Prin. of Music. Ed)	3
Music 67 (Pageantry)	3

PE 142 (Plays and Games)	1
PE 16 (First Aid)	1

JUNIOR YEAR

Semester I

Psychology	3
Speech 16	2
Philosophy 21	3
Education 41	3
PE 56 (Kinesiology)	3
Major or Electives	1 or 2
	14 to 16

Semester II

Speech 16	2
Speech 19 (may be taken 2nd semester of senior year)	3
Philosophy 25	3
Education 90	2
Major or Electives	4 to 6
	14 to 16

Suggested Major Studies

Music 31 (History)	2
PE 163 (Gymnastic Therapeutics)	4

PE 45 (Swimming Technique)	1
PE 81 (Camp Leadership)	2
Music 31 (History)	2

SENIOR YEAR

Semester I

Art History 51	3
PE 146 (Theory of the Dance)	3
PE 165 (Dance Composition)	2
PE 90 (Teaching and Adaptation)	2
PE 19 (Supervised Teaching)	2
Thesis	2
Major or Elective	1 or 2
	15 to 16

Semester II

Art History 52	3
PE 19 (Supervised Teaching)	2
Thesis	2
Major or Electives	7 to 9
	14 to 16

Suggested Major Studies

Music 65 (Appreciation)	1
Music 67 (Pageantry)	4

PE 80 (Comm. Recreation)	2
Music 65 (Appreciation)	1

GENERAL REQUIREMENTS - See. Page 1 (Item II).

The above document was forwarded to the Faculty of the College of Letters and Science at the University of Wisconsin-Madison by Margaret H'Doubler and Blanche Trilling on 8 June, 1926. Following the College's initial approval, the document was returned to the Faculty of the School of Education for their approval. Document #34 of the College of Letters and Science (academic year 1926 - 1927), resubmits the curricular plan and cites approval of the Specialized Major in Dancing by the School of Education on 11, October, 1926. The introduction to Document #34 reads as follows:

The Department of Physical Education recommends to the Faculty of the College of Letters and Science the following course in Dancing to be offered as a specialized major within the Course in Physical Education for Women. This course was approved by the School of Education at its meeting on Monday, October 11, 1926.

The specialized Major in Dancing was approved by the University Regents in November 1926, and first majors were accepted into the program for the spring semester 1927.

(College of Letters and Science Document 34: 1926 - 1927.)

Appendix B
Formal Structures and Affiliates of the
American Physical Education Association in 1934

The following provides a sense of the range of interest in the field for dance and physical education in the early 1930's. These were the organizational structures of the American Physical Education Association shortly after formally acceptance of the National Section on Dancing in 1932.

Committees:
>　Committee on Constitutional Matters
>　Honor Awards Committee
>　Necrology Committee
>　Committee on Resolutions
>　Committee on Educational Policy

Sections:
>　Public Schools Section
>　Recreation Section
>　Research Section
>　Teacher Training Section
>　Therapeutic Section
>　Women's Athletic Section
>　Men's Athletic Section
>　Dancing Section
>　Camping Section
>　Men's College Physical Education Section
>　Health Education Section

Affiliated Organizations:
>　Administrative Directors' Society
>　American Academy of Physical Education
>　College Physical Education Association
>　National Association of Directors of Physical Education
>　　　for College Women
>　National Collegiate Athletic Association
>　Society of State Directors
>　Women's Division, N.A.A.F.
>　Y.M.C.A. Physical Directors' Society
>　Y.W.C.A. Physical Directors' Society

(as referenced in Chapter 7, endnote 2 - Williams and Brownell 1934: 44.)

Appendix C
Council of Dance Administrators:
Standards for Dance Major Curricula

Throughout the 1970's standards for dance major curricula were of increasing concern to administrators of dance major programs in higher education. As discussed in Chapter 10, the Council of Dance Administrators worked to develop standards in the late 1970's. The following document was considered by Council members at their November 24 - 25, 1977 meetings. From this draft emerged the *Standards for Dance Major Programs* publication of 1979.

November 1977

I. *Undergraduate Program*

Curriculum
The undergraduate dance major should include:
1. A range of courses covering the various aspects of dance discipline (body of knowledge) including Technique, Choreography, Dance Notation, History of Dance, Philosophy of Dance, Music for Dance (analysis, literature, and accompaniment), Anatomy/Kinesiology for Dance, Dance of other Cultures, and Dance Theater Production/design.
2. Four years of dance technique (modern/ballet) with a minimum of 1 1/2 hour daily experience.
3. A minimum of two years of Choreography (including improvisation) in a class situation.
4. Performance experience including repertory in a variety of situations.
5. A four-year program with some options--probably in the senior year.

Dance Requirements
The dance major must have:
1. Breadth courses in general education (areas other than dance).
2. Experience in related arts as a part of the breadth study.
3. Forty percent (minimum) of the degree units in dance courses.

Admissions Practices
1. Selection procedures should include consideration of the student's ability to successfully complete the major program in dance.
2. Number of students admitted annually should be controlled in terms of faculty and space available. Careful consideration should be given to faculty/student ratio.

Faculty

1.　　The major program must be supported by five (5) full time faculty positions.　There must be a core of at least three full time continuing faculty, with additional full or part-time appointments according to curricular needs.　(This does not include teaching assistants.)

2.　　Selection of faculty should ensure that:

　　a.　All faculty are qualified to teach their specific assignments. This means that each instructor should have in-depth preparation in his area of teaching.

　　b.　Studio classes are taught by teachers who are or have been practicing artists and have ability to communicate and teach effectively.

　　c.　Faculty (especially core faculty) have ability to accomplish creative and/or scholarly work.

3.　　Appointments (including salary scales) and advancement of dance faculty must be based on the same criteria used in the institution for all academic faculty.　Creative activity must be accepted as equivalent to scholarly writing and experimental research.

4. *Faculty Schedule*

　　1.　Scheduled contact hours should be consistent with the guidelines used by the institution (15 contact hours as a maximum).

　　2.　Time should be provided in the schedule for maintaining technical proficiency and/or creative/scholarly work.

Musicians

1.　　There must be one full-time musician appointed as faculty or as staff.

2.　　A competent musician must be provided for all technique classes and be available for other studio classes.

3.　　A musical director should be provided for all concerts.

Production Staff

1.　　All concerts in performing spaces should be provided adequate technical support staff (costuming, lighting, technical director, stage manager, and promotion).

Staff

The major program must be supported by adequate secretarial and support staff.

Facilities and Equipment

1. Provision for space and facilities should support the enrollment.
2. Minimum of two large studios. Each studio should have unobstructed space with a minimum of 2400 sq. ft., ceiling height of at least 18 ft., resilient floors, windows and adequate lighting and ventilation. Studio equipped with mirrors and barres for ballet classes.
3. Appropriate classroom and rehearsal space, in addition to scheduled studio class space.
4. Piano in each studio.
5. Video, film, and slide projector, record players and tape recorders as needed to support the instructional program.
6. Variety of percussion instruments available for studio and music classes.
7. A theater or well-equipped studio theater available for concerts and for a class laboratory.
8. Appropriate dressing and shower facilitates for students and faculty.
9. Adequate office space for faculty located in close proximity to studio and classrooms.
10. Administrative office space and equipment appropriate to the needs of the program.
11. Adequate storage space for equipment, video, film projector, etc.
12. Adequate space for costume construction and storage.

Budget
The major program should be supported by adequate funding for the full operation of the major program.
1. Faculty
2. Visiting artists
3. Staff
4. Production
5. Equipment and supplies
6. Library and curricular resources

Advising
1. Advisor should have regularly scheduled conferences with students and be available at other times.
2. Each student should be kept informed about his/her progress in the dance major.
3. Each student folder should include records related to curricular progress.
4. Advising procedures should include concern for the student's long-range plan and assistance with undergraduate courses that provide appropriate preparation for advanced study.

5.	Students should be provided with information about specialization's available at the graduate level and about career possibilities.

Library
Adequate library holdings in dance related fields should be available to the dance major--including films, video tapes and records.

Publications
Catalogs and other literature representing the dance major must reflect accurately the faculty and program offered by the institution.

II. *Graduate-Master's Degree Program*

Curriculum
1.	Graduate programs must provide for breadth and depth in the discipline (body of knowledge) that extends the student's understanding beyond the scope of the undergraduate curriculum as set forth in this document.
2.	Master's degree curriculum must provide for a substantial number of graduate level content courses. In addition, there should be opportunity for independent research and creative work.
3.	Master's degree plan, in contrast to the undergraduate curriculum, should provide flexibility that allows the individual in consultation with an advisor to design a program of study appropriate to his needs and talents.
4.	Concentrations offered in different areas of the discipline should be supported by an adequate number of courses which ensure comprehensive understanding of the specialization.

Degree Requirements
1.	Sixty percent of the credits required for the master's degree should be in the graduate level dance courses and open only to graduate students.
2.	A thesis should be considered as an integral part of the degree requirements. This requirement may be met though a research oriented project or creative work in choreography and or performance. The creative thesis, in addition to the theater presentation, must include documentation in written thesis format. This written statement and the video or film must be filed.
3.	The MFA degree should include additional credit hours and residency beyond that required for the MA degree.

Admission

344

1. An undergraduate dance major or equivalent experience must be a requirement for admission to the master's program.
2. Admission criteria should include critical evaluation of the applicant's competence in dance as well as academic achievement and ability to work independently.
3. Number of students admitted should be controlled in relation to available faculty and space.
4. Undergraduate courses that are prerequisite to the given undergraduate major program should not be used for credit towards the master's degree.
5. Students who are admitted with undergraduate deficiencies which must be met should not be permitted to use those course for degree credit.

Faculty
1. A graduate curriculum must be supported by a sufficient number of qualified faculty. This means that additional faculty should be appointed beyond the minimum required for the undergraduate major. Institutions should not undertake a master's degree program unless this criteria can be met.
2. Faculty should include individuals who have had advanced study in academic institutions (MA degree as a minimum) as well as artists with professional experience.
3. Faculty must include persons who are qualified to supervise both research and creative theses.
4. The teaching load of faculty should reflect the time required for individual work with students such as independent study and thesis.
5. Appointments and advancement of dance faculty must be based on the same criteria used by the institution for all academic faculty. Creative activity must be accepted as equivalent to scholarly writing and experimental work.

Library
Institutions offering a graduate program should have library funds and resources substantially in excess of those which are provided for the undergraduate program. These should include films, video tapes, and records.

PREPARED BY:
Members of CODA

Appendix D
The Council of Dance Administrators:
Organizational Culture and Group History

As stated in Chapter 10, the creation of a National Association of Schools of Dance caused members of the Council of Dance Administrators to reflect on the group's place and reason for being in the organizational environment. The Council's mission was clear enough during its first ten years of function 1970 - 1980; the Council was a forum for participants to discuss the state of dance as an academic discipline, and to discuss the role of Council members as managers of major programs in dance. But now that a federally recognized accreditation agency existed, what was the purpose of CODA? In response to the creation of the new organization, Council members sought to clarify the group's internal sense of mission by inviting new institutional members to join, and by offering new services to dance administrators.

In 1988 - 1989, I conducted a study of the Council of Dance Administrators titled, "The Council of Dance Administrators: A Sociological Analysis of Group Culture," parts of which are included here. The story of how some of CODA's members understood their history and group culture is added because it permits individual "voices" to portray cultural and historical aspects of a very important group for dance in higher education. CODA members, through their professional activities, and through their work at their respective universities, shaped the landscape for dance in the American university in the 1970's and 1980's as surely as did Martha Hill, Mary Josephine Shelly, and colleagues in the 1930's.

To analyze the Council's organizational culture I used traditional field research methodologies of participant interview, document analysis, and observation of the group in session. Four founding members of CODA were interviewed for their personal recollections. Data collected from interview responses were then compared with data culled from a comprehensive review of CODA documents 1966 - 1989. Interview and document data were juxtaposed with data that emerged from observation of the Council at an annual meeting. The story that unfolded painted a portrait of the group's culture and process, and their attention to the issues that affected dance in higher education spanning a 23 year period.

One part of the study involved identifying the nature and frequency of issues that the Council addressed at regular meetings. Topics for issues included: administration, curriculum, the dance program as part of the college or university, the dance program as an academic entity, and the organization of the Council itself. The frequency of reference to issues under each overarching topic, as these appeared in CODA documents, was calculated to provide a hierarchical portrait of Council attention to these issues. I include data for the period 1966 - 1977 because these years represent the first decade of significant development for independent dance programs in American higher education. Council concerns in each of the topic categories include:

Administration: Issues were related to clarifying the role of the dance administrator in higher education. Council members often referred to themselves as dance educators who suddenly found themselves "administrating."

Curriculum: Issues were related to the development of standards for dance major programs in higher education. The need for clarification in this matter was viewed as a paramount concern.

The Dance Program as part of the College or University: Issues were related to the educational prerequisites necessary for recognition for an independent dance major program. This was linked to the idea of standards for the field. The concern being that the dance major program have a well-defined, academically "sound" curricular design.

The Dance Program as an Academic Entity: Issues were related to the effectiveness of individual programs as represented by national reputation, recognition, and productivity. The original members of CODA took a great pride in their individual accomplishments. A "national reputation" for quality was very important to them, even if "reputation" was determined among themselves.

The Organization of the Council of Dance Administrators: Issues were related to the experience of each individual member. The small, informal nature of CODA was important to members as they spent time identifying the unique problems each faced. Having the opportunity to explain their particular circumstances and have these reflected on by the group as a whole was greatly valued by individual members. The range and disparity of administrative-curricular issues and pressures underscored the need for discipline based standards.

With CODA's commitment to participate with the JCDTA in 1980, there was discussion about the future for both organizations. But, matters of academic survival for dance, issues that threatened the discipline throughout the 1980's, may have delayed a true discussion regarding CODA's future. During observation of the group in session in 1988, I witnessed what one founding member referred to as "our first real discussion about the future." Group members were in discussion when one Council participant raised her hand and commented "I just covered this topic at NASD last month, why am I here talking about it again?"

The answer to this question was partially addressed in a subsequent free - flowing, and very open conversation. Council members considered the intellectual and practical overlap of their work with that of NASD, yet they also found clear ways to contextualize the unique aspects of CODA's process: an intuitive process of dialogue; a small, intimate, group setting; a strong cultural history; no pressure to produce or comply. The Council continued to address the essence of the "why are we here?" question over the next few years, and continues to reassess its value to its members regularly. Perhaps this is a unique attribute of an organization founded solely on shared interest; the Council's members are women and men committed to the quality and success of dance as a vital part of the American university.

**The Council of Dance Administrators Organizational Culture and Group
History: Selected Responses to Questions**

Following observation of the Council, I asked selected, founding members
to respond to a set of 10 questions. The juxtaposition of multiple responses
provides an interesting portrait of organizational process, group dynamics, and
historical events. It also allows the reader to "hear" the individual voices of some
of CODA's founders. Respondents are identified by assigned numbers, 1 - 4.

1.   How would you describe the Council of Dance Administrators as a formal
        organization?

        #1:   CODA is only formal in that it meets regularly, has elected offices,
                and bylaws. The membership supplies the President with agenda
                items. Discussion in the group is informal. The membership has
                been kept small to facilitate an informal format and exchange. I
                believe the smallness of our group has facilitated our ability to act.
                Larger groups have not been able to do what CODA has, as an
                example consider the initiation of NASD.

        #3:   CODA exists primarily as a forum. In the past it was discussed
                and the group optioned to make a distinction between being a
                service organization and a forum. The group does, however, render
                valuable services: the 1978 Standards for Dance Major Guidelines,
                the 1985 Conference on Dance Administration at the University of
                Illinois at Urbana-Champaign. CODA renders services as any
                important organization does. Our members resisted formalization
                for some time. I admit to being the one who said, "The day we
                formalize, I quit." Yet I also admit to being the one who wrote up
                the documents of formalization. I see the annual meetings as a two
                day seminar. CODA remains informal in that it does not become
                bogged down in bureaucratic mechanics.

2.   What were the circumstances surrounding the Council's origins?

        #1   Alma Hawkins received a government grant to hold two
                conferences on the development of dance in education. Leaders in
                the arts and education were invited. The second conference was
                expanded to include philosophers, artists, and teachers. New
                dance administrators felt they needed to get together alone and
                decided to meet the following year in Washington D.C. (1968). At
                this meeting we discussed mutual problems we faced in
                administration. No one really knew how to make a dance major

program work. We decided to meet annually and for a number of years had no name, offices, or formal organization. In the beginning we were not administrators, we were educators who suddenly found ourselves with newly created departments, suddenly administrating.

#4:   In 1966 Alma Hawkins initiated the first developmental conferences on dance. This event was one of the most important ever held for the professional and academic dance worlds. It was the first time leaders from both arenas sat across from one another and spoke freely and frankly. It was a time when professional dance, through government grants and sponsorship, was exploding. At the same time dance educators were separating themselves from programs in physical education and joining programs in fine arts, music, theater, or moving into their own department. The conferences evoked a new freedom of thought and a confidence that did not exist before. The conferences provided the impetus for many of the attendees to return to their institutions and establish dance as an independent artistic and educational medium.

3.   What might you cite as examples of the routine function of the Council at its annual meeting?

#1:   We discuss current problems relevant to dance in education. Some problems change from year to year (like student enrollments), but others remain more constant (curriculum). Some problems are always being reviewed and others are related to the times.

#4:   To discuss the creation of quality dance programs. To accomplish this it was imperative that dance be separate from physical education. We struggled as a group to develop dance programs. This was not easy because of the negative reaction to separation by physical educators. In a number of cases all communication between the disciplines stopped. All our members had problems finding space, acquiring materials and funding, locating secretarial help and getting a commitment from the registrars office to actively list dance as a major. Most of the individuals who made up this first group were not prepared as administrators to accept and deal with the challenges surrounding the formation of independent dance programs. Today's Council operates in a much more sophisticated manner although it is still an informal group. Topics and issues are now on a world scale. We must dig deeper, as our topics demand in depth study. It is such a fast moving and changing world. Our 1988 meetings were a real turning point for the group. As new

350

members form the bulk of the membership new challenges emerge to spark provocative discussions out of which emerges a new momentum.

4.   How did the Council's meaning and mission evolve? Has it always been clear what the group's reason for being is?

#2   The mission evolved out of the first meeting. That mission has remained central however, as we have grown we have extended our areas of concern. The group's reason for being has been clear throughout.

#3   The developmental conferences prompted a need for meeting. We were all fighting the same battles and dealing with the same issues. It wasn't as if we could come up with one answer that everyone could use. We left our meetings feeling that the solutions we had discussed could be applied to each person's unique administrative context. The group was really trying to build a central vision of professional dance training in the academy. As time passed CODA began to do more in the area of outreach. Our reason for being has been clear until recently. The recent lack of clarity is not a threat, it is a sign of growth. Some of the group's members have been puzzled as to their place within this and other organizations. Active NASD members new to CODA often ask what the purpose of CODA is. The President of CODA asked, at the inception of NASD, "Is there a need for CODA?" We decided there was a special need CODA fulfills. As CODA gets larger, new members question what CODA is all about, this is good albeit rigorous.

5.   Please cite examples of events in the group's history that feel are significant in the Council's evolution.

#1   The decision to meet annually. The creation of the Standards for Dance Major programs document. The Administrative Conference of 1985. The initiation of NASD for accreditation purposes.

#3   For a time CODA didn't have a name. I remember sitting at a table at the Santa Ynez Inn and laughing with another member about the name we had just chosen.   The formalization of the Council changed us.   The accomplishment of the Standards, the 1985 · Conference, both of these were accomplishments that achieved some level of sophistication. The year we decided to take on new members and formalize our rules was quite significant.

6.   Does the Council work with other organizations to accomplish goals?

    #1   When we were involved with creating NASD we were given a lot of
          assistance from the National Association of Schools of Music
          (NASM). However CODA, for the most part, works alone.

    #2   The only close work we have done with an organization is our
          relationship with Mr. Sam Hope and NASD and the certification of
          dance programs. We decided not to be the organization to do this
          so we invited Mr. Hope to meet with us. He organized another
          group of artists and educators to discuss the creation of a NASD.

7.   What do you feel are the Council's greatest accomplishments?

    #2   The creation of a network of leaders clarifying and developing
          quality dance programs in higher education. The Standards for
          undergraduate and graduate programs. The week long Conference
          on Administration shared with other leaders in dance education,
          especially the young leaders in new programs.

    #4   Publication of the Standards document. The International
          Conference on Dance Administration. The initiation of NASD.
          The consistency of the membership and its vitality and vision.
          Maintaining great respect for one another.

8.   Has an increase in group membership affected the Council's function?

    #1   As new members come into the group there is a tendency for them
          to identify with one of the old guard. New members come and go.
          New members often just listen, it takes several years for new
          members to lead a discussion.

    #3   Very definitely the group is different. It is time to recognize this, it
          is a part of growth. It is good. We are not that small intimate
          group sharing similar experiences. Second and third generation
          administrators have changed this. While CODA is more formal it is
          beautifully informal.

    #4   CODA has remained small for several reasons. A large group
          prohibits intimate discussion. We did not want to repeat
          processes, we wanted to move on. We did not want to consider
          ourselves a formal group. We didn't want to get tangled up in
          formal rules and regulations. We came together by choice and we
          paid to do what we wanted to do. Our intent has always been

more important than the elitist or Dance Mafia tags. New people caused us to go over previously covered territory. Some new members are shy and have often felt uncomfortable. Others have been so eager they have monopolized conversations, but I feel new members have added to the group's strength and have broadened the process for all of us.

9.   Whom would you identify as a significant organizational figure?

#1   Alma Hawkins.

#2   Different members have played different roles. A remarkable feature of the organization is the lack of competition.

#3   Alma Hawkins is without a doubt the most significant figure. Alma is the core, the spine, and the vision of CODA.

#4   Alma Hawkins, an unusual leader. I doubt there is anyone who is as objective, and able to set the stage for dialogues, able to masterfully summarize scattered discussion, and spark the vision of what dance can mean in education. She is one of a kind, a very unusual woman, and very rare.

10.   In your opinion what is the Council's greatest resource?

#1   New membership.

#2   The group's commitment to dance as an art and discipline and their willingness to work against many odds to achieve quality.

#3   The membership. They are a repository of experience, a wonderful blend of the old and the new. A great human resource for the profession.

Bibliography

Abelson, P. *The Seven Liberal Arts: A Study in Medieval Culture.* New York: Teachers College Press, 1906.

American Association for Health, Physical Education, and Recreation. *DANCE DIRECTORY.* Washington, D.C: American Association for Health, Physical Education, and Recreation, 1966.

American Association of Colleges for Teacher Education. "No One Model." *Journal of Teacher Education* 24, no. 4 (1973): 264-265.

American College Dance Festival Association. "Celebrating 25 Years of Excellence." College Park, Maryland: American College Dance Festival Association, 1998.

And, Metin. *Dance Perspectives 3.* Edited by A. J. Pischl and Selma Jean Cohen (Summer 1959). New York: *Dance Perspectives* Inc., 1959.

Anderson, Jack. "Monsters and Prophets: Ted Shawn: Father of American Dance by Walter Terry." *DanceScope* 11, no. 2 (Spring/Summer 1977): 38-43.

Anderson, Jack. *The American Dance Festival.* Durham, North Carolina: Duke University Press, 1987.

Andrews, Gladys. "A Study to Describe and Relate Experience for the Use of Teachers Interested in Guiding Children in Creative Rhythmic Movement." Ph.D. diss., University of Wisconsin-Madison, 1952. Abstract in *Dissertation Abstracts International* 12-A (1953): 3183.

Baird, Henry M. *Rise of the Huguenots of France.* New York: Charles Scribner's Sons, 1900.

Baker, G. C. "Multicultural Imperatives for Curriculum Development in Teacher Education." *Journal of Research and Development in Education* 2, no. 1 (1977): 70-83.

Baker, Robb. "Frisbees and Unicycles Versus the Politics of Paternalism." *Dance Magazine* 47, no. 6 (June 1973): 62-63.

Banes, Sally. *Terpsichore in Sneakers: Post-Modern Dance.* Boston: Houghton Mifflin Company, 1980.

_____. *Democracy's Body: Judson Dance Theatre 1962 - 1964*. Durham, North Carolina: Duke University Press, 1993.

_____. *Greenwich Village 1963: Avant Garde Performance and the Effervescent Body*. Durham, North Carolina: Duke University Press, 1993.

_____. *Writing Dancing in the Age of Post-Modernism*. Hanover, New Hampshire: University of New England Press, 1994.

_____. "Feminism and American Postmodern Dance." *Ballett International* 6 (June 1996): 34-41.

Bauman, M. Garrett. "Liberal Arts for the Twenty-First Century." *Journal of Higher Education* 58, no. 1 (January/February 1987): 38-45.

Beckman, Cathy. "Performance and Education." *DanceScope* 15, no. 2 (1981): 26-33.

Beiswanger, George W. "Physical Education and the Modern Dance." *Journal of Health and Physical Education* 9, no. 32 (1936): 413-415, 463.

Beiswanger, George W. "The Dancer and Today's Needs." In: *Modern Dance in America: The Bennington Years*, edited by S. A. Kriegsman. Boston: G. K. Hall & Company, (1981): 280-283.

Bird, Bonnie. "Report of Annual CORD Membership Meeting." Edited by Anne Schley Duggan. *CORD News* 1, no. 1 (April 1969): 1-8.

Blair, Frederika. *Isadora: Portrait of the Artist as a Woman*. New York: McGraw- Hill, 1986.

Bloomer, Ruth H. "Bennington School of the Dance-Summer 1937." *Dance Observer* 4, no. 7 (August/September 1937): 73-74, 83-84.

Bloomer, Ruth H. "Four Summers at Bennington." *Dance Observer* 4, no. 7 (August/September 1937): 76, 83.

Blum, John M., William S. McFeely, Edmund S. Morgan, Arthur M. Schlesinger, Jr., Kenneth M. Stampp, and C. Vann Woodward. *The National Experience: A History of the United States* (7th edition). San Diego: Harcourt Brace Jovanovich Publishers, 1989.

Boas, Franz. *Primitive Art* . New York, Dover: (original publishing 1927), 1955.

Bonbright, Jane M. "Dance Education 1999: Status, Challenges, and Recommendations." *Arts Education Policy Review* 101, no. 1 (September/October 1999): 33-39.

Bossman, David M. "Cross Cultural Values for a Pluralistic Core Curriculum." *Journal of Higher Education* 62, no. 6 (November/December 1991): 661-681.

Boyce, Johanna, Ann Daly, Bill T. Jones, and Carol Martin. "Movement and Gender: A Roundtable Discussion. *"The Drama Review: A Journal of Performance Studies* 32, no. 4 (Winter 1988): 18-19.

Brennan, Mary A. (ed.) *Research in Dance III.* Reston, Virginia: National Dance Association (Stock # 243-29662), 1982.

_____. "Where Have all the Scholars Gone?." Reston, Virginia: National Dance Association, *Spotlight on Dance* 2, no. 3 (May 1985): 6-7.

_____. Untitled: "Scholar's Address-1985." In: *Lectures by NDA Scholars 1977- 1987.* Reston, Virginia: National Dance Association, (1987): 63-72.

_____. Telephone conversation with the author regarding developments in dance at the University of Wisconsin-Madison: 1987-1994. Mary Alice Brennan, Professor and Chair, Dance Program, University of Wisconsin-Madison, Madison, Wisconsin. 22 October, 1999.

Brown, Irving. "Report of Annual CORD Membership Meeting-Part I": September 21, 1969, edited by Anne Schley Duggan. *CORD News* 1, no. 1 (April 1969), : 4-8.

Carter, Curtis L. "Intelligence and Sensibility in Dance." *Arts in Society: Growth of Dance in America* 13, no. 2 (1976): 210-221.

Cetron, Marvin J., Soriano, Barbara, and Gayle, Margaret. "Schools of the Future," *The Futurist.* 19, no. 4 (August 1985): 18-23.

Chalif, Louis H. *The Chalif Textbook of Dancing.* New York: Isaac Goldman Coy. 1916.

Chatterjea, Ananya. "Towards Creating a Variegated, Multilayered Fabric." *Impulse: The International Journal of Dance Science, Medicine, and Education* 3, no. 3 (1995): 148-158.

Child, John. "Culture, Contingency and Capitalism in the Cross-National Study of Organizations." In: *Research in Organizational Behavior*, edited by B. Staw and L.L. Cummings, (1981): 303-356.

Chin, Daryl. "Books: Yvonne Rainers' Work 1961-1973." *DanceScope* 9, no. 2 (Spring/Summer 1975): 50-64.

Church, Marjorie. "The Bennington Dance Festival." *Dance Observer* 3, no. 7 (August/September 1936): 73, 77.

Cicero, Marcus Tullis. *M. Tvlli Ciceronis: Orationes.* "Pro Murena" 6(15), edited by Albert Curtis Clark. London: Clarendon Press. 1908.

Code, Grant. "Dance Theatre of the Works Progress Administration: A Record of National Accomplishment." *Dance Observer* 7, no. 3 (March 1940): 34-35.

Cohen, Barbara Naomi. "Modern Americanized Ballet." *DanceScope* 14, no. 3 (1980): 29-36.

Cohen, Selma Jeanne and A.J. Pischl. "Index to Dance Perspectives and Current Bibliography for Dance, 1959." New York: *Dance Perspectives* Inc., (1960): i.

Colby, Gertrude K. *Natural Rhythms and Dances.* New York: A. S. Barnes & Co. 1922.

Cole, R. E. *Work, Mobility and Participation: A Comparative Study of American and Japanese Industry.* Berkeley: University of California Press, 1979.

Conrad, C.F. and J. C. Wyer. "Liberal Education in Transition." *Higher Education Research Report #3.* Washington, DC: American Association for Higher Education, 1980.

Congress on Research in Dance. "Mission Statement." Mission statement included in *Dance Research Journal* and CORD publicity materials.

Cooper, Elizabeth. "Tamiris and the Federal Dance Theatre 1936 - 1939: Socially Relevant Dance Amidst the Policies and Politics of the New Deal Era." *Dance Research Journal* 29, no. 2 (Fall 1997): 23-48.

Council of Dance Administrators. "Summary Notes-Developmental Conference on Dance." 25 - 28 May, 1968. TMs. (photocopy). In the hands of the author.

_____. "Agenda and Summary Notes." 24 - 25 November, 1972. TMs. (photocopy). In the hands of the author.

_____. "Agenda." 24 November, 1976. TMs. (photocopy). In the hands of the author.

_____. "Summary Notes." 23 - 25 June, 1977(a). TMs. (photocopy). In the hands of the author.

_____. "Summary Notes." 25 - 26 November, 1977(b). TMs. (photocopy). In the hands of the author.

_____. "Summary Notes." 24 - 25 November, 1978. TMs. (photocopy). In the hands of the author.

_____. "Summary Notes." 23 - 24 March, 1979. TMs. (photocopy). In the hands of the author.

_____. "Summary Notes." 24 - 26 May, 1980. TMs. (photocopy). In the hands of the author.

_____. "Summary Notes." 27 - 28 November, 1981. TMs. (photocopy). In the hands of the author.

_____. "Summary Notes." 20 - 21 November, 1983. TMs. (photocopy). In the hands of the author.

_____. "Summary Notes." 11 - 12 November, 1984. TMs. (photocopy). In the hands of the author.

_____. "Summary Notes." 24 - 25 November, 1985 TMs. (photocopy). In the hands of the author.

_____. "Summary Notes." 9 - 10 November, 1986. TMs. (photocopy). In the hands of the author.

_____. "Summary Notes." 8 - 9 November, 1987. TMs. (photocopy). In the hands of the author.

_____. "Summary Notes." 4 - 5 November, 1989. TMs. (photocopy). In the hands of the author.

Cremin, Lawrence R. *The Transformation of the School: Progressivism in American Education 1876 - 1957.* New York: Vintage Books, 1961.

Cushing, Maxine. "The Bennington Record: July 2 - August 13, 1938." *Dance Observer* 5, no. 7 (August/September 1938): 104-105.

Dalbotten, Ted. "The Teaching of Louis Horst." *DanceScope* 8, no. 1 (Fall/Winter 1973/74): 26-41.

Daly, Ann. "Unlimited Partnership: Dance and Feminist Analysis." *Dance Research Journal* 23, no. 1 (Spring 1991): 2-5.

Daly, Lowrie J. *The Medieval University 1200 - 1400.* New York: Sheed and Ward, 1961.

Dell, Cecily. "Far Beyond the Far Out." *DanceScope* 1, no. 1 (Winter 1965): 13-18.

de Mille, Agnes. "Agnes de Mille Speaks to Congress on the State of the Arts: Her Statement and Questions and Answers before the House Select Subcommittee on Education." *Dance Magazine* 44, no. 5 (May 1970): 34 - 35, 80-85.

_____. *Martha: The Life and Work of Martha Graham, A Biography.* New York: Random House, 1991.

de Vries, Herbert . *Physiology of Exercise.* 84. Dubuque, Iowa: William C. Brown Co., 1980.

Dewey, John. *An Introduction to the Philosophy of Education.* New York: Macmillan & Co., 1916.

_____. *Dewey on Education,* edited by Martin S. Dworkin with introduction and notes by Martin S. Dworkin. New York: Teachers College Press, 1959.

_____. *John Dewey on Education,* edited by Reginald D. Archimbault. Chicago: University of Chicago Press, 1964.

_____. "Experience and Education." *Kappa Delta Phi,* 1938 (as it appeared in · Collier-Macmillian, (1957): 1-23. In: *ASHE Reader on Academic Programs in Colleges and Universities,* edited by Clifton F. Conrad, Lexington, Massachusetts: Ginn Press, (1987): 113-119.

Doll, E. "Foundations for a Post-Modern Curriculum." *Journal of Curriculum Studies* 21, no. 3 (1989): 243-253.

Dougherty, M. Frances. "Dance and Physical Education." *The Dance Encyclopedia*, edited by Anatole Chujoy and P. W. Manchester. New York: Simon and Schuster, (1967): 248-251.

Duncan, Donald, (ed.) "PressTime News." *Dance Magazine* 38, no. 1 (January 1964): 3-4.

Duncan, Isadora. *My Life*. New York: Liveright, 1927.

_____. *The Art of the Dance*. New York: J. J. Little and Ives Company, 1928.

_____. *Isadora Speaks*, edited by Franklin Rosemont. San Francisco: City Lights Books, 1981.

Dunkel, Elizabeth. "Putting Dance in its Place." *Journal of Health and Physical Education* 9 (September 1938): 419.

Durkheim, Emil. *The Evolution of Educational Thought.* 2nd ed. London: Routledge & Kegan Paul, 1969.

Duryea, E. D. "Evolution of the University." In: *The University as an Organization* edited by James A. Perkins. Carnegie Foundation for the Advancement of Teaching, New York: McGraw Hill, 1973.

Emery, Lynne Fauley. *Black Dance: from 1619 to Today.* Dance Horizons. Princeton, New Jersey: Princeton Book Co., 1988.

Erdman, Jean. "Dance in Education: Statement I." In: *Dance: A Projection for the Future,* edited by Marian Van Tuyl. San Francisco: Impulse Publications Inc., (1968): 65-69.

al Faruqi, Lois Ibsen. "Dances of the Muslim People." *DanceScope* 11, no. 1 (Fall/Winter 1976/77): 43-52.

Findlay, Elsa. "Dalcroze: The Nature of Rhythm." In: *Focus on Dance II: Dance as Movement Conference Proceedings 1961.* Washington, D.C: National Section on Dance, American Association for Health, Physical Education, and Recreation, (1962): 7-10.

Foley, Kathy. "My Bodies: The Performer in West Java." *The Drama Review : A Journal of Performance Studies* 34, no. 2 (1990): 62-80.

Fortin, Sylvie. "Content Knowledge in Dance Education." In: *Dance in Higher Education*. Reston, Virginia: American Alliance for Health, Physical Education, Recreation and Dance, (1992): 33-34.

Foster, Susan Leigh. *Reading Dancing: Bodies and Subjects in Contemporary American Dance*. Berkeley: University of California Press, 1986.

Fraleigh, Sondra Horton. *Dance and the Lived Body*. Pittsburgh: University of Pittsburgh Press, 1987.

Francis, Sandra T. "Exploring Dance as Concept: Contributions from Cognitive Science." *Dance Research Journal* 28, no. 1 (Spring 1996): 51-67.

Gates, Paul Wallace. *Dictionary of American History,* definition of "Morrill Act." 27. edited by James Truslow Adams and R.V. Coleman. New York: Charles Scribner's Sons, 1940.

Gere, David, Lewis Segal, Patrice Clark Koelsch, and Elizabeth Zimmer (eds.) *Looking Out: Perspectives on Dance and Criticism in a Multicultural World.* New York: Simon and Schuster Macmillan, 1995.

Gibb, Sara Lee. Telephone conversation with the author regarding her attendance at the American Dance Symposium, August 20-23, 1969, Wichita State University, Wichita, Kansas. Sara Lee Gibb, Professor and Chair, Department of Dance, Brigham Young University, Provo, Utah. 10 January, 1999.

Ginn, Victoria. *The Spirited Earth: Dance, Myth, and Ritual from South Asia to the South Pacific*. New York: Rizzoli International Publication, 1990.

Glassow, Ruth B. Interview by Laura Smail, February 1976. 60. TMs. (photocopy). In the hands of the author. Madison, Wisconsin: University Archives-Oral History Project. Department of Physical Education and Dance, 1982.

Glenny, Lyman A. "Demographic and Related Issues for Higher Education in the 1980's." *The Journal of Higher Education* 51, (July/August 1980): 363-380.

Gordon, Lonny Joseph. "Dancing in Japan." *DanceScope* 15, no. 2 (1981): 13-28.

Grande, Peter C. "The 1990s Challenge-Leadership or Survival." *Journal of Physical Education, Recreation, and Dance* 61, no. 5 (1990): 65-67.

Gray, Judith A. *Dance Technology: Current Applications and Future Trends.* Reston, Virginia: National Dance Association, 1989.

_____. "Dance Education In the Future-Trends and Predictions." *Journal of Physical Education, Recreation, and Dance* 61, no. 5 (1990): 50, 53.

_____. (ed.) *Research in Dance IV: 1900-1990.* Reston, Virginia: National Dance Association, 1992.

Gray, Judith A. and Dianne S. Howe. "Margaret H'Doubler: A Profile of Her Formative Years 1898 - 1921." *Research Quarterly for Exercise and Sport, Centennial Issue.* (1985a): 93-01.

_____. "The H'Doubler Idea of Dance and its Effect on the Physical Education Curriculum: 1919 - 1927." TMs. (photocopy). In the hands of the author. University of Wisconsin-Madison, Department of Physical Education and Dance, 1985(b).

Hagood, Thomas K. "The Council of Dance Administrators: A Sociological Analysis of Group Culture." University of Wisconsin-Madison, Department of Physical Education and Dance, 1989.

_____. "The Organizational Sociology of Dance: An Analysis, Comparison, and Environmental Description of Primary Organizations Advocating Dance in Higher Education." Ph.D. diss., University of Wisconsin-Madison, 1990. Abstract in *Dissertation Abstracts International* 51/04-A (1991): 1156.

_____. "Defining an Organizational Ecology for Dance." In, Proceedings: *Retooling the Discipline: Research and Teaching Strategies for the 21st Century,* compiled by Linda J. Tomko. University of California-Riverside, (1994a): 53-61.

_____. "Studies in the Sociology of Dance: The Organization and Culture of the Wisconsin Dance Council." *Impulse: The International Journal of Dance Science, Medicine, and Education* 2, no. 2 (April 1994b): 106-121.

_____. "Report to the Future Directions Task Force." National Dance Association. March 23, 1998.

Haley, Bruce. *The Healthy Body and Victorian Culture*. Cambridge, Massachusetts: Harvard University Press, 1978.

Hall, G. Stanley. *Educational Problems*. 2. vol. New York: Appleton, 1911.

Hanna, Judith Lynne. *To Dance is Human*. 8-9. Austin, Texas: University of Texas Press, 1979.

Hanstein, Penelope. "Educating for the Future-A Post-Modern Paradigm for Dance Education." *Journal of Physical Education, Recreation, and Dance* 61, no. 5 (May/June 1990): 56-58

Hartshorne, Joan and Tom. "Jolly Black Minstrels Need Not Apply." *DanceScope* 3, no. 2 (Spring 1967): 17-23.

Haskins, James. *Black Dance in America: A History through its People*. New York: Harper Trophy, A Division of Harper Collins, 1990.

Hausler, Barbara. "The Influence of Francis W. Parker on Doris Humphrey's Teaching Methodology." *Dance Research Journal* 28, no. 2 (Fall 1996): 10-22.

Hawkins, Alma M. *Modern Dance in Higher Education*. New York: Teachers College, Columbia University Bureau of Publications, 1954: v-vi.

Hawkins, Alma M. "Introduction." In: *Dance: A Projection for the Future,* edited by Marian Van Tuyl. San Francisco: Impulse Publications Inc., (1968): v-vi.

Hawkins, Alma. M. Letter to members of the "Dance Administrators Council." TMs. (photocopy). In the hands of the author. Council of Dance Administrators, 12, July 1973.

Hayes, Elizabeth R. "The Dance Teacher and the Physical Education Administrator." *Journal of the American Association for Health, Physical Education, and Recreation.* (December) 1954. In: *"Selected Articles from the Journal of Health, Physical Education, and Recreation,"* edited by Gertrude Lippincott (August) 1958. Reston. Virginia: American Alliance for Health, Physical Education, Recreation, and Dance. (1958): 26-28.

_____. "The Education, Training, and Development of Dance Educators in Higher Education-1978." In: *Lectures by NDA Scholars 1977 - 1987.* Reston, Virginia: National Dance Association. (1987): 1-6.

H'Doubler, Margaret N. *A Manual of Dancing*. Madison, Wisconsin: Tracy and Kilgour, 1921.

_____. *The Dance and its Place in Education*. New York: Harcourt, Brace and Co., 1925.

_____. *Dance: A Creative Art Experience*. New York: Appleton-Century Crofts, Inc., 1940.

_____. "A Way of Thinking. " TMs. (photocopy). In the hands of the author. University of Wisconsin-Madison, Department of Physical Education and Dance, 1948.

_____. "Personal Data Sheet." TMs. (photocopy). Stencil # 25-54. In the hands of the author. University of Wisconsin-Madison, Department of Physical Education and Dance, 1971.

_____. Interview by Carl Gutknecht, 3 June, 1972. TMs. (photocopy). In the hands of the author. University of Wisconsin-Madison, Department of Physical Education and Dance, 1972a.

_____. Interview by Mary Alice Brennan, 8 October, 1972. TMs. (photocopy). In the hands of the author. Reston, Virginia: American Alliance for Health, Physical Education, Recreation, and Dance-Archives. 1972b.

Hecht, Robin Silver. "Reflections on the Career of Yvonne Rainer and the Values of Minimal Dance." *DanceScope* 8, no. 1 (Fall/Winter 1973/74): 12-25.

Henderson, Algo D. and Jean C. *Higher Education in America: Problems, Priorities, and Prospects*. San Francisco: Jossey-Bass, 1974.

Hering, Doris. "The Peerless Princess Turns to Dance." *Dance Magazine* 42, no. 11 (November 1968): 71-75.

Heymann, Jeanne Lunin. "Dance in the Depression: The WPA Project." *DanceScope* 9, no. 2 (Spring/Summer 1975): 28-41.

Hill, Martha. "Report of the Committee on Percussion Accompaniment for Dance." Bennington, Vermont. Bennington School of the Dance, Summer, 1934. TMs. (photocopy). In the hands of the author. Wichita State University, Alice Bauman Archives-Ablah Library, 1934.

Hills, Dolores. "The Major Event of the Year." *Wichita Sunday Eagle*, 23 June, (1968): 1G.

Hodes, Stuart. "Artistic Future of Dance." Paper presented at the annual meeting of the National Association of Schools of Dance, 17 September, 1988. Reston, Virginia: National Association of Schools of Dance, 1988.

Hofstadter, Richard and Wilson Smith, (eds.) *American Higher Education: A Documentary History.* vol. 1, Chicago: University of Chicago Press, 1961.

Howe, Dianne S. (ed.) "Dance, 1990 and Beyond-Future Trends." *Journal of Physical Education, Recreation, and Dance* 61, no. 5 (1990): 49.

Howe, Eugene C. "What Business Has the Modern Dance in Physical Education." *Journal of Health and Physical Education* 8 (March 37): 131- 133, 187- 188.

Jencks, Christopher, and David Riesman. *The Academic Revolution.* Garden City, New York: Doubleday Books, 1968.

Joel, Lydia. "The Kennedy's at the Ballet" *Dance Magazine* 35, no. 7 (July 1961): 30-31.

_____. "Ford Foundation Controversy-Pros and Cons." *Dance Magazine* 38, no. 2 (February 1964): 34-37, 81-82.

_____. "The Impact of IMPACT: Dance Artists as Catalysts for Change in Education." *DanceScope* 6, no. 2 (Spring/Summer 1972): 6-26.

Johnson, Lyndon. Speech announcing the creation of the National Foundation for the Arts and Humanities, 29 September, 1965. In: *Dance Magazine* 39, no. 11 (November 1965): 34.

Jowitt, Deborah. *Time and the Dancing Image.* New York: William Morrow and Company, Inc., 1988.

Kaepler, Adrienne L. "Method and Theory in Analyzing Dance Structure with an Analysis of Tongan Dance." *Ethnomusicology* 16, no. 2 (1972): 173-217.

Kahlich, Luke. "Conduit or Gate? Mover or Museum?: The Future of Performance in Dance Education." *Journal of Physical Education, Recreation and Dance* 61, no. 5 (1990): 54-55.

Kahlich, Luke. "Educating Dance Educators-What Next?" In: Bulletin of the Council for Research in Music Education, School of Music, University of Illinois, Urbana-Champaign, (1993): 136-151.

Kamata. S. *Japan in the Passing Lane.* New York: Pantheon, 1982.

Kealiinohomoku, Joann. "An Anthropologist Looks at Ballet as a Form of Ethnic Dance." In: *Impulse 1970,* edited by Marian Van Tuyl. San Francisco: Impulse Publications Inc., (1970): 24-33.

_____. "Field Guides." In: Proceedings, New *Dimensions in Dance Research: Anthropology and Dance-The American Indian.* CORD Research Annual VI, edited by Tamara Comstock. New York: Committee on Research in Dance (CORD), (1974): 245-260.

_____. *Theory and Methods for an Anthropological Study of Dance.* Ann Arbor, Michigan: University Microfilms. 1970.

Kendall, Elizabeth. *Where She Danced.* New York: Alfred A. Knopf, Inc., 1979.

Kerr-Berry, Julie A. "Bursting the Eurocentric Bubble: African American Contributions to 20th Century Dance History." In: Proceedings, *Of, By, and For the People: A Joint Conference with the Congress on Research in Dance,* compiled by Linda J. Tomko, University of California-Riverside, (1993): 131-138.

Kiester, Gloria J. "Total Education: Arts Balance the Analytical with the Aesthetic." *Music Educators Journal* 72, no. 2 (October 1985): 24-27.

Kinderfather, Kathleen. "...And Beyond." *Journal of Physical Education, Recreation, and Dance* 61, no. 5 (1990): 64.

Kirby, Michael. "Post-Modern Dance." *The Drama Review* 19, no. 1 (1975): iii-iv.

Kirstein, Lincoln. *Dance; A Short History of Classic Theatrical Dancing.* 3rd ed., 353. Brooklyn, New York: Dance Horizons, 1974.

Klassen, F.J. and D. M. Gollnichs (eds.) *Pluralism and the American Teacher.* Washington, D.C: American Association of Colleges for Teacher Education, 1977.

Kotler, Philip, and Murphy, Patrick. "Strategic Planning for Higher Education." *The Journal of Higher Education* 52 (September/October 1981): 470-489.

Kraus, Richard. *History of the Dance in Art and Education.* Englewood Cliffs, New Jersey: Prentice Hall, 1969.

_____, Sarah Chapman-Hilsendager, and Brenda Dixon. *History of the Dance in Art and Education.* 3rd ed., 305. Englewood Cliffs NJ: Prentice Hall, 1991.

Kriegsman, Sali Ann. *Modern Dance in America: The Bennington Years.* Boston: G. K. Hall & Co., 1981.

Langer, Suzzane K. *Feeling and Form: A Theory of Art Developed from Philosophy in a New Key.* New York: Charles Scribner's Sons, 1953.

_____. *Philosophy in a New Key.* 3rd ed., Cambridge, Massachusetts: Harvard University Press, 1957.

LaPointe-Crump, Janice D. "The Future is Now-An Imperative for Dance Education." *Journal of Physical Education, Recreation, and Dance* 61, no. 5 (May/June 1990): 51-53.

Larkin, Joseph M. and Christine E. Sleeter (eds.) *Developing Multicultural Teacher Education Curricula.* Albany, New York: State University of New York Press, 1995.

LaSalle, Dorothy. Letter from Dorothy LaSalle to Gladys Andrews Fleming: "The Organizing of the Section." April, 1969. TMs. (photocopy). In the hands of the author. Reston, Virginia: American Alliance for Health, Physical Education, Recreation, and Dance-Archives. 1969.

Lee, Mabel. Letter to Dorothy LaSalle and Ruth Murray: "The Formation of a Committee to Report on Dancing at the 1931 American Physical Education Association Meeting." TMs. (photocopy). In the hands of the author. Reston, Virginia: American Alliance for Health, Physical Education, Recreation, and Dance-Archives, 1931.

_____. "A Synopsis of the Development of the National Section on Dancing." TMs. (photocopy). In the hands of the author. Reston, Virginia: American Alliance for Health, Physical Education, Recreation, and Dance-Archives, 1973.

_____. *A History of Physical Education and Sports in the U.S.A.* New York: John Wiley & Sons, 1983.

Lee, Ronald T. "The Expanding Role of the Arts in Education." *Music Educators Journal* 72, no. 2 (October 1985): 28-33.

Lekas, Lisa. "The Origin and Development of Ethnic Caribbean Dance and Music." Ph.D. diss., University of Wisconsin-Madison, 1955. Abstract in *Dissertation Abstracts International* 16/06, (1956): 1126.

Levy, Fran J. *Dance Movement Therapy: A Healing Art.* Reston, Virginia: National Dance Association. 1988.

Limón, José. "The Universities and the Arts." *DanceScope* 1, no. 2 (Winter 1965): 23-28.

Limón, José. "Dance in Education-Statement IV." In: *Dance: A Projection for the Future*, edited by Marian Van Tuyl. San Francisco: Impulse Publications Inc., (1968): 77-81.

Lippincott, Gertrude. "Aesthetics and the Dance: A Study of Some Problems in Dance Theory Presented for the Dancer." TMs. (photocopy). In the hands of the author. M.A. thesis, New York University, School of Education, 1943.

_____. "A Bright Future for Dance." *DanceScope* 1, no. 1 (Winter 1965): 10-13.

_____. "Report of the Arts." In: *Impulse: Dance and Education Now,* edited by Marian Van Tuyl. San Francisco: Impulse Publications, Inc., (1965): 8.

_____. Letter to the field, 6, November 1979. TMs. (photocopy). In the hands of the author. Dance Department, Mills College, Oakland, California, 1979.

Lloyd, Margaret. *The Borzoi Book of Modern Dance.* Brooklyn, New York: Dance Horizons, 1949.

Lockhart, Aileene. "Dance in Academe-1986." *Lectures by NDA Scholars 1977-1987.* Reston, Virginia: National Dance Association, (1987): 73-79.

Loewenthal, Lillian. *The Search for Isadora: The Legend & Legacy of Isadora Duncan.* Pennington, New Jersey: Dance Horizons-Princeton Book Co., 1993.

Lomax, Alan. *Folk Song and Structure.* Washington D.C: American Association for the Advancement of Science, 1968.

Lorber, Richard. "The Problem with the Grand Union." *DanceScope* 7, no. 2 (Spring/Summer 1973): 33-35.

Mallet, Charles Edward. *A History of the University of Oxford: Vol. 1, The Medieval University and the Colleges Founded in the Middle Ages.* London: Methuen & Co., 1924.

Marett, R.R. *The Threshold of Religion*. 2nd ed. London: Methuen & Co., 1914.

Marks, Joseph E. III. *The Mathers on Dancing. Including: An Arrow Against Profane and Promiscuous Dancing Drawn out of the Quiver of the Scriptures*, by Increase Mather (1685). Brooklyn, New York: Dance Horizons, 1975.

Marsh, Carol G. "Dancing in the Millennium: An International Conference" Call for Proposals and Conference Announcement. Copy in the hand of the author, 1999.

Marsh, Agnes L. and Lucile. *The Dance in Education.* New York: A.S. Barnes and Company, 1924.

Marsh, Lucile. "The New Dance Era." *Journal of Health and Physical Education* 3, no. 10 (1932): 22-24, 59-60.

Martin, John. *America Dancing: The Background and Personalities of the Modern Dance.* New York: Dodge Publishing, 1936.

_____. *Introduction to the Dance.* New York: W. W. Norton & Co., 1939.

_____. *Introduction to the Dance.* Brooklyn, New York: Dance Horizons, 1965.

_____. *The Modern Dance.* Brooklyn, New York: Dance Horizons, 1965

_____. "The Developmental Conference on Dance." Letter written 9 May, 1968. TMs. (photocopy). In the hands of the author. Council of Dance Administrators

Mattingly, Kate. "Deconstructivists Frank Gehry and William Forsythe: De-Signs of the Times." *Dance Research Journal* 31, no. 1 (Spring 1999): 20-28.

Maynard, Olga. "Eugene Loring talks to Olga Maynard." *Dance Magazine* 40, no. 7 (July 1966a): 35-39.

_____. "Eugene Loring Talks to Olga Maynard-Part II." *Dance Magazine* 40, no. 8 (August, 1966b): 52-54, 72-4.

_____. "College Controversy: The University of California at Irvine." *Dance Magazine* 40, no. 9 (September 1966c): 62-65.

McDonagh, Don. *Martha Graham.* 100. New York: Praeger Publishers Inc., 1975.

McLaughlin, John. "Advocating for Dance Education in the Nineties." *Journal of Physical Education, Recreation, and Dance* 61, no. 5 (1990): 62-63.

McMillan C. J. *The Japanese Industrial System.* Berlin: Walter de Gruyter, 1984.

Meigs, Anna. "Multiple Gender Ideologies and Statuses." In: *Beyond the Second Sex: New Directions in the Anthropology of Gender.* Philadelphia: University of Philadelphia Press, 1990.

Minton, Sandra and Karen McGill. "A Study of the Relationships between Teacher Behaviors and Student Performance on a Spatial Kinesthetic Awareness Test." *Dance Research Journal* 30, no. 2 (Fall 1998): 39-53.

Montague, Mary Ella. "Beliefs, Fears, Biases: Status of Dance as Revealed in the Catalogues of Selected Colleges and Universities-1987." *Lectures by NDA Scholars 1977 - 1987.* Reston, Virginia: National Dance Association, (1987): 81-85.

Moomaw, Virginia. Letter to author regarding 1961 Conference on Movement (National Section on Dance), and the 1965 Dance as a Discipline Conference (Dance Division of the American Association for Health, Physical Education, and Recreation), October, 1994.

Moore, Ellen. "A Recollection of Margaret H'Doubler's Class Procedure: An Environment for Learning Dance." *Dance Research Journal* 8, no. 1 (Fall/Winter 1975-1976): 12-17

Moore, William. "The Other Dance." *DanceScope* 3, no. 2 (Spring 1967): 26-30.

Morgan, Clyde. "Art Had a Power Then." *DanceScope* 3, no.2 (Spring 1967): 23-26

Morrison, Jack. *The Rise of the Arts on the American Campus*. New York: McGraw-Hill Book Company, 1973.

Murray, Ruth. "Petition to Form a Dance Section in the American Physical Education Association." 16 February, 1931. TMs. (photocopy). In the hands of the author. Reston, Virginia: American Alliance for Health, Physical Education, Recreation, and Dance-Archives, 1931.

Murray, Ruth. "The Dance in Physical Education." *Journal of Health and Physical Education* (January 1937): 10-14, 59.

National Association of Schools of Dance. Brochure Describing the Function of the Association. Reston, Virginia: National Association of Schools of Dance, March, 1985.

Neal, Nelson D. "Early Television Dance." *DanceScope* 13, no. 2 & 3 (Winter/Spring 1979): 51-56.

Nesbitt, Dorothy. "North Carolina Leads the Way: A State School for the Arts." *DanceScope* 1, no. 2 (Spring 1965): 15-19.

Nesbitt, Richard C. *Wisconsin: A History*. 426. Madison, Wisconsin: University of Wisconsin Press, 1973.

"New School Series." *Dance Observer* 1. no.6 (August 1934): 68.

Nikolais, Alwin. "Dance in Education-Statement II." In: *Dance: A Projection for the Future*, edited by Marian Van Tuyl. San Francisco: Impulse Publications Inc., (1968): 69-75.

Novack, Cynthia J. *Sharing the Dance: Contact Improvisation and American Culture*. Madison, Wisconsin: University of Wisconsin Press, 1990.

O'Donnel, Mary P. "Petition to the American Physical Education Association." 9 March, 1932. TMs. (photocopy). In the hands of the author. Reston, Virginia: American Alliance for Health, Physical Education, Recreation, and Dance-Archives. 1932.

_____. "Martha Hill." *Dance Observer* 3, no. 4 (April 1936): 37, 44.

Ouchi W. A. *Theory Z: How American Business Can Meet the Japanese Challenge*. Reading, Massachusetts: Addison-Wesley, 1981.

Page, Barbara. "Contemporary Exponents of the Modern Dance." *Journal of Health and Physical Education* 6 (April 1935): 11.

Paprock, Dara. Telephone conversation with the author regarding M.A studies in dance in the Department of World Culture and Arts at the University of California-Los Angeles. 22 October, 1999.

Parker, Ellen. "Image of Dance in Academe." *DanceScope* 15, no. 2 (1981): 22 - 26.

Pascale, R. and A. Athos. *The Art of Japanese Management.* New York: Warner Books, 1981.

Paulsen, Frederich. *The German Universities: Their Character and Historical Development*", introduction by Nicholas Murray Butler. London: Macmillan and Co., 1895.

Pease, Esther. "Oral History-1986." Reston, Virginia: American Alliance for Health, Physical Education, Recreation, and Dance-Archives, 1986.

Phillips, Patty. "The View from Florida: Dancers in Cap and Gown-Part Three." *Dance Magazine* 58, no. 9 (September 1994): 58-61.

Povall, Richard. "Dance and Technology: Technology Is With Us." *Dance Research Journal* 31, no 21 (Spring 1998): 2-4.

Prevots, Niama. *American Pageantry: A Movement for Art and Democracy.* Ann Arbor, Michigan: UMI Research Press, 1987.

_____. "University Courses in Pageantry and American Dance: 1911 - 1925." In: Proceedings, *Eleventh Annual Conference of the Society of Dance History Scholars,* compiled by Linda J. Tomko. University of California-Riverside, (1988): 237-247.

_____. *Dance for Export: Cultural Diplomacy and the Cold War.* Hanover, New Hampshire: University of New England Press-Wesleyan University Press, 1998.

Rashdall, Hastings. *The Universities of Europe in the Middle Ages.* Vol. 1 and vol. 2., Oxford: The Clarendon Press, 1895.

Remley, Mary Lou. "The Wisconsin Idea of Dance: A Decade of Progress 1917 - 1926." *Wisconsin Magazine of History* 58, no. 3 (Spring 1975): 179-195

Rice, Emmett A. *A Brief History of Physical Education.* New York: A.S. Barnes and Company, 1926.

Roemer, Robert E. "Vocationalism in Higher Education: Explanation from Social Theory." *The Review of Higher Education* 23, no. 2 (Winter) 1981: 23-46. In: *ASHE Reader on Academic Programs in Colleges and Universities,* edited by Clifton F. Conrad, 155-169. Lexington, Massachusetts: Ginn Press, 1987.

Rosaldo, Remato. "Others of Invention: Ethnicity and its Discontents." *Village Voice,* Literary Supplement, February (1990): 27-28.

Rose, Ruth June. "The Wisconsin Dance Idea." 40. B.A. thesis, University of Wisconsin, 1950.

Rowe, Patricia. "Comments from the Chairman of CORD." *CORD News* 2, no. 1, (April 1970): 1.

_____. "Report from the Chairman." *CORD News* 3, no. 1 (1971): 4-5.

Rudolph, Frederick. *Curriculum: A History of the American Undergraduate Course of Study Since 1636.* 1. San Francisco: Jossey-Bass, 1977.

Russell, Carroll. "John Martin on Audiences; A Conversation with Carroll Russell." *Impulse,* edited by Marian Van Tuyl. San Francisco: Impulse Publications. (1962): preface, 1, 8.

Ruyter, Nancy Lee Chafla. *Reformers and Visionaries: The Americanization of the Art of Dance.* Brooklyn, New York: Dance Horizons, 1979.

Sachs, Curt. *World History of the Dance.* 245. New York: W. W. Norton, 1937.

Sayle, M. "The Yellow Peril and the Red-Haired Devils." *Harpers.* (November 1982): 23-35.

Schachner, Nathan. *The Medieval Universities.* New York: Frederick A. Stokes & Co., 1938.

Schmitz, Nancy Brooks. "Key Education Issues-Critical to Dance Education." *Journal of Physical Education ,Recreation, and Dance* 61, no. 5 (May/June 1990): 59-61.

Shah, Purnima. "Transcending Gender in the Performance of Kathak." *Dance Research Journal* 30, no. 2 (Fall 1998): 2-18.

Shapiro, Judith. "Dancing in China" *DanceScope* 15 no. 2 (1981): 1-13.

Sheets, Maxine L. "The Phenomenology of Dance." Ph.D. diss., University of Wisconsin-Madison, 1962. Abstract in *Dissertation Abstracts International* 24/04-A, (1963): 1559.

Shelly, Mary Josephine. "Art and Physical Education-An Educational Alliance." *Journal of Health and Physical Education* (October 1936): 476-477, 529 - 531.

_____. "Facts and Fancies about the Dance in Education." *Health and Physical Education* 9, no. 1 (1940): 18-19, 56-57.

Sherman, Jane. *The Drama of Denishawn Dance*. Middletown, Connecticut: Wesleyan University Press, 1979.

_____. "Denishawn Oriental Dances." *DanceScope* 13, no. 2&3 (Winter/Spring 1979): 33-44.

Siegel, Marcia B, (ed.) *DanceScope* 1, no.1 (Winter 1965): 2.

_____. "Education of a Dance Critic." *DanceScope* 15, no. 1 (1981): 16-22.

_____. *Days on Earth: The Dance of Doris Humphrey*. New Haven and London: Yale University Press, 1987.

Simpson, Douglas J., and Michael J. B. Jackson. *Educational Reform: A Deweyan Perspective*. New York: Garland Publishing Inc., 1997.

Sloan, Douglas. "Harmony, Chaos, and Consensus: The American College Curriculum." *Teachers College Record* 73 (1971): 221-251.

Smith, Nancy, (ed.) "Introduction: Dance as a Discipline." In: *Focus on Dance IV*. Washington D.C: American Association for Health, Physical Education and Recreation, (1967): v.

Smith-Fichter, Nancy, compiler. *Survey of Colleges*: TMs. (photocopy). In the hands of the author. Council of Dance Administrators, 1976.

_____. "The Future of Dance in Higher Education." Paper presented at the annual meeting of the National Association of Schools of Dance [?]. TMs. (photocopy). In the hands of the author. Reston, Virginia: National Association of Schools of Dance. [?]: 1-9.

Soares, Janet Mansfield. *Louis Horst: Musician in a Dancers World.* Durham, North Carolina: Duke University Press, 1992.

Soares, Janet Mansfield. "Barnard's 1932 and 1933 Dance Symposiums: Bringing Dance to the University." In: Proceedings, *Reflecting our Past; Reflecting on our Future: Society of Dance History Scholars,* compiled by Linda J. Tomko. University of California-Riverside, (1997): 191-202.

Society of Dance History Scholars. "Mission Statement." Mission statement included in SDHS publicity materials, 1999.

Sommer, Sally R. "Trisha Brown Making Dances: Choreograms from Trisha Brown's Notebook." *DanceScope* 11, no. 2 (Spring/Summer 1977): 7-10.

Sorell, Walter. *Hanya Holm: The Biography of an Artist.* Middletown, Connecticut: Wesleyan University Press, 1969.

Sparrow, Patricia. "The Choreographic Devices: Their Nature and Function as Related to the Principle of Opposition." Ph.D. diss., University of Wisconsin-Madison, 1962. Abstract in *Dissertation Abstracts International* (1963).

Spencer, Herbert. *Education: Intellectual, Moral, and Physical.* New York: Appleton, 1896.

Spiesman, Mildred C. "Dance Education Pioneers: Colby, Larson, H'Doubler." *Journal of Health and Physical Education* (January 1960): 25-27.

Stanley, S.C. and D.M. Lowery. *Manual of Gymnastic Dancing.* New York: Association Press, 1920.

St. Denis, Ruth, and William H. Bridge. "The Dance in Physical Education." *Journal of Health and Physical Education* (January 1932): 11-14, 61.

Stebbins, Genevieve. *Delsarte System of Expression.* 6th ed. Unabridged reproduction of 6th ed. Originally published by Edgar S. Werner Publishing and Supply Inc., New York, 1902. Brooklyn, New York: Dance Horizons, 1977.

Stewart J. R., and D. G. Dickason. "Hard Times Ahead." *American Demographics* (June 1979): 23

Sticklor, Susan Reimer. "The Spirit of Denishawn: Klarna Pinska." *DanceScope* 11, no. 2, (Spring/Summer 1977): 43-47.

Stillman, Benjamin, (ed.) "Original Papers in Relation to a Course in Liberal Education." *The American Journal of Science and Arts* 15 (January 1829): 297-351.

Stodelle, Ernestine. "College of Career for Dancers: Bennington's Answer." *Dance Magazine* 38, no. 9 (September 1964): 40-45.

_____. "College or Career? The University of Arkansas." *Dance Magazine* 40, no. 2 (February 1966a): 56-58.

_____. "College or Career? The University of Illinois." *Dance Magazine* 40, no. 4 (April 1966b): 52-54.

Swisher, Viola Hegyi. "PressTime News." *Dance Magazine* 42, no. 4 (April 1968): 3.

Terry, Walter. *Isadora Duncan: Her Life, Her Art, Her Legacy*. New York: Dodd, Mead & Co., 1963.

_____. "New Spirit In the Colleges.'" *New York Herald Tribune*, Sunday Magazine. 11 July, (1965): 30.

_____. *Miss Ruth: The "More Living Life" of Ruth St. Denis*. New York: Dodd, Mead & Co., 1969.

_____. *I Was There*. New York: Audience Arts-A Division of Marcel Dekker Inc., 1978.

Thorpe, Edward. *Black Dance*. Woodstock, New York: The Overlook Press, 1990.

Topaz, Muriel. Untitled. Paper presented to the annual meeting of the National Association of Schools of Dance, September 1984. TMs. (photocopy). In the hands of the author. Reston, Virginia: National Association of Schools of Dance, 1984.

Toulmin, S. *The Return to Cosmology*. Berkeley: University of California Press, 1982.

Trilling, Blanche. *History of Physical Education for Women at the University of Wisconsin 1898 - 1946*." TMs. (photocopy). In the hands of the author.

University of Wisconsin-Madison, Department of Physical Education and Dance, 1951.

"The Trustees of Dartmouth College v Woodward." Reports of Cases argued and decided in the Supreme Court of the United States, IV (Newark, New Jersey, 1882), 625-654; first published in 4 Wheaton, (1819): 625-654.

University of California-Los Angeles. Information taken from the website, Http://www.campaign.ucla.edu/programs/wac.htm. October 22, 1999.

University of Wisconsin-Madison. College of Letters and Science, Document # 33: 8, June 1926, TMs. (photocopy). In the hands of the author. University of Wisconsin-Madison, University Archives-Memorial Library, 1926.

_____. College of Letters and Science, Document # 34: 13, October 1926, TMs. (photocopy). In the hands of the author. University of Wisconsin-Madison, University Archives-Memorial Library, 1926.

_____. "Mission Statement." Interarts and Technology Program (IATECH) TMs: (photocopy). In the hands of the author. School of Education-Dance Program, 1992.

Van Tuyl, Marian. "Creative Dance Experience and Education." *Impulse! 1951.* San Francisco: Impulse Publications Inc., (1951): 10-12.

_____, (ed.) "Manifesto." *Dance: A Projection for the Future.* San Francisco: Impulse Publications Inc., (1968a): 7.

_____, (ed.) "Dance Department-Minimum Standards." *Dance: A Projection for the Future.* San Francisco: Impulse Publications Inc., (1968b): 129.

Vesey, Laurence. "Stability and Experiment in the American Undergraduate Curriculum." In: *Content and Context: Essays on College Education,* edited by Carl Keysen, 1-63. McGraw-Hill, Carnegie Foundation for the Advancement of Teaching, 1973.

Vissicaro, Pegge. "Cross-Cultural Dance Education: Diminishing Boundaries." In: Proceedings, *Eighteenth Annual Conference of the Society of Dance History Scholars,* compiled by Linda J. Tomko. University of California-Riverside, (1995): 287-289.

Wagner, Ann. *Adversaries of Dance: From the Puritans to the Present.* Chicago: University of Illinois Press, 1997.

Wilde, Patricia. "Dance in Education-Statement II." *Dance: A Projection for the Future,* edited by Marian Van Tuyl. San Francisco: Impulse Publications Inc., (1968): 75-77.

Wilkinson, William Cleaver. *The Dance of Modern Society.* New York: Funk and Wagnalls, 1884.

Williams, Charles H. "The Hampton Institute Creative Dance Group." *Dance Observer* 5, no. 8 (October 1937): 97-98.

Williams, Jesse Fiering and Clifford Lee Brownell. *The Administration of Health and Physical Education* , frontispiece and pgs. 19, 28-31, 42-43. Philadelphia and London: W. B. Saunders Co., 1934.

Williams, Julinda Lewis. "Book Notes: Aspects of Ethnic Dance." *DanceScope* 13, no. 4 (Summer 1979): 60-67.

_____. "Black Dance: A Diverse Unity" *DanceScope* 14, no. 2 (1980): 54-64.

Wilson, John M. "The Thought of Margaret H'Doubler." TMs. (photocopy). Unpublished monograph. Copy in the hands of the author. University of Arizona-Tucson,1981.

_____. "Education and Training Issues: Curricular and Instructional Practices." Paper presented at the annual meeting of the National Association of Schools of Dance, St. Paul, Minnesota, 1 October, 1983. TMs. (photocopy). In the hands of the author. Reston, Virginia: National Association of Schools of Dance, 1983.

Wimmer, Shirley. "Gertrude Prokosch Kurath." In: Proceedings, *New Dimensions in Dance Research: Anthropology and Dance-The American Indian.* Research Annual VI, (CORD),Third Conference on Research in Dance, March 26-April 2, 1972, University of Arizona- Tucson and the Yaqui Villages of Tucson. Committee on Research in Dance, (1974): 31-34.

Wooten, Betty Jane, (ed.) *Focus on Dance II; An Interdisciplinary Search for Meaning in Movement".* Washington D.C: National Section on Dance, American Association for Health, Physical Education and Recreation, 1962.

INDEX

American School of Dance, 198, 199. *See also* Loring, Eugene
Amherst College, 192
An American in Paris (the movie), 180
Anderson, John Murray, 106. *See also* Graham, Martha; Greenwich Village Follies; John Murray Anderson-Robert Milton School of the Theater
Anderson, William G., 51, 52, 53, 54, 59
Brooklyn Normal School, 52
Brooklyn School of Physical Education, 52
Andrews, Gladys, 285
Annual Dance Symposium, 113. *See also* Barnard College
APEA. *See* American Physical Education Association
Arizona, University of, 254
Arts and Humanities Bill, 185. *See also* Federal Arts Advisory Council; Morehead, William; Pell, Claiborne. *See also* 9 n 3
Association of Land Grant Colleges, 192
At Dawn (the dance), 117
Atlanta Civic Ballet, 179, 188
Auctioneer (the play), 64
Baby Boom, 175, 218, 219, 249, 255, 284
Babylon (the movie). *See* Griffith, D. W.
Baker, Robb, 225
Balanchine, George, 180, 186, 188, 288. *See also* New York City Ballet
Ballet Girl, The (the play). *See* St. Denis, Ruth
Ballet Society, 187, 188. *See also* Ford Foundation; Kirstein, Lincoln; New York City Ballet
Barbarossa, Frederick, 14
Habita, 14
Barnard College, 78, 112, 113, 161
Battle Creek Michigan, 113

Bauman, Alice, 215, 216. *See also* American Dance Symposium, 1968
Kansas Dance Councils Inc., 214
Mid-America Center for the Dance, 216
Sherbon, Elizabeth, 215
Wichita, State University of, 214
Beaman, Jeanne, 302. *See also* Pittsburgh, University of
Beecher, Catherine, 28
Beegle, Mary Porter, 55, 92
Beiswanger, Professor George W., 133, 134, 297
Monticello College, 133
Belasco, David, 64, 65
Bennington College, 7, 50, 104, 110, 111, 112, 113, 115, 116, 117, 118, 119, 120, 121, 122, 123, 125, 127, 129, 133, 134, 135, 138, 139, 140, 141, 144, 150, 152, 153, 173, 174, 197, 201, 203, 210, 215, 239, 255. *See also* Graham, Martha; Hill, Martha; Holm, Hanya; Horst, Louis; Humphrey, Doris; Martin, John; Shelly, Mary Josephine; Tamiris, Helen Tamiris; Weidman, Charles
Bennington Experience, 199
Bennington Farm, North, 113
Bennington School, 117
Big Four of, 118, 119, 120
Board of Trustees for, 113, 116
Curriculum, 118. *See also* 5 n 42
Faculty, 118
Gymnasium Circuit, 119, 174
Horst, Louis, 121, 123
Jennings, Mrs. Frederic B., 113
Kirstein, Lincoln, 123
Kriegsman, Sali Ann, 111, 112, 114, 118, 119
Lauterer, Arch, 123
Leigh, Robert D., 112, 113, 116

Standards for Dance Major Curricula, 234

Council on Post Secondary Accreditation, COPA, 234, 237

Court Cases. *See* United States Supreme Court

CPAT. *See* Center for Performing Arts and Technology

Cremin, Lawrence R., 44

Crusades, 14

Cumnock School of Expression, 106. *See also* Graham, Martha

Cunningham, Merce, 288
  Merce Cunningham Studio, 232
  Winterbranch, 289

Dalcroze, Emile-Jacques, 41, 85, 117
  Dalcroze Eurythmics, 40, 41, 69, 70, 110, 151
  Dalcroze System, 43
  Findlay, Elsa, 110

Daly, Augustin, 60, 63

Dance Administrators Council. *See* Council of Dance Administrators, CODA

Dance and the Child International, 306
  United States Chapter, 306

Dance and Theater Accreditation, Joint Commission for, 237
  JCDTA, 234, 235, 237, 238, 239, 240, 241

Dance as a Discipline Conference, 1965, 192, 193, 195, 196, 204, 205, 295. *See also* 9 n 16

Dance Boom, 218, 219, 221, 225, 228, 284. *See also* 10 n 4

Dance Critics Association, 306

Dance Directory. *See* National Section on Dance

Dance Division of AAHPER, 156, 193, 194, 195, 232, 284, 307

Dance Dynamics. See Journal of Physical Education, Recreation, and Dance

Dance Magazine, 111, 180, 187, 188, 197, 198, 207, 224, 225, 273, 276, 311

Dance Notation Bureau, 191, 282, 306

Dance Observer, 128, 129, 165, 273, 274, 278. *See also* Bennington College; Horst, Louis

Dance of Steam (the dance), 54

Dance of the Future, The (the lecture). *See* Duncan, Isadora

Dance Perspectives, 274, 275, 282. *See also* Cohen, Selma Jeanne; Pischl, A. J.

Dance Repertory Theatre, 110, 111. *See also* Tamiris, Helen Tamiris

Dance Scope, 192, 278. *See also* Siegel, Marcia B.

Dance Theater of Harlem, School of the, 232

Dance Therapy, 91, 221. *See also* 12 n 12
  American Dance Therapy Association, 306

Dancing in the Millennium Conference, 2000, 306

Dancing, Natural. *See* Natural Dancing

Dartmouth College v Woodward, case from 1817. *See* United States Supreme Court

Darwin, Charles, 43

Darwinism, Social, 43. *See also* Hall, G. Stanley; Spencer, Herbert

Davis, Lynda, 311

Dawson, Dr., 92. *See also* H'Doubler, Margaret

de Laban, Juana, 215, 277

de Medici, Catherine, 18
  St. Bartholomew's Day Massacre, 18

de Mille, Agnes, 198

Degrees, in dance
  BA, 231, 262, 266, 267, 300
  BFA, 167, 219, 231, 258, 261, 264, 267

Joel, Lydia, 188
Lowry, W. McNeil, 187, 188
National Ballet of Washington, 188
New York City Ballet, 186
Pennsylvania Ballet, 188
San Francisco Ballet, 187, 188
Utah Ballet, 188
Fort Hays State Teachers College. *See*
Hill, Martha
Fortin, Sylvie, 314
Francis, Parker. *See* Dewey, John
Franklin, Benjamin, 20, 21. *See also*
Philadelphia, College of; Smith,
Reverend William
Frederick II, 17. *See also* Gregory IX
Free Corporation, 16. *See also*
Universitas
Frelighuysen, Peter (congressman), 193
Frolic, The. See Colby, Gertrude
Frost, Robert, 54
Fuller, Loie, 60. *See also* Duncan,
Isadora; Paris Exposition, 1900
Fundamentals. *See* H'Doubler, Margaret
Future Directions Task Force. *See*
National Dance Association
Garrison, Clayton, 200, 201, 202, 203.
See also Irvine, University of
California at
General School. *See* Studium Generale
German/Germany. *See also* lehrfreiheit;
lernfreiheit
Contemporary Dance Movement, 109
German Gymnastics, 315
German Idea of Physical Culture, 29
German influence on the University,
26
German philosophy, 26
German School of Dance, 210
German Universities, 26
Gymnasium Movement, 28
Idea of Physical Culture, 28, 55
Jahn, german gymnastics, 28
Turner Halls, 29

Turnvereine, 29, 55
GI Bill, GI Bill of Rights, 162, 179
Gibb, Sara Lee, 308
Gilbert, Melvin. *See* H'Doubler,
Margaret
Gilbert, Melvin B., 53
Glassow, Ruth. *See* H'Doubler, Margaret
Glenny, Lyman, 248, 251, 265
Graduate, The (the movie), 221
Graham, Martha. *See also* Bennington
College; Hill, Martha; Holm,
Hanya; Horst, Louis; Humphrey,
Doris; Shawn, Ted; Tamiris,
Helen Tamiris; Weidman, Charles
48th Street Theatre, 107
Anderson, John Murray, 106
Bennington College, 118
Cumnock School of Expression, 106
Dance Repertory Theater, 111
Denishawn, 105, 106
Eastman School of Music, 106
Graham, George and Jane "Jennie"
(parents), 105
Graham, Georgia "Geordie", 105
Graham, Mary, 105
Greenwich Village Follies, 106
Horst, Louis, 107
John Murray Anderson-Robert
Milton School of the Theater,
114
Klaw Theatre in New York, 114
Letter to the World, 122
Martha Graham School of
Contemporary Dance, 232
Phaedra, 193
Santa Barbara High School, 1913, 106
Xochitl, 106
Gray, Judith A, 302
Gray, Miriam, 194
Great Depression, 104, 119, 124, 176
Great Society Programs. *See* Johnson,
Lyndon

Frederick II, 17
Germanic, 14
Hoover, Herbert, 124
Hope, Samuel, 237, 240. *See* Council of
    Dance Administrators, CODA;
    Joint Commission of Dance and
    Theater Accreditation; National
    Association of Schools of Dance
Hopkins University, Johns. *See* Johns
    Hopkins University
Horst, Louis, 105, 107, 109, 116, 118,
    121, 123, 129, 130, 174, 227,
    273, 278. *See* Bennington
    College, *Dance Observer*,
    Denishawn; Graham, Martha;
    Tamiris, Helen Tamiris
    48th Street Theatre, 107
    Collegiate plastique, 121
    Craft of choreography, 118
    Dance Observer, 129
    Denishawn, 107
    Influence on Alwin Nikolais, 121
    Soares, Janet, 121
    Vienna, 107
Horton, Lester, 126
House Un-American Activities
    Committee, HUAC, 126, 176.
    See also Dies, Martin; Thomas,
    J. Parnell
Houston Ballet. *See* Ford Foundation
Howe, Dianne S., 295
Howe, Eugene C,, 140, 141
Howe, Eugene C., 138, 139
HPE. See Health and Physical Education
HUAC. *See* House Un-American
    Activities Committee
Huguenot, Protestant Scholars, 18
Humphrey, Doris, 105, 107, 108, 109,
    112, 116, 118, 119, 120, 121,
    122, 123, 146, 172, 174, 212,
    239. *See also* Bennington College;
    Denishawn; St. Denis, Ruth;

Tamiris, Helen Tamiris;
    Weidman, Charles
Hinman, Mary Wood, 92, 108.
Humphrey-Weidman School, 109
New Dance, 122
Partnership with Charles Weidman,
    107
Humphrey-Weidman Company, 108,
    172, 212
Hurok, Sol, 188
Huxley, Thomas, 27
IATECH. *See* Interarts and Technology,
    IATECH
ICFAD. *See* International Council of
    Fine Arts Deans
IEA. *See* Legislation, Education Acts
Illinois Industrial University, 25. *See*
    also Morrill-Land Grant Act of
    1862
Illinois, University of, 25
Imperial Bull of 1158. *See Habita*
Impulse, 172, 173, 174, 175, 189, 190,
    192, 205, 208, 233, 274, 275. *See*
    also Van Tuyl, Marian
    Dance:A Projection for the Future,
    205
    Halprin-Lathrop students, 172
    West Coast Annual, 173
Incense (the dance). *See* St. Denis, Ruth
Indiana University, 286
Indiana, Butler University in. *See* Butler
    University
Innocent IV, Pope, 15, 16, 17. *See also*
    Free Corporation; Universitas
    Papal Bull of 1243, 15, 16
Interarts and Technology, IATECH, 300
International Association for Dance
    Medicine and Science, 307
International Association of Blacks in
    Dance, 306
International Council of Fine Arts
    Deans, 234

International Education Committee of
YMCA's, 53
Intolerance (the movie). *See* Griffith, D.
W.
Iowa, University of, 215
Iran Hostage Crisis, 245
Irey, Charlotte, 194, 213
Irvine, University of California at, 198.
See also Garrison, Clayton;
Loring, Eugene; Penrod, James
Isis, Egyptian goddess, 64
Jackson, Andrew (US President), 23
Jacksonian Democracy, 24
Jacksonian egalitarianism, 6
Jahn, Freidrich Ludwig, 28. *See also*
German/Germany
James, William, 45. *See also* Columbia
University; Dewey, John
Japan culture, Asian culture. *See also* 11
n 26
Japan, culture, Asian culture, 265
JCDTA. *See* Dance and Theater
Accreditation, Joint Commission
for
Jennings, Mrs. Frederic B.. *See*
Bennington College
Joel, Lydia, 188
John Murray Anderson-Robert Milton
School of the Theater, 114
John the Baptist, 77
Johns Hopkins University, 27
Johnson, Lyndon (US President), 185,
186
Education Acts, 275
Johnson Administration, 218
National Arts and Humanities
Foundation, 185
Joos, Kurt, 109
JOPER. See Journal of Physical
Education and Recreation
JOPERD. See Journal of Physical
Education, Recreation, and Dance
José Limón Company. *See* Limón, José

Journal of Higher Education, 248
Journal of Physical Education, 111
Journal of Physical Education and
Recreation, 169, 174, 175, 274
Journal of Physical Education,
Recreation and Dance, 290
Journal of Physical Education,
Recreation, and Dance, 295
Dance Dynamics, 295
Juba (the dance). *See* Hampton Institute
Creative Dance Group
Judson Church, 226, 288. *See also*
Rainer, Yvonne
Julliard School, 207
Jus Ubique Docendi, 15
Kahlich, Luke, 314, 315
Kansas Dance Councils Inc.. *See*
Bauman, Alice
Kansas, University of, 215
Kant, Immanuel. *See* Duncan, Isadora
Kealiinohomoku, Joann, 304
Kellogg School for Physical Education,
113, 114. *See also* Hill, Martha
Kennedy Cultural Center for the
Performing Arts, 192
Kennedy, Charlotte Moton. *See*
Hampton Institute Creative
Dance Group
Kennedy, Jaqueline, 184
Kennedy, John F. (US President), 184
assassination of, 185, 217
Education Acts, 275
Robert Frost Library at Amherst
College, 192
Kerr, Clark, 189
Kilpatrick, Professor. *See* Columbia
University
Kinesthetic sense. *See* H'Doubler,
Margaret
King, Bruce, 215
Kinsley, Professor Richard. *See* Yale
Report, The of 1828

392

National Endowment for the Humanities, 185, 310. *See also* Federal Arts Advisory Council

National Foundation for the Arts and Humanities Act, Title 13, 280

National Geographic Society, 38

National Section on Dance, NSD, 158, 159, 169, 190, 191, 192, 193, 218. *See also* 9 n 16

Conference on Movement, 190

Dance as a Discipline Conference, 192

Dance Directory, 218

National Section on Dancing, NSD, 7, 111, 153, 155, 156, 157, 158, 159, 161, 169, 307. *See also* La Salle, Dorothy; Lee, Mabel; Maroney, F. W.; Murray, Ruth; O'Donnell, Mary P.

Hernlund, President of APEA, 161

Natural Dancing, 56, 70, 71, 72, 73, 75, 76, 77, 78. *See also* Colby, Gertrude

Natural Gymnastics, 53, 56. *See also* Gulick, Luther; Wood, Thomas D.

Natural Rhythms and Dances. See Colby, Gertrude

Nature Friends Dance Group, 176

Nautch (the dance). *See* St. Denis, Ruth

NDA. *See* National Dance Association

NDEO. *See* National Dance Education Organization

NEA. *See* National Endowment for the Arts

Nebraska, University of, 152, 157. *See also* Lee, Mabel

New Dance (the dance). *See* Bennington College; Humphrey, Doris

New Dance Group, 176

New Deal, 124, 126, 246. *See also* Roosevelt, Franklin (US President)

New Haven. *See* Yale University

New School for Social Research, 110, 164. *See also* Hill, Martha; Martin, John

New York City Ballet. *See* Ford Foundation

New York City Center of Music and Drama, 187

New York City Cultural Affairs Office, 193

New York State College Dance Festival. *See* Erdman, Jean

New York Times, 107, 110, 130, 214. *See also* Downes, Olin; Findlay, Elsa; Martin, John

New York University, 111, 112, 113, 115, 207, 208, 213, 277, 285, 286. *See also* Barnard college; Committee on Research in Dance; Erdman, Jean; Rowe, Patricia

New York University Summer School of Physical Education. *See* Gulick, Luther

New York World, 32

New York, State University of, 184

College at Purchase, 207, 213

New York, State University of College at Purchase, 230

Nietzsche, Fredrich Wilhelm. *See* Duncan, Isadora

Nikolais, Alwin, 121, 208, 210, 211, 212, 288. *See also* Developmental Conference on Dance; Holm, Hanya; Louis, Murray

philosophy of, 210

Soares, Janet, 121

Nixon, Richard (US President), 217, 242

No Manifesto. See Rainer, Yvonne

North Carolina, University, 190, 286

North Dakota

first state to regulate physical training and hygiene, 29, 54

Turner Movement, 29
Turner, Jonathan Baldwin. *See* Morrill-
Land Grant Act of 1862
Turnvereine. See German/Germany
United States Supreme Court, 22
Chief Justice John Marshall, 22
Constitution, United States, 22
Universitas, 6, 13, 16, 17. *See also* Free
Corporation; Innocent IV; Papal
Bull of 1243
University of California
at Berkeley. *See* Berkeley, University
of California at
at Irvine. *See* Irvine, University of
California at
at Los Angeles. *See* Los Angeles,
University of California at
at Riverside. *See* Riverside, University
of California at
at San Diego. *See* San Diego,
University of California at
University of Chicago. *See* Chicago,
University of
University of Colorado. *See* Colorado,
University of
University of Iowa. *See* Iowa,
University of
University of Kansas. *See* Kansas,
University of
University of Maryland. *See* Maryland,
University of
University of Michigan. *See* Michigan,
University of
University of Nebraska. *See* Nebraska,
University of
University of North Carolina. *See* North
Carolina, University of
University of Oregon. *See* Oregon,
University of
University of Paris. *See* Paris,
University of
University of Pennsylvania. *See*
Pennsylvania, University of

University of Pittsburgh. *See* Pittsburgh,
University of
University of Southern California, 286
University of Utah. *See* Utah,
University of
University of Wichita. *See* Wichita,
University of
University of Wisconsin. *See* Wisconsin,
University of
University of Wisconsin at Madison. *See*
Wisconsin, University
Utah Ballet. *See* Ford Foundation
Utah, University of, 170, 201, 207, 213,
230
Van Hise, Charles. *See* Wisconsin,
University of
Van Tuyl, Marian, 173, 174, 175, 225.
See also Impulse; Mills College
Vassar College, 42, 112
Vaudeville House. *See* St. Denis, Ruth
VEA. *See* Legislation, Education Acts
Vienna, Austria, 14
Vietnam Conflict, 217, 218
Vietnam War, 226
Vocational Education Act. *See*
Legislation, Education Acts
Von Laban, Rudolf, 109
Wagner, Ann, 3, 37
Wagner, Richard. *See* Duncan, Isadora
Wallack, Miss Hazel. *See* Shawn, Ted
Warren, Gretchen, 311, 312
Watergate, 226, 228, 242, 245
Watson, Thomas, 278
WCTU. *See* Women's Christian
Temperance Union
WDC. *See* Wisconsin Dance Council
Weber, Lynne, 302. *See also* Technology
Weidman, Charles, 105, 107, 108, 109,
116, 122, 174, 212, 215, 239. *See
also* Bennington College;
Denishawn; Humphrey, Doris
Quest, 122

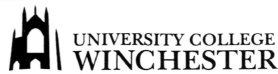